# Narratives, Health, and Healing

∾

## Communication Theory, Research, and Practice

# LEA'S COMMUNICATION SERIES
### Jennings Bryant/Dolf Zillmann, General Editors

Selected titles in Applied Communication
(Teresa L. Thompson, Advisory Editor) include:

**Braithwaite/Thompson** • *Handbook of Communication and People With Disabilities: Research and Application*

**Greene/Derlega/Yep/Petronio** • *Privacy and Disclosure of HIV in Interpersonal Relationships: A Sourcebook for Researchers and Practitioners*

**Hummert/Nussbaum** • *Aging, Communication, and Health: Linking Research and Practice for Successful Aging*

**Nussbaum/Coupland** • *Handbook of Communication and Aging Research, Second Edition*

**Segrin/Flora** • *Family Communication*

**Socha/Diggs** • *Communication, Race, and Family: Exploring Communication in Black, White, and Biracial Families*

**Thompson/Dorsey/Miller/Parrott** • *Handbook of Health Communication*

**Vangelisti** • *Handbook of Family Communication*

**Williams/Nussbaum** • *Intergenerational Communication Across The Life Span*

# Narratives, Health, and Healing

∾

## Communication Theory, Research, and Practice

*Edited by*

**Lynn M. Harter**
*Ohio University*

**Phyllis M. Japp**
*University of Nebraska-Lincoln*

**Christina S. Beck**
*Ohio University*

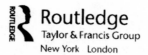

Routledge
Taylor & Francis Group
New York   London

Transferred to Digital Printing 2008

First published by Lawrence Erlbaum Associates, Inc., Publishers
10 Industrial Avenue
Mahwah, New Jersey 07430

Reprinted 2008 by Routledge
Routledge
Taylor & Francis Group
270 Madison Avenue
New York, NY 10016

Routledge
Taylor & Francis Group
2 Park Square
Milton Park, Abingdon
Oxon OX14 4RN

Cover design by Sean Sciarrone

**Library of Congress Cataloging-in-Publication Data**

Narratives, health, and healing : communication theory, re-
    search, and practice / edited by Lynn M. Harter, Phyllis
    M. Japp, Christina S. Beck.
        p.  cm. — (LEA's communication series)
Includes bibliographical references and index.
ISBN 0-8058-5031-7 (cloth : alk. paper)
ISBN 0-8058-5032-5 (pbk. : alk. paper)
1. Social medicine. 2. Physician and patient. 3. Discourse
    Analysis, Narrative. 4. Narration (Rhetoric). I. Harter,
    Lynn M. II. Japp, Phyllis M. III. Beck, Christina S. IV.
    Series.

RA418.N365 2005
362.1'042—dc22
                                                2004057531
                                                CIP

*In Dedication ...*

*I dedicate this book to my parents Rich and Bev Harter. Dad, I have learned how to live by watching you re-story your life in light of multiple myeloma. Bev, I have learned how to give by watching you care for others during sickness and health.*

*—Lynn*

*I dedicate this book to my grandchildren, Brendan and Rachel Japp. You've enriched my life beyond measure.*
*—Phyllis*

*I dedicate this book to the memory of my grandfather, George Groscost, who went home to be with the Lord as we finished this book. Thanks for always being so proud of me!*
*—Christie*

# Contents

∿

# Foreword—
# Stories By and About Us

℺

**Arthur W. Frank**
*University of Calgary*

Books like this one become increasingly necessary, because the weave of stories about health and illness has become dense. Two trends have intensified in the last 10 years, both affecting what stories people tell. One is the increasing separation of health from illness, bringing about a new species of health stories. People have always talked about their ailments. A good case can be made that now people are talking in new ways about their health, and we are only beginning to question how these health stories affect illness stories. Illness stories have also proliferated during the last decade, told from an increasing variety of perspectives, as more groups have some stake in what illness is and how it is regarded. All of these stories—health and illness stories together—constitute a formless but formative framework of interpretive effects that structures people's sense of what events and actions are worth telling stories about and how these stories are to be understood, including what actions follow from them.

Health, increasingly distinct from illness, comprises its own practices, professional practitioners, discourses, and institutional delivery sites. Practices include but are hardly limited to fitness, diet, diverse uses of complementary medicine, and a variety of medical enhancement technologies (Ellott, 2003; Parens, 1998; Rothman & Rothman,

2004), including pharmacology (Prozac, Viagra, Ritalin), surgery (ever-expanding uses of cosmetic surgery and adjunctive techniques), and a veritable promised land of possibilities for health and commerce, with genetics receiving the greatest hype. Enhancement medicine pushes people to think of the body as a collection of parts, to be upgraded as one desires and can afford (Frank, 2002c). Products from skin cream to foods to clothing (e.g., fabrics with sun protection) are sold under a rubric of *health*. Complementary medical services claim to improve the body's structural alignment, enhance the immune system, detoxify, tone, stimulate, and rejuvenate. These practices are variously offered, taught, or sold by professionals from the highly credentialed (physicians) to the marginally certified (store "consultants"). Like all practices, products, and professionals, each implies a story about what a body can and ought to be, and how a life can and ought to be lived to make that desired body possible. People tell stories about how they have used or refused these services, and what sorts of lives have followed from these decisions.

Illness stories are told within a dense weave of stories people tell about their own bodies and stories from elsewhere, told (usually from a stance of expertise) about the ill bodies of other people, including both patients (the currently ill) and bodies at risk (the virtually ill). This weave is denser—there are simply more stories, from more sources, about more bodies—than it was in 1991, when my story of my several years of serious illness, *At the Will of the Body* (Frank, 2002a), was published. I was attempting to write a story that could be a sort of companion to other ill people, allowing them to compare experiences and observations. The story was my own, yet even then I drew on narrative resources going back hundreds of years (see Frank, 2002b), as any storyteller inevitably must draw on such resources. The boundaries of anyone's own story have always frayed at the edges, but it becomes increasingly difficult to find any boundary at all.

In *The Wounded Storyteller* (Frank, 1995), I contrast the predominate type of story that institutional medicine teaches patients to tell about themselves—and prefers that they tell—with a story people learn to tell for themselves. Medicine prefers the *restitution story* that projects a future of the patient being restored to her condition prior to illness. Ill people learn to tell the *quest story*, in which illness is understood as a source of some insight that needs to be shared with others. But quest stories are hardly less culturally conditioned than restitution stories: their discursive tradition goes back to epic heroes—Inanna, Gilgamesh, and jumping forward many centuries, Parzival. These heroes suffer, learn to submit to suffering, and eventually achieve greater power through suffering. That narrative tradition generates possibilities and parameters for present stories. Because stories are always already there, narrative traditions affect what any person selects, from the flux of his or her life, to count as experience. Yet for all the embeddedness of stories within narrative traditions, any one person's quest story remains that person's own, reenacted as if for the first time, just as each person suffers for the first time. Suffering has no regard for how many have suffered such illnesses or injuries before; it is always original, and so are stories of that suffering.

Many of the chapters in this volume work to sustain a delicate balance: to acknowledge the personal authenticity of the individual story, while recognizing how that story is embedded in a proliferation of stories telling people what it is to be healthy, on one hand, and how to respond to illness, on the other hand. Stories about health and illness are told by diverse government agencies, by corporations, by professional associations, by advocacy groups, by politicians running for office, and by entertainers trying to get a laugh or a tear from an audience. Collectively, these stories constitute a social *pedagogy*— they teach people who we can expect to be, who we should want to be, and what we ought to do (and not do) to fit the identity templates that different stories project. As we—because all of us are caught in this web—tell our own stories, we are expected and we expect ourselves to take up identities projected by this pedagogy: to narrate our lives as if we feel the desires that the stories tell us we have, as if the practices those stories invoke are natural to us, and as if we embrace a self that is the very picture of what the stories from elsewhere imagine us to be.

Thus I am suggesting that this much-used phrase, *narrative identity* (e.g., Bruner, 2002) is, at least from a social scientific perspective, a pedagogy in narrative that circumscribes identity. This pedagogy is both dense—the stories refer to multiple aspects of our lives and reach us constantly, through multiple media—yet also loosely connected. The sources of these stories are not linked in demonstrable ways; analysts would search in vain for an central, organizing agency that orchestrates these stories. The pedagogy of stories from elsewhere is not an ideology—its sources are too diverse in their interests—yet it shapes our ideas about how our stories can be told and lived.

Scholarly studies of narrative seek to sustain the necessary complementarity of two recognitions. First, to recognize the storyteller's practical and moral know-how: her awareness of what shapes her own life, her care for those she tells her story to, and her aspiration to truth (MacIntyre, 1981). Second, to help to sort out the effects of us all being inundated with stories from elsewhere that shape how we tell our own story. This book takes on a major task for those who study health, illness, and narrative. How do professional students of people's stories achieve the subtlety, tact, and respect necessary when dealing with how any person talks about his or her life, while recognizing that no life is ever anyone's own? Stories entwine and tell each other, yet each story is no less unique for that.

# Preface and Acknowledgments

*No story sits by itself. Sometimes stories meet at corners and sometimes they cover one another completely, like stones beneath a river.*

—(Albom, 2003, p. 10)

As the reader might anticipate, the story of this volume intersects with the lived stories of many individuals, people we wish to recognize and honor. Narrative inquiry always takes on a multi-layered, nested quality including stories told, co-constructed, and eventually narrated in research texts. The authors, research participants, and editors of this volume form a textured space of knowing and being that we believe greatly expands ways of remaining healthy in the world. Some individuals, for reasons of time and space, we met only through their writings or stories—distant yet kindred spirits who inspired us to imagine possibilities of narrative theory, research, and practice for enhancing health communication. Thanks to everyone who co-constructed stories that grace the pages of this book.

This book offers intersections between health communication and other sub-disciplines of communication by spanning three broad context areas—public discourse, organizational communication, and interpersonal communication. As such, we hope arguments advanced in this collection will be interesting and and informative to scholars beyond those individuals with a central focus on health communication issues. Further, because of the interesting attention on narrative in disciplines such as medical anthropology and medical sociology, this book targets readers in related fields as well. We hope researchers, teachers, students, and practitioners of health communication find the theoretically rich essays valuable for their personal and professional journeys.

We remain grateful to Linda Bathgate at LEA, Teri Thompson, Jim Query, and anonymous reviewers of our original book proposal. Their belief in the theoretical and practical value of our vision was instrumental in securing a contract for the book. We deeply appreciate Linda's professionalism, expertise, creativity, and editorial advice. We also wish to thank Paul Overmeyer and Sara Scudder for supervising the production stage of the book, including copyediting and typesetting.

We thank each and every chapter contributor. Over the span of 2 years, this volume came to fruition due to their efforts. We are grateful that these authors initially submitted top-notch work, revised their work in response to our reflections, and always worked in a timely and professional manner. The theoretical value of their work emerged in exciting ways that we had not anticipated and that we proudly showcase in this volume. Most important, their transformative ideas about narrative and health continue to renew and inspire us.

The School of Communication Studies and the College of Communication at Ohio University provided invaluable resources toward the completion of this book. We thank Kathy Krendl and Greg Shepherd for their allocation of financial resources for subject indexing and reference work. Many thanks to Michaela Meyer for her diligence in compiling the reference section and to Teodora Carabas for her careful attention to detail in subject indexing. We also thank Jennifer Scott for her assistance with line editing.

Lynn thanks her husband, Scott, and daughter, Emma Grace, both of whom patiently heard this book read aloud on many occasions. You both remain central to the plot of my life, scholarly and otherwise. I appreciate my colleagues at Ohio University and elsewhere who provided support for this project. Erika Kirby, Beth Graham, Arvind Singhal, Gayle and Raymie McKerrow, and Bill Rawlins generously fueled my enthusiasm for this project. Phyllis and Christie, I have appreciated this opportunity to learn with you and further develop our shared passions for narrative and health communication.

Phyllis thanks her family for their interest and support, her colleagues at University of Nebraska for encouragement and willingness to talk over ideas, former and current graduate students for a continuing supply of ideas and intellectual challenges. She is especially grateful to Lynn and Christie for the opportunity to work together. Co-editing this book has been a wonderful experience and I've learned so much from both of you. Thanks so much for your intellectual stimulation as well as your personal support and caring. You're the best!

Christie thanks the many people who have enriched her personal and professional narratives.... Although a tad ironic, I remain grateful for my own health experiences that opened my eyes to the human dramas that unfold every minute of every day in hospitals, health care facilities, and homes. Encounters with health care providers and seekers, often strangers to me before our paths intersect, inspire me to explore the ways in which they construct those mundane yet life-altering moments, and I thank them for raising my awareness and passion for understanding health narratives. Further, I am so appreciative of my many colleagues in the discipline who encourage me in this work, especially Lynn and Phyllis. Your words of support humble me, and they mean more than you can ever know. Finally, completing this book would ring hollow without the intimate co-participants in my personal life journey, individuals who ground me and remind me that family and true friends will always be more important than work. Michelle, Corinne, Shari, and Carolyn have shared my life stories for nearly 30 years. My "sampler platter" of children—Brittany (17), Chelsea Meagan (9), and Emmy (3)—enrich my journey daily as I watch them interact with their own friends and enjoy special moments of success and accomplishment. I praise God for blessing me with riveting life and health experiences, dedicated friends, smart and talented children and, perhaps most of all, my husband, Roger. He remains the absolute best life partner that any one could hope to have. He will always be the "wind beneath my wings."

As we close these acknowledgments, we herald the collaborative nature of this endeavor. This project reminded the three of us how much fun it can be to work together toward common goals. We value the insights, diversity of thought, and synergy that emerges from collaboration.

*—Lynn, Phyllis, and Christie*

# I

# Overview of Narrative
# and Health Communication Theorizing

ᐭ

## INTRODUCTION

**Phyllis M. Japp**
*University of Nebraska-Lincoln*

**Lynn M. Harter**
*Ohio University*

**Christina S. Beck**
*Ohio University*

*Samantha is a sweet, chubby, kissable 8-month old, with huge blue eyes and a topper of fuzzy blond hair. Sammie is nourished through a feeding tube and spends most of her time on a respirator to aid her breathing. Most days she is too weak and lethargic to kick, raise her head, or do any of the things an active 8-month-old loves to do. Today, her eyes track the visitor who is talking to her but there is little spark in the blue eyes and no answering smile. "She does smile," her mother assures, "she's just too tired today." Her parents, Brad and Joyce, do not believe Sammie is mentally impaired but at this early age it is hard to tell. What is wrong with Sammie? Medically, there is nothing wrong with Sammie. Her digestive system is "normal"*

I

*although without the feeding tube she is unable to retain enough food to nourish her body. Her respiratory system is "normal" although she has difficulty breathing without assistance. Physicians can find no markers of any known disease that would explain her muscle weakness. Sammie's parents, an attractive suburban couple with two other children, are frantic to find a diagnosis and hopefully a cure for Sammie. They are telling Sammie's story for two reasons: to raise funds to take Sammie to an eastern medical center that specializes in children's diseases, a visit for which their insurance will not pay because Sammie has no identifiable illness, and in the hope that someone, somewhere, will hear about Sammie and provide the answers they so desperately need. Although frustrated with their managed-care system, and disappointed with physicians who seem to lose interest when they cannot provide answers, Brad and Joyce retain their faith in the miracles of modern medicine. Surely there is a cure somewhere, if only they can find a diagnosis. "When they know what it is," Brad declares, "they'll know how to fix it." Meanwhile they struggle on physically exhausted and emotionally drained and on the brink of bankruptcy. Joyce smiles bravely and hugs Sammie as the news segment ends.*[1]

As we began work on this volume, we quickly realized that we were blessed with three different but compatible perspectives on narrative and health communication. Narrative inquiry in communication studies, as is true in other disciplines, tends to be theorized and researched within intradisciplinary "boxes," the subareas in which we each have been trained to think and work. Health communication transcends those boxes, yet in this area as well, scholars tend to work with what they know best. Interpersonal scholars focus on health narratives as chronicles of disrupted personal lives, threatened relationships, and spoiled identities in need of narrative readjustment and repair. Viewed as a personal narrative, Sammie's story gives us entry into the world of pain, confusion, and hardship caused by the illness of a child, in this case an illness with no name and therefore no possibility of closure. Organizational scholars naturally gravitate toward institutional narratives, those stories constructed within and constrained by the collective consciousness of the individuals and groups within their domain. Framed within these interests, Sammie's story is not only a personal narrative of dealing with illness; it is a saga of encounters with medical personnel, organizations, and institutions. How can Sammie be so sick and yet not be classified in any known category of disease? Why do we have a health care system so dependant upon classification that insurance will not pay for treatments of illnesses that cannot be defined? Public communication scholars will invoke the social and political metanarratives, often disseminated via media, within which Sammie's story is constructed, realizing that they necessarily embody the matrix of assumptions, expectations, and values common to our public cultural narratives. Sammie's story appeared on the evening news, sandwiched between weather reports, bulletins from Iraq, baseball scores, and the fate of a family of ducklings who fell into a culvert on their way to the lake for their first swim. Why, these scholars ask, are stories of personal illness frequently part of our daily "bulletin" of what is going on in our world? What does it mean when personal illness stories are presented on the pages of newspapers, in magazines, on television news, news magazines and documentary dramas? What ends—whose ends—do they serve?

Sammie's story illustrates that no narrative is solely personal, organizational or public; stories necessarily bleed across the artificial boundaries of discrete areas of knowledge. Personal stories cannot escape the constraints of institutional interests, nor can they fail to engage the assumptions, expectations, and values encoded in public narratives. Conversely, narratives constructed and circulated in the public domain are built upon personal and institutional narratives, drawing from the experiences and understandings of those within their domain. The sections in this book, then, serve as different "ways of seeing," alternate standpoints on the integrated and interconnected process of human narrativity.

Personal narratives become the building blocks of public knowledge. More and more, mediated and public dialogue, from legislative testimony to newscasts to public health promotion, rely on individual stories to embody problems, shape arguments and engage emotions, as well as to persuade, evaluate, reward, and punish. Personal stories increasingly provide a "face" for any issue, a convention of reality-making in news, advertising, promotional campaigns, or entertainment. If Sammie is eventually diagnosed with a rare disease, her story may become the impetus for support groups to help care-giving parents and/or it may serve as a centerpiece for efforts to secure attention and funding for research. If she is cured, she can be featured as proof of the miracles of modern medicine; if not, she may serve as a reminder that medical science has not yet conquered the mysteries of the human body and mind.

Although it is evident that personal narratives energize public narratives, it is often less obvious that the cumulative force of public narratives shapes and constrains personal narratives. Personal stories can never be constituted independently from public narratives, those pervasive patterns that provide the language, structure, and formulas that shape our ways of thinking and our collective understandings. As we watched Sammie's story unfold, we noted the reporter's difficulty in deciding which familiar narrative pattern fit best for this story. Sammie's was not a "restitution" story, that formula so beloved of media and public discourse (Frank, 1995), wherein health is restored and all is well. Think of the story that can be told if doctors find a miracle cure and Sammie's good health returns!

However restitution evades Sammie, at least at the moment. Nor can Sammie's story be a "quest" story, an equally beloved and inspiring formula that demonstrates how all involved have learned and grown from dealing with adversity (Frank, 1995). Brad and Joyce are not conceptualizing, at least at this point, the good that can come from this tragic problem. Yet, Sammie's parents seem aware of the familiar narrative formulas. Brad invoked restitution in his assurance that "they'll know how to fix it," and Joyce reflected, at the interviewer's prompt, that Sammie's illness has taught her not to be so independent but to ask others for help when necessary. Sammie's story most closely resembles a chaos narrative, a sense of disconnected events characterized by lack of closure and day-to-day uncertainty. Although, as Frank (1995) noted, such stories often are too incoherent to be told and too painful to hear, Sammie's story smacks of chaos as it reveals the frightening limbo of caring for a beloved child with an undiagnosed illness; its depiction of Sammie's exhausted parents and confused siblings provides us with little sense of a satisfactory narrative ending.

Between the public and the private are, of course, the groups, institutions, and organizations that always mediate between personal experience and public knowledge in a complex society. In sum, any personal story is constituted in dialogue with relevant public and institutional narratives, whether in confirmation, denial, or challenge. Embedded in Sammie's story are the assumptions and values of bio-medicine, family and community life, health economics, and politics. Likewise, her story reveals the power of health organizations to refine personal constructions of health and illness, as well as to constrain and direct public dialogue. Both personal stories and public dialogue encapsulate the narratives of those institutions, their personnel, their definitions and practices. For Sammie, we hope her visit to the famous medical center will result in a diagnosis and cure so that her story can move from the category of *medical mysteries* to that of *medical miracles*, and a satisfying institutional (as well as personal and public) story can emerge.

Like Sammie's story, the chapters in this volume embody the hopes, dreams, fears, and frustrations of individuals as they deal with traumas of health and healing. Authors demonstrate how the personal, public, and institutional dimensions of narrativity intertwine in the search for knowledge and understanding of the health problems of our time. These chapters can be engaged from a variety of perspectives; here we emphasize the interconnectedness of narrative activity. Some authors focus on the relational work performed by narrative activity. Others take a broader, more critical, look at institutional and cultural parameters of narrative forms and repertories. In various ways, the chapters give clear voice to actors-in-context—often including the author—conceptually developing micro-, meso-, and macroperspectives on narrativity. Consequently, the volume is arranged in five parts: (I) Overview of Narrative and Health Communication Theorizing; (II) Personal Narratives and Public Dialogues; (III) Narrating and Organizing Health Care Events and Resources; (IV) Narrative Sensemaking About Self and Other; and (V) Continuing the Conversation: Reflections on Our Emergent Scholarly Narratives. These sections remain necessarily approximate as many chapters possess overlapping themes. Collectively, these authors and chapters introduce readers to the diverse corpus of work related to health communication and narrative theorizing and articulate agendas for future communication theory, research, and practice.

The chapters in Part I position narrative theorizing about health and healing in the broader landscape of the communication discipline. In chapter 1, we synthesize literature about narrative activity, health, and healing and articulate four key problematics that often remain unarticulated yet are pervasive in the way scholars engage in narrative theorizing and research. In fleshing out these problematics, we illustrate the aspirations of narrative theory to comprehend key problematics of life: knowing and being, continuity and disruption, creativity and constraint, and the partial and indeterminate. Chapter 2, authored by Austin Babrow, Kimberly Kline, and William Rawlins, juxtaposes narrative theorizing with central claims of health communication theory including meaning making and being human, meaning making and context, meaning making and temporality. Babrow and colleagues beautifully illustrate the heuristic potential of integrating problematic integration theory and narrative theory to understand how health communicators embrace possibilities, address contingencies, engage in sensemaking, and, when feasible, make health care decisions.

We continue our discussion of each chapter in the introductions to main sections of the volume. We end the volume with a consideration of what might come next. We offer extended reflections on how health and healing are co-constructed through narrative activity, examine points of convergence and divergence across this collection of essays, and articulate unspoken undercurrents that merit further attention by scholars, across disciplines, interested in narrative constructions of health and healing. We hope this collection conveys the fascinating, complicated, and pragmatic nature of narrative work and points the way toward work left to do. Most essentially, the readings offer a sense of hopefulness that narrative activity, although often difficult, can accomplish something: make sense of health and healing, (re)construct identities in light of the disruption of illness, organize health care events and resources, and personalize otherwise distant public dialogues. The readings do not necessarily offer easy answers or clear resolutions to health care dilemmas. However, we hope they offer useful guidance for how to think about and enact health care from one's own local conditions and more global, collective standpoints. Like narrative itself, the ideas in *Narratives, Health, and Healing: Communication Theory, Research and Practice* are not finalized or finalizable—they remain partial and indeterminate. We invite you, the reader, to critique and extend the issues raised throughout the volume, expanding voices and ways of voicing.

## NOTE

1. Sammie is at its core a true story that we have extended into a case to illustrate our discussion. We have altered names, locations, and a number of other details for two reasons: First the story is pieced together from a media account and comments of friends of the family, thus some details remain unclear and some undoubtedly are not factually accurate. Second, by using it as an explanatory case, we are changing the narrative purpose of the original story and using it for our own ends. Thus we feel it essential that it not be associated with any real people, anywhere.

# 1

# Vital Problematics of Narrative Theorizing About Health and Healing[1]

~

**Lynn M. Harter**
*Ohio University*

**Phyllis M. Japp**
*University of Nebraska*

**Christina S. Beck**
*Ohio University*

An increasing number of scholars across disciplines envision narrative as a new frontier for advancing health-related theory, research and practice. Rhetoricians (e.g., Fisher, 1984, 1985b), medical anthropologists (e.g., Mattingly, 2000, 2001), sociologists (e.g., Frank, 1995, 1997, 2004; Riessman, 2000), physicians (e.g., Charon, 2001; Kleinman, 1988), psychologists (e.g., Bruner, 2002; Polkinghorne, 1988) and communication scholars (e.g., Bochner, 2002; Carbaugh, 2001; Langellier & Peterson, 2004) assert that narrative facilitates emergent social selves, relational identities, and co-cultural understandings. This interest has evolved not only from the linguistic turn in the social sciences, but also from shifts toward postmodern ways of envisioning the world. Indeed, as Morris (1998) noted, "One infallible sign that you have entered the gravitational field of postmodernism is a swerve toward narrative" (p. 250). This book features work that engages narrative forms and practices as constituting complex and sophisticated knowledge of individuals, as well as the lived sociocultural and political contexts in which agents construct, share, and revise stories. Narratives are especially appropriate means of examining issues of health and healing because they wrestle with complexities that face contemporary health care participants: identity construction, order and disorder, autonomy and community, fixed and fluid experiences.

In talking about how to organize this introductory chapter, we considered several alternatives. First, we considered rehearsing key *functions* served by narrative, such as identity construction and community building (see Sharf & Vanderford, 2003; Sunwolf & Frey, 2001). We also considered highlighting key *grammars* of narrativity, such as emplotment, characters, and temporality (see Polkinghorne, 1988), or *types* of narrative, progressing from microcontexts, ontological narratives, to macrocontexts, institutional and societal narratives (see Somers, 1994). Each of these frameworks could usefully organize the chapters in this volume and permit meaningful readings; and throughout this chapter, we do address functions, grammars, and types of narrative activity. However, we weave these concerns in the broader fabric of vital problematics that are engaged in different ways and to different ends by narrative scholars interested in health and healing.

Scholars constitute a "disciplinary matrix," a community of sorts, when they share a set of assumptions (i.e., problematics) about the study of phenomena (Mumby & Stohl, 1996). This sharing does not imply a consensus on every issue, but rather that diverse scholars approach the study of experience and behaviors in light of similar concerns. Narrative theorizing involves complex issues that defy simplistic sets of propositions that scholars can embrace and perfectly embody in practice. Instead, we assert that engaging in narrativity requires scholars to delve more deeply into murky, cluttered, and complicated interrelationships between sometimes incompatible issues. Narrative theory propels scholars into inherently messy domains, especially in this postmodern era. Because our contemporary lives challenge us to juxtapose multiple (and sometimes competing) social selves (Gergen, 1991), understandings of narrative co-constructions often extend from wrestling through tensions and concerns that challenge individuals as they enact their everyday lives. Narrative theorists implicitly struggle with such vital problematics in defining and delimiting their particular area of research. Yet, in our examination of extant narrative theorizing, we find these problematics operating in the background without explicit acknowledgment. In this chapter, we bring these issues to the forefront, highlighting them as core dimensions of narrative theorizing. By articulating these problematics, we not only synthesize narrative and health literatures, we explore possibilities for more empowering ways of understanding and enacting health and healing.

Collectively, these vital problematics of narrative theorizing bespeak a concern for humans as symbol (mis)using creatures and storytellers (Burke, 1969; Fisher, 1984, 1985b, 1987), stories as both mundane and extraordinary ritual symbolic forms, stories as sites for action and agency, and stories as occasions for the act of acknowledging (Heidegger, 1972). They include (a) the problematic of knowing and being, (b) the problematic of continuity and disruption, (c) the problematic of creativity and constraint, and (d) the problematic of the partial and the indeterminate. What unifies many narrative scholars is not how we engage these problematics, but rather the recognition of and continual struggle with these abiding tensions and concerns. The problematics are not mutually exclusive, nor are they exhaustive. We distinguish them here in this form for analytical purposes—to distill common theoretical and methodological assumptions that often remain unarticulated yet are pervasive in the way scholars do narrative work. Throughout this chapter, we articulate these problematics and illustrate how narrative scholars in general and authors in this volume specifically engage these issues in theory, research and practice. Especially for scholars of health communication, a rich theoretical understanding of narrative experiences can prompt fruitful insight into the lived realities of health care participants.

## KNOWING AND BEING

There is no such thing as an intuitively obvious and essential self to know, one that just sits there ready to be portrayed in words. Rather, we constantly construct and reconstruct our selves to meet the needs of the situations we encounter, and we do so with the guidance of our memories of the past and our hopes and fears for the future.

—Bruner, 2002, p. 64

Narrative as representation has long been respected as an optional vehicle for teaching preestablished truths (e.g., the case study or story example that supplements and personalizes information). Even so, understanding the epistemological and ontological power of narrative is a vital direction for health communication researchers to pursue. Garro and Mattingly (2000) argued, "Narrative is a fundamental human way of giving meaning to experience. In both telling and interpreting experiences, narrative mediates between an inner world of thought–feeling and an outer world of observable actions and states of affairs" (p. 1). The problematic of knowing and being foregrounds how we narratively construct and understand what we call our lives, creating ourselves in the process and shaping our existence in particular ways. We rely on narrative to engage in sense-making (Query, Kreps, Arneson, & Caso, 2001; Weick, 1995) and to figure out how to be in the world, how to live our lives in meaningful ways (Coles, 1989). Accordingly, we organize our discussion of narrative knowing and being around issues of identity construction and dialogic activity.

## Identity Construction

Narrating is a central feature of communication between providers and patients, in the relationships enacted in health organizations, and in the mediated world of health-related persuasion, information, and entertainment. As scholars interested in narrative as a way of knowing and being within micro- and macrocontexts, we are less concerned with defining what a narrative is and more so with what the process of narrating does. Labeling some form of communication as a *narrative* (i.e., when frozen under the microscope it corresponds to predetermined characteristics of narrative) matters less than how that form of communication viewed as *narrating* provides us with knowledge of the realities people presuppose in defining themselves and enacting their social and relational identities. Narrating is a discursive, social, and relational process that constitutes knowledge of self and others (Gergen, 1991).

Identity construction inevitably is entangled in a meandering, discursive web of narrative (Brockmeier & Carbaugh, 2001). Through our narrative activity, we embody what we call our self and its actions, reflections, thoughts, and place in the world. Narratives, or what Somers (1994) termed "ontological narratives," are used to "... define who we are. This in turn can be a precondition for knowing what to do. This 'doing' will in turn produce new narratives and hence, new actions; the relationship between narrative and ontology is processual and mutually constitutive" (p. 618).

Narratives simultaneously work as agents of *self-discovery* and *self-creation* (Bruner, 1990, 2001, 2002), a primary communicative practice through which the author's identity evolves, is enacted, and put to use. In true Burkean (1969) spirit, we hold that humans tell stories and also that humans are storied. We live stories in and through our being—embodied performances—and within and through the tensions constituted by our memories of the past and anticipations of the future.

Self-making depends heavily on the symbolic systems in which it is situated, as individuals engage in a performative struggle of sorts over the meanings of health and healing (Langellier, 2001). In the telling of

particular stories in particular ways, narrators and others are constituted as participants whose subjectivities emerge through a symbiosis
of the performed story and the social relations in which it is embedded.
Key questions for narrators include: What are the consequences my
story produces? What kind of person does it shape me into? What new
possibilities does it introduce for being in this world? How does "my"
story position readers? (Eco, 1994; Ellis & Bochner, 2000).

As authors argue throughout this book, narratives become especially consequential for ever-emergent relationships between various
health care participants. Through their ongoing participation in (and
shaping of) health narratives, health care participants demonstrate
and construct their orientations to medical situations, personal and
relational identities, and even "ownership" of the narrative (i.e., "this is
my story as opposed to your story"). In chapter 3, Beck enters the public conversation about Cathy Hainer's (a writer for *USA Today*) journey
through diagnosis of and treatment for breast cancer. Hainer refused
to accept the narrow label of *reporter with cancer*, opting instead for
complex, narrative embodiments of her multifaceted, ever-evolving,
identity as a woman grieving for unborn children, wife, daughter, journalist, and so on. Ultimately, Beck draws our attention to how "personal" stories are always co-constructed and increasingly, in postmodern times, negotiated in public dialogues about health and healing
(see also Morris, 1998).

## Narrative as Dialogic

We further position *narrativity* as a social, communicative process
that is inherently dialogic. Rather than representing only the inner
state of a narrator, meaning is always co-constructed in the liminal
space (Turner, 1980) between participants. Meaning, thus, lies in the
interface between stories, not in the mind or the words of any sole participant. Rawlins (2003) beautifully captured the essence of dialogue in
his discussion of hearing voices:

> Hearing others is not a passive enactment of being-in-conversation.
> Hearing *voices*, it says something about you that is critical ... this speak-
> ing constituted by your listening matters only if you actually do hear, only
> if you allow the other person's voice and stories to reach you, to change
> you. (p. 122)

We create possibilities (or fail to) for knowing and being together in the
moment-to-moment dialogue with others that marks the flow of
human, ongoing interaction (Bakhtin, 1984a; Hyde, 2004).

It is difficult to resist the conclusion that the nature and shape of
selfhood are as much matters of culture as individual concern

(Gergen, 1991). As Claude Levi-Strauss (1966) suggested, we are *bricoleurs*, beneficiaries of society's stock plots yet improvisers in the stories we tell of ourselves. Identity construction depends upon co-constructed, shared meanings and depends also on dialogically performed modes of discourse (i.e., narratives) for negotiating differences in meanings and interpretations. "The very shape of our lives—the rough and perpetually changing draft of the autobiography that we carry in our minds," argues Bruner (1990), "is understandable to ourselves and to others only by virtue of those cultural systems of interpretation" (p. 33).

In her 2001 book, Beck details a health care crisis. However, her story encompasses more than information about medical procedures and complications, and her personal journey through illness and wellness. Her travels include passing interactions with emergency medical workers and ongoing dialogues with innumerable health care professionals and a diverse collection of family members and friends. Although individuals may bodily experience the agony of a broken bone or the discomfort of chemotherapy, health care challenges are inherently relational. Implicitly, each individual shares his or her own health experience with an array of others as she or he crosses paths with others traveling their own trails, with their own frustrations, orientations, concerns, perspectives, and so on. Many authors in this volume privilege explorations of emergent, co-constructed health narratives and their implications for individual and relational identities and for the accomplishment of health care and social support. For example, Bill Rawlins (chap. 9) presents a compelling account of his father's "calling" to be a patient-centered physician committed to understanding others' health in and through their lived stories. Dr. Jack Rawlins is a storyteller, healer, expert diagnostician, and *co-constructor* of his patients' stories—interconnected aspects of narrative competence that form the essence of the life of one called to heal.

To view physician–patient interviews as the co-construction of narrative knowledge—interactions that both parties and others will use to understand and explain the physical, psychological, and spiritual status of the patient—is a new way of envisioning the delivery of health care (Hunter, 1991). A family's or group's ongoing struggle to deal with a seriously ill member can be understood as the co-construction of a group story that allows them to cope with changes in identities, relationships, and duties imposed by an illness (Adelman & Frey, 1997). From this perspective, health organizations serve not only the repositories of stories but constitute stories themselves (i.e., co-constructed sociopolitical narratives that impact both those within and outside the organization). Advertising, news and entertainment use discrete stories that, taken collectively, compose a cumulative story about health and illness in our culture, our common expectations and fears, and beliefs in causes and cures.

From a dialogic perspective, narrative methodology expands as well, inviting alternative considerations of narrative form, structure, function, and content. Rather than treating narratives merely as containers of concepts or themes, scholars can engage issues of *narrative selection* and *variation*, directing attention to what stories are told and retold in particular contexts until they become taken-for-granted as knowledge, or, alternatively, how stories evolve and change across time and space as various constituencies render their experience in alternate stories (see chap. 14, this volume, by Miller, Geist-Martin, & Cannon). Scholars can direct attention to *narrative voice*, who participates as active agents in the co-construction of stories (see chap. 10, this volume, by Morgan-Witte), as well as *narrative auditors*—to whom the stories are told, locating the anticipated audience in stories (see chap. 8, this volume, by Singhal, Chitnis, & Sengupta). Equally important are *narrative silences*, the gaps in stories, the unmentioned or unmentionable, as well as the absence of certain stories altogether (see chap. 7, this volume, by Carabas & Harter, and chap. 4, this volume, by Harter, Kirby, Edwards, & McClanahan). A dialogic perspective also permits attention to *narrative ideologies*, the values and morals embodied in the form and structure of the narrative (see chap. 15, this volume, by Sharf, and chap. 5, this volume, by Japp & Japp). Narratives, like other linguistic genres, represent what Bakhtin (1981) termed *dialogized heteroglossia*—struggles among sociolinguistic systems and ideological points of view. Scholars can and should deal with the life and behavior of narrative in a contradictory and multilanguaged world.

Narrative scholars attempt to make sense of co-constructed social life. We collaborate with participants to understand how human experience is endowed with meaning. Stories do not merely present themselves to us. We actively construct important aspects of narratives, from the formulation of research questions and the identification of a research "problem" to the drawing of conclusions (see also Boje, 2001; Cheney, 2000; Czarniawska, 1998). Scholars ought to be aware of the processes by which we interpret social activity. In narrative work, the researcher's reflexivity is not only allowed for, it is encouraged, perhaps even summoned. Authors in this volume remain keenly aware of their power in co-constructing stories with participants. Keeley and Kellas (chap. 17) poignantly reveal how narrative works to construct individual and relational identities during final conversations between loved ones, allowing individuals to come to terms with their own life trajectories (including death) and reaffirm, celebrate, and in some cases, recapture relationships with others. Keeley's personal experiences with final conversations flavor how the authors embody final conversations. Likewise, Bosticco and Thompson (chap. 18) position *bereavement* as disruption, a call for stories, and grieving individuals as storytellers making sense of their malaise, taking control of events formerly beyond their power or influence, and restoring coherence in their lives. Cecilia's riveting narrative as a still-grieving mother who lost a child invites readers in and encourages them to understand bereavement as co-constructed by Cecilia and other grieving parents.

## CONTINUITY AND DISRUPTION

There always remains an unrealized surplus of humanness; there always remains a need for the future, and a place for this future must be found.

—Bakhtin, 1981, p. 37

The problematic of continuity and disruption concerns disorder and the human desire for coherence. Philosophers from Aristotle to Kenneth Burke have noted that the primary impetus to narrative is expectations gone awry. Narrativity involves characters embedded in the complexities of lived moments of struggle, heroes or victims who resist or accept the intrusions of disruption and chaos, preserve or restore continuity, and re-story meaning in their lives in the face of unexpected blows of fate. Although such complexities resound throughout history, the postmodern condition confounds our quest for stability. As Gergen (1991) details, "social saturation furnishes us with a multiplicity of incoherent and unrelated languages of the self. For everything we 'know to be true' about ourselves, other voices within respond with doubt and even derision" (pp. 6–7). Amid the blur of conflicting truths, abundant social and relational options, and massive technological advances, individuals seek answers (although perhaps not absolutism), identities (although likely fragmented), and understanding (although quite certainly incomplete). We make stories to come to terms with the surprises and oddities of the human condition and our imperfect grasp of that condition (Bruner, 2002). Indeed, as Bruner suggests, "The narrative gift seems to be our natural way of using language for characterizing those deviations from the expected state of things that characterize living in a human culture" (p. 85). Making stories is deeply about human plight. This being so, in this section we discuss narrating as emplotting and locating, and illness as a call for stories.

### Narrating as Emplotting and Locating

A central feature of narrative is its ability to deal simultaneously with the canonical and the unexpected (Bruner, 1986, 1990, 2002). Narratives recount human plans gone off course, what Aristotle in *Poetics* termed *peripeteia*, and conventionalize the common forms of mishap into genres (e.g., comedy, tragedy, romance, and irony). Burke's (1969) theory of symbolic action, often called *dramatism*, also emphasizes expectations gone awry. Well-formed stories, argues Burke, reveal the source or force of action, *the agent*; the nature of action, *the act*; the context in which action take place, *the scene*; the manner or means of action, *the agency*; and the ultimate goals that propel that action, *the purpose*. It is the conversion of "Trouble" with a capital "T" (in Burke's sense) into narrative plight that makes human drama so powerful, comfortable, dangerous, and culturally essential (see chap. 6 by Workman in this volume). Trouble consists of imbalance among elements of Burke's pentad, and involves moral values, commitments, and consequences. Given such threats to the coherence of our experiences, stories achieve meaning, in part, by emplotting deviations from the ordinary in comprehensible form.

*Narrating* as *emplotting* refers to how characters and actions are organized in a temporal trajectory that determines action and implies movement toward a point or goal (Ricouer, 1981b). Ricouer describes a story as:

> A sequence of actions and experiences of a certain number of characters, whether real or imaginary. These characters are represented in situations which change ... [to] which they react. These changes, in turn, reveal hidden aspects of situations and the characters, giving rise to a new predicament which calls for thought or action or both. The response to this predicament brings the story to its conclusion. (p. 277)

Narrative usually embodies implicit or explicit opposition. Without conflict—overt or implicit, actual or potential—some argue, no narrative exists (e.g., Somers, 1994). A story implies that differences exist, even the fundamental opposition of "I" and "you," or "now" and "then," and that such differences have the potential to influence outcomes. The process of emplotting often defines the loci of difference, and determines how relationships are developed and differences engaged (or avoided). Characters, or sites of action, are designated and articulated; these loci of action may be people, ideas, institutions, or other elements that propel the story in time, ground it in space, and drive it toward some sort of resolution (Burke, 1969).

*Narrating* as *locating* involves the process of placement, constructing boundaries of time and space (Somers, 1994). Narrative theorists posit the fundamental process of narrating as the "and then," the constructing of a sequence of elements with all of the implications and evaluations involved in temporal ordering. As one narrates, he or she constructs and weighs the past/present/future flow of continuity and disruption to give force to some understanding of the distinction between "now" and "then." Other theorists point out that narrative also constructs an "and there," the placement of elements in juxtaposition to each other spatially or relationally (e.g., Holstein & Gubrium, 2000). Thus, distinctions of "here/there," "in/out," or "we/they," for example, are spatial, relational indicators of closeness and distance equally as important as temporal placements. Narrative action, then, occurs within this co-constructed locus. As Holstein and Gubrium (2000) noted, "it is important to remember that narrative practice does not simply unfold within the interpretive boundaries of going concerns but constructs the definition of those boundaries" (p. 107).

Although characters' lives are necessarily temporally bound, they are not inherently linear (Ricouer, 1981b). Indeed, especially in a health context, individuals "recover" and "suffer relapses." Health conditions fluctuate. Amid physical changes, advances, and setbacks, the trajectory ensues as individuals enact their physical, emotional, spiritual and professional selves. Trajectories may clash as others judge, label, and stereotype (see chap. 13, this volume, by Buzzanell & Ellingon). Can we "move on" if others "lock us in?" Thus, narrative theorizing must grapple with the incompatibility of stories in light of time, place, and space.

Narrating, emplotting and locating, provides a ready and supple means of dealing with unexpected outcomes or unintended consequences of our plans, anticipations, and hopes (Giddens, 1979). The efficacy of narrative for sense making becomes especially consequential when the continuity of our lives is disrupted by illness, violence, or trauma. Yet, narrative is not an instant cure—it cannot make pain go away, and things do not always make sense. We cannot always package stories into neat and organized accounts of experiences that wreck havoc on our existence and life as we knew it before the disruption of illness.

## Illness as a Call for Stories

In his foundational work, *The Wounded Storyteller*, Arthur Frank (1995) positions illness as a call for stories and ill individuals as wounded storytellers. Individuals with serious illness have lost a central resource that most storytellers depend on—a sense of temporality. Individuals can use narration to (re)create a sense of where one is in light of bodily malfunction and change. For example, Gibbs and Franks (2002) illustrated how women narrate their experiences with cancer and draw on metaphorical patterns of thought that are inherently temporal (e.g., life as a journey, life as a gamble). Of course, not all metaphors or narratives are equal in their transformative power and ability to enable women to restory their lives in light of the disruption of cancer. Vanderford and Smith (1996) also illustrated how women engage in narrative sensemaking when faced with the disruption of immune-related illnesses due to breast implants, relying on support groups, interactions with health care providers, and public dialogues to manage uncertainty and restore continuity to their lives.

Importantly, Frank (1995) argued that stories are not just *about* the body—they are told *through* a wounded body:

> The stories that ill people tell come out of their bodies. The body sets in motion the need for new stories when its disease disrupts the old stories. The body, whether still diseased or recovered, is simultaneously cause, topic, and instrument of whatever new stories are told. (p. 2)

Telling a story through the body is part and parcel of the human problem of authorship, and the desire of individuals to preserve voice and agency (Charmaz, 1995; Ellis, 1995; Ellis & Bochner, 2001; Langellier, 2001; Langellier & Peterson, 2004). Seeking medical care too often involves what Frank describes as *narrative surrender*—with individuals following prescribed regimens and embodying their "story" using the vernacular and practices of the dominant biomedical model (see also Geist & Dreyer, 1993; Kleinmann, 1988; Mishler, 1984; Morris, 1998).

Fortunately, medical journals attest that physicians are increasingly cognizant of narrative, not in opposition to science but as an integral and necessary aspect of health and healing (e.g., Charon, 2001b; Elwyn & Gwyn, 1999; Garro, 1994; Greenhalgh, 1999; Jones, 1999). If health unfolds as a storied experience, healing, too, can be usefully understood as narrative activity. The rise of "narrative medicine" as co-constructed by "narratively competent" health care seekers and providers may signify fundamental changes in the experience of illness (Charon, 2001b). Charon (2001b) described *narrative medicine* as that which is "practiced with the competence to recognize, interpret, and be moved to action by the predicaments of others" (p. 83).

White and Epston (1990) reenvisioned the work of psychiatry as inherently narrative and popularized the therapeutic value of narrative. By helping patients to reframe key moments and characters around which people organize their lives, new, liberating, co-constructed stocks of knowledge emerge that allow individuals to restory their lives. Likewise, Mattingly (2000, 2001) encouraged physical therapists and other health care providers to envision therapy as a punctuated moment in the patient's longer life story. Therapy itself becomes an occasion for individuals (with the help of providers) to remake life stories that can no longer continue as they once did when a disability was absent, or less serious. In this volume, Ragan, Mindt, and Wittenberg-Lyles (chap. 12) emphasize the value of narrative pedagogy in the professional socialization of medical students, particularly in introducing students to palliative care. In doing so, Ragan and her colleagues outline ways that medical schools address the narrative structure of medical knowledge and health care delivery by (a) requiring students to study and analyze fiction and nonfiction illness narratives, and (b) requiring students to write their own narratives.

Many authors in this book recognize the power of narrative to empower and enable women and men, health care providers and seekers, to account for continuity and disruption across their lifespans. Sharf (chap. 15, this volume), well-known for her scholarly work on patient empowerment and health citizenry (e.g., 1990, 1997, 2001), poignantly shares how her personal road toward patient autonomy and clinical partnership during hip replacement therapy was detoured by pain, fatigue, and the still-dominant biomedical model. O'Hair, Scannell and Thompson (chap. 19, this volume) foreground how people with cancer can exert agency through narrative in managing the cancer care environment. O'Hair and his colleagues encourage health care seekers and providers to co-construct narrative emplotments of the cancer experience, including treatment protocols. Carabas and Harter (chap. 7, this volume) share testimonials of former political prisoners and deportees in Romania, drawing attention to the degenerative role that the censoring of storytelling plays in the lives of people who suffered from state-induced illness. Their participants' narratives poignantly capture how their "forbidden stories" increased their psychological trauma. If storytelling allows individuals to cope with the disruption of trauma, and indeed it can, then the absence of the narrative act deepens the sense of turmoil, loss, and discontinuity.

Noticeably absent from this volume and interdisciplinary writing about narrative and health more generally is the chaos story—an incoherent pastiche of observations and characters that is often uncomfortable to witness. Unlike the reassuring restitution narratives imbued with faith in modern medicine's progress and promise, chaos narratives reveal human vulnerability, the futility and impotence of science, and an inability of the human body and spirit to overcome adversity (Frank, 1995). O'Hair and his colleagues (chap. 19, this volume) aptly argue that the "wounded storyteller" may be unable to exercise agency through narrative due to physical, social, relational, and structural forces. Likewise, Ragan and her colleagues (chap. 12, this volume) question the extent to which students' empathic skills can be honed by witnessing illness narratives that, for the most part, are polished, edited, and complete. Authors often edit literary narratives to produce a coherent and compelling chronology of events and emotions, with competent and articulate narrators and characters. In reality, individuals' stories are often incoherent bits and pieces that must be stitched together to make sense.

We believe that social, political, and economic forces coalesce in ways that often inhibit the telling and witnessing of chaos stories. It is difficult to *hear* stories in which wounds remain raw, bodies and spirits broken. Frank (1995) suggested:

> Hearing is difficult not only because listeners have trouble facing what is being said as a possibility or a reality in their own lives. Hearing is also difficult because the chaos narrative is probably the most embodied form of story. If chaos stories are told on the edges of a wound, they are also told on the edges of speech. Ultimately, chaos is told in the silences that speech cannot penetrate or illuminate. (p. 101)

We yearn for emplotments that redeem disruptions in orderly ways. Restitution narratives provide happy endings, reassuring consumers, among other things, that technology can triumph over nature. Moreover, when we as scholars focus on the agency of narrative, we privilege stories of successful empowerment, preferring to believe in the efficacy of communication. Yet, it is also our moral obligation to recognize and honor chaos as part of life and to witness chaos stories as shared by others. We agree with Rawlins (2003) who argued, "Listening and hearing honors the gift of self that is speaking: it renders voice meaningful" (p. 121).

## CREATIVITY AND CONSTRAINT

> A self-making narrative is something of a balancing act. It must, on the one hand, create a conviction of autonomy, that one has a will of one's own, a certain freedom of choice, a degree of possibility. But it must also relate the self to a world of others—to friends and family, to institutions, to the past, to reference groups … we seem virtually unable to live without both, autonomy and commitment, and our lives try to balance the two. So do the self-narratives we tell ourselves.
>
> —Bruner, 2002, p. 78

The problematic of creativity and constraint foregrounds the human struggle to be individuated (i.e., assert creativity) and still identify with a group (i.e., respond to social and institutional constraints). Berger and Luckmann (1966) argued that societies are constructed as people act in patterned ways—routines that, over time, are taken for granted

as "reality." In other words, most of what we take for granted in communal life is constructed through symbolic interactions. Across time
and space, routines develop and people amass a general knowledge of
"how things are done." Social life, then, involves an unresolvable tension between creativity and constraint; individuals co-construct social
reality and become constrained by those constructions (Giddens,
1979, 1984). Moreover, simultaneous desires for individualism and
community represent a fundamental tension of liberal pluralistic societies (deTocqueville, 1835/1956; Locke, 1690/1975). We examine this
struggle as embodied in narrative activity. We believe that narrativity
involves the moment-to-moment negotiation of tensions between individual creativity and social constraints (see also Eisenberg & Goodall,
2004; Harter, 2004). In this section, we explore connections between
the personal and the cultural, and the ideological and political nature
of narrative activity including creative resistance to social constraints.

### The Personal and the Cultural

Numerous scholars have contributed to our understanding of the interconnectedness of the personal and the cultural (e.g., Bakhtin, 1981,
1984b; Burke, 1969; Bruner, 1991, 2001, 2002; Dewey, 1922; 1984;
Foucault, 1975; Giddens, 1979; Goffman, 1959; Wittgenstein, 1953).
For example, Dewey (1922) positioned experience as both personal and
social. People are individuals and need to be understood as such, but
they cannot be understood only as individuals (see also Blumer, 1969;
Mead, 1934). Self is always in relation to others, always in social context
(Gergen, 1991). Goffman, too, reminds us that individuals create and
enact their roles as scripted, in part, by larger social forces. Bakhtin
draws our attention to *intertextuality*—how narratives of all sorts draw
meaning, in part, from their relation to other texts. Individuals config-
ure events into stories, ordering experiences by intermixing various elements of their cultural repertoire of sedimented stories. We lead storied
lives on storied landscapes. Collectively, these scholars encourage us to
consider simultaneously the personal and the cultural, and the enabling
and constraining aspects of narrativity.

To participate as a member of a culture, individuals must possess a
general knowledge of signifying systems and their situated meanings.
Cultures maintain collections of normative meanings in their myths,
fairy tales, histories, and other stories. Our personal experiences are
shaped within these discursive parameters, including enveloping
macronarratives ranging from stories of one's family to institutional
stories of the workplace, church, government, and nation (Somers,
1994). We live our lives within a series of intersecting social systems
that may be thought of as stories, each characterized by plotlines,

characters, genres, and themes. These master narratives, or what Somers calls *metanarrativity*, provide a wider circle of narrative patterning that incorporates and shapes personal and public narratives. Master narratives are often subsumed in a word or phrase that evokes the repository of stories, metaphors, and images that coalesce around what Burke (1969) called "god terms," such as individualism, progress, enlightenment, equality, and so on. For example, Conrad and Millay (2001) foregrounded conservative politics and libertarian, free market ideology in their analysis of the enactment of the first Patient's Bill of Rights by the Texas legislature. They illustrate the powerful rhetoric of free-market romanticism, and how it flavors the American political psyche and health care reform rhetoric.

Of course, cultural stocks of meaning are not static; they are added to by new members, and atrophy by lack of use. Narrative scholars explore the experiencing of life in the here and now as well as experiences throughout life trajectories—people's lives, institutional lives, lives of things. Our lives are embedded within larger narrative landscapes, times and spaces that shape our lives and the stories we tell of them. The construction of individuals as storytellers, characters, or witnesses comprises a contextual feature of particular material, social and historical moments, and is explored as such by numerous narrative scholars (see Workman, chap. 6, and Beck, chap. 3, this volume).

## The Ideological and Political Nature of Narrative Activity

Public discourses of health and healing are narratively constructed. The social world is a world of narrative forms and formulas people use to construct meanings of self and others. These narratives draw on and reinforce personal and organizational narratives and function as public "mindsets," the boundaries within which health and healing are interpreted and discussed. Such master narratives embody sociocultural beliefs, values, hopes and fears. Indeed, narrative is one of the principal symbolic forms through which ideology and power structures are expressed and constituted (Mumby, 1987). Narrative—in all its forms—does ideological work that shapes our relationships to the world in ways that are not always apparent to us.

Scholars who direct attention to the ideological and political aspects of narrative ask why narratives are framed as they are, how stakeholders negotiate them within social contexts of action, and how emergent narratives enable and constrain the human spirit. These questions, once raised, lead scholars to speculate about how narratives could be constructed differently, recontextualizing key issues and concerns. Harter and Japp (2001), for example, positioned Western medical dramas as texts to be read for dominant meanings of health and health care. In doing so, they highlighted how these discourses serve to reinforce the dominance and legitimacy of technological medicine (i.e., the biomedical model) even as they sometimes appear to question it. In this volume, Morgan-Witte (chap. 10) similarly positions the contemporary nurse's station as a web of storytelling. Health care providers create and maintain ideologies of the biomedical model as they tell stories, gossip, crack jokes, and play pranks.

Morris (1998) also positions the biomedical model as a grand narrative: an ongoing structure of values and beliefs; a hierarchy of characters; a past, present, and future; sacred spaces; goals and purposes; manners and means. The long dominant biomedical narrative reduces disease to a biological mechanism of cause and effect that can be effectively diagnosed and treated through science and technology. But doing so privileges the "voice of medicine" and marginalizes the "voice of the lifeworld" (Mishler, 1984). Arthur Kleinman (1988, 1995), a psychiatrist and medical anthropologist, among others (e.g., Brody, 1980, 1987; Geist & Gates, 1996; Vanderford, Jenks, & Sharf, 1997), has worked to disrupt the dominance of a biomedical approach as the primary means of understanding health and healing. Yet, interweaving the voice of medicine and the voice of the lifeworld in a dialogue that transforms individuals and helps them to navigate through preventative care, diagnosis of particular ailments and treatment regimens is difficult, in part, because we continue to exist in a world of binaries: illness versus wellness, disease versus illness, biology versus culture.

Constructing a counternarrative to the still-dominant biomedical model involves, among other things, a postmodern perspective of health that escapes the dualism that we are either sick or well. According to Morris (1998, p. 243), "A postmodern perspective on health opens when we imagine that—except at the extremes of terrible illness and perfect comfort—most people live within a trajectory exposing them to intermittent trauma and even chronic damage."

In this counternarrative, health and health care are reenvisioned as the manners in which we live *well* despite our inescapable illnesses, disabilities, and trauma. For example, in this volume Buzzanell and Ellingson (chap. 13) problematize the limiting nature of entrepreneurial narratives of maternity in the workplace that reproduce the binary of ill versus well—narratives that associate pregnancy with deviance, unreliability, and disability. Moreover, they urge communication scholars–practitioners to create counternarratives that present bodily variation and fluctuation as normative and give voice to the diverse experiences of pregnant workers. "Stories must be told for awareness," argue Buzzanell and Ellingson, "and retold in counternarratives until they impact cultural and organizational delusions of ideal bodies and perpetuation of the sick/well dichotomy."

As illustrated by our discussion of the biomedical model, stories of any sort are not innocent; rather, they embody worldviews and biases—they have a spin. Narratives are shaped within certain beliefs and value systems, and serve to reinforce or challenge those systems as they are constituted in social interaction. Three decades ago, feminist scholars declared that "the personal is political," meaning among other things that personal experience is inescapably social and social experience is inescapably political. In narrative as well "the personal is political." We construct personal experience within social contexts, bounded and constrained by the identities and relationships of the social group. Further, these identities are positioned in ongoing negotiations within that society. To empower a group is to legitimate its story of who its members are; to silence a group (or person) is to refuse to hear or accept its story.

Master narratives thereby embody the ideological concerns and political conflicts of a culture and are powerful in their ubiquity and familiarity. As Lindemann-Nelson noted (2001):

> Master narratives retain their tenacious hold on a culture for a number
> of interconnected reasons: they are organized ensembles that grow and
> change, they constitute a world view, and they assimilate oppositions. In
> addition, oppressive master narratives are often epistemically rigged.
> Taken in combination, these features produce a formidable resiliency.
> (pp. 157–158)

Social narratives (de)legitimate certain modes of culture, consciousness, and practice. Yet, narratives emerge as contested terrains, open to challenge by those who seek to reshape perceptions of health issues and construct alternate narratives. Indeed, "postmodernism" loosely represents challenges to the domination of master narratives (e.g., science as progress), favoring instead local storytelling and the ability of people to use resources at their disposal to make sense of their lives (Lyotard, 1984). For example, feminist political struggles across borders of nations and states crucially involve new ways of perceiving and retelling a nation's history (Harding, 1998; Narayan, 1997).

Just as we may accede to habitual responses and environmental forces, we also have the capacity to deliberate and decide which stories we will tell and live, and whether we will imagine and enact alternative emplotments. The realm of meaning making possesses plasticity (Bakhtin, 1981). Bruner (2002) aptly argued:

> Stories are a culture's coin and currency. For culture is, figuratively, the
> maker and enforcer of what is expected, but it also, paradoxically, com-
> piles, even slyly treasures, transgressions. Its myths and its folktales, its

dramas and its pageants memorialize both its norms and notable violations of them. (p. 15)

Stories are not mere instantiations of the canonical; they often evolve
as terrains of struggle and political contestation, embodying what
Bruner calls the dialectic of the established and the possible. A group
or society can disrupt hegemonic forces and construct an alternative
story that is more equitable and inclusive.

Master narratives may appear monolithic but because they are a brico-
lage of components, they have tensions, fissures, and gaps that can be ex-
ploited by those who want to challenge their power (Lindemann-Nelson,
2001). The recommendation of Conrad and Millay (2001) is a case in point:

> Instead of casting [health care] reform as a story that competes with the
> narrative of a self-correcting free market, an approach that has typified
> past [failed] efforts at both the federal and state levels ... proponents can
> instead operate within free market ideology, searching for fissures and
> contradictions, and arguing that reform can strengthen and purify the
> free market system. (pp. 166–167)

Social, political, and economic conditions sometimes coalesce in
ways that create spaces where counternarratives can take hold. For
example, individuals share personal narratives of AIDS within the
boundaries of public and societal narratives that determine social
meanings and attributions of the disease (Sontag, 1988). These personal narratives are often used in the service of negotiating awareness, demanding justice, and seeking resources, as well as
challenging the public narratives of "placement" of the disease and its
victims. Personal narratives, thus, function as powerful tools in efforts to enact both social understanding and political recognition.
Some narratives, like those of people with AIDS or cancer, have direct
political utility as they are used to advocate for protective legislation
or funding for research.

Personal narratives enacted in local or interpersonal settings are no
less political. These narratives assert both a right to proclaim publicly
(to even a few others) one's identity and the need to define one's experience as relevant. Such stories also testify to the opportunities and constraints of operating within the ideologies of the public, master
narratives available in a culture. Whether in acceptance of or opposition to the larger narratives, they embody prevailing attitudes and beliefs about illness and understandings of the institutions and
structures of health care.

Many authors in this volume envision narratives as sources of both
creativity and constraint. Japp and Japp (chap. 5) focus attention on
one genre of illness narratives—stories told by individuals (mainly

women) with "biologically invisible illnesses" (BII). They illustrate how women's stories of BII reside in and are connected to a broader network of narratives (e.g., master narrative of bio-medicine) that both enable and constrain women in their attempts to legitimize their experiences. Workman (chap. 6), guided by Burke's (1969) notion of the representative anecdote, argues that the "death story" of Scott Kruger, an upper class student at MIT, worked to frame binge drinking as a public health problem. Although the death story served to raise awareness of heavy episodic drinking, Workman illustrates how it also criminalized and victimized particular individuals. He offers alternative stories for framing binge drinking that concentrate on more salient harms to college students such as embarrassment, regret, academic failure, or legal liability. In examining the narrative construction of age-related infertility (ARI), Harter, Kirby, Edwards, and McClanahan (chap. 4) argue that the technical rationality of expert voices (e.g., reproductive endocrinologists) shapes the way women narrate their experiences with ARI—what they include (e.g., time, technology, meritocracy) and exclude (e.g., husband's influence, possibility for adoption) in their storytelling. At the same time, they present alternative stock plots that capture the systemic nature of how reproduction is embodied symbolically, biologically, materially and in networks of relationships.

## THE PARTIAL AND THE INDETERMINATE

> We enter the conversation after it has already started; we try to get the hang of it; we leave it, just as we are catching the drift of it; after us, it goes on.
>
> —Cheney, 2000, p. 21

Whenever we use language to narrate our experiences, slippage, inexactness, and indeterminancy remain (Burke, 1969; Wittgenstein, 1953). Concomitantly, every narrative is embedded in a lived context of interaction, uncertainty, intention, and imagination (see Babrow, Kline, & Rawlins, chap. 2, this volume). As situations and standpoints shift, new and different stories emerge. The problematic of the partial and the indeterminate recognizes that stories are discretely bounded (and as such always partial), and cumulatively ongoing (and as such always indeterminate). Likewise, any scholarly performance ought to be understood as situated, contingent, partial, and subject to revision. Narrativity and narrative scholarship are inherently open-ended; a good story and a good study ought to conclude with questions as well as tentative answers. In this section, we explore the situated and shifting nature of narrative knowledge.

## Situated Knowledge

In narrative thinking and other "language games" context matters
(Wittgenstein, 1953). Narrativity always occurs in particular situations
as storytellers draw on the resources of language and cultural, relational, material and physiological conditions to perform narrative. We
require contextual knowledge to make sense of any person, event, experience, and emplotment. Moreover, because we construct meaning
in the fragmented contexts and subjectivities of our lives (Gergen,
1991), any story or interpretation is always partial.

Narrative scholars explore how varied contexts give rise to particular stories and performance practices, directing attention to how resources in a particular situation make storytelling possible. Narrative
scholars explore the places and spaces in which narratives are performed and how storytelling reveals the social conditions of its production. Babrow, Kline, and Rawlins, (chap. 2), emphasize that a narrative
perspective foregrounds two contextual forms: the setting of the narrative, or the *lived context* of the storied events, and the setting of the telling itself, or the *living context* of the storytelling. Meaning-making
emerges in the symbolic space or liminal space (Turner, 1980) between
lived and living contexts, and between narrators, emplotments, and
audience. "Meaning is understood to take shape—for different critics
in different ways and to different degrees," argued Chambers and
Montgomery (2002), "in the symbolic space that reader, text, and other
elements create during the reading process and does not exist without
the subjective activity and the contextual element brought to the text by
each reader" (p. 87). In sum, storytelling informs and is informed by
temporal, relational, and spatial contexts.

Bakhtin's (1981, 1984b) work usefully positions narrative as interactive and contextually rooted. Bakhtin envisions narrative as dialogue, a *heteroglossia* of different voices, a continuous and shifting
struggle within and among discourses representing ideological belief
systems and competing views of the word:

> The living utterance, having taken meaning and shape at a particular his-
> torical moment in a socially specific environment, cannot fail to brush up
> against thousands of living dialogic threads, woven by socioideological
> consciousness around the given object of an utterance; it cannot fail to
> become an active participant in social dialogue. (p. 276)

Bakhtin's work encourages us to consider the range of multiple languages, voices and understandings present in any particular "text" or
reading, and reminds us that narrative knowledge is always situated
and always partial. For example, research texts constitute stories, usu-

ally presented as complete yet always open to diverse consumption (Ellis & Bochner, 2000). Readers enter scholarly narratives from the perspective of their own standpoints, become co-performers, and, ultimately, (re)consider themselves through the narrative text.

In the mutual interplay of telling and listening, the question of authorship and individual participation in meaning-making becomes critical. A dialogic perspective permits us to move away from a message production standpoint (i.e., emphasis on storyteller as sole "owner" of a singular story) toward one that recognizes how narratives are fluid, co-constructed, meaning-centered (re)productions of experience always achieved in particular contexts and subject to frames of intelligibility (see also Zook, 1994). Many authors in this volume operate from a dialogic perspective. Beach and Mandelbaum (chap. 16), in their careful conversation analysis of a medical interview, foreground the locally situated, interactional accomplishment of narrative between a health care provider and patient. As illustrated by Beach and Mandelbaum, what gets expressed, understood, and accepted (and what remains untold or underdeveloped) depends as much on the context of the interaction as on the desires of the participants. Sunwolf, Frey, and Keranen (chap. 11) draw our attention to the therapeutic importance of "story sharing" for tellers and listeners. Sunwolf and her colleagues position story sharing as a dynamic and transformational process through which individuals (re)construct individual and communal identities.

## Shifting Knowledge

Meaning-making is not static; rather, it shifts through the ongoing exigencies of relational work and as individuals continuously reconfigure experiences through reflection and recollection (Polkinghorne, 1988; Rawlins, 2003). We privilege the term *narrativity* to emphasize the open-ended, ongoing process of narrating rather than fixed and frozen texts conveniently designated as narratives (see also Langellier & Peterson, 2004; Somers, 1994). People live stories, and in the living of these stories, reaffirm them, modify them, and create new ones. For example, while our self-making stories accumulate over time and may even pattern themselves after conventional genres, they shift not just because we get older or wiser but because our stories need to fit new circumstances, relationships, and enterprises (Bruner, 2002).

Our narratives, scholarly and otherwise, are always tentative, always open to revision. Contemporary perspectives on history, for example, take history not as an already written narrative of the past, but as actions in the continuing process of living and being within community (White, 1981). Narrative seeks to keep the past alive in the present, showing us that meanings and significance of the past are incomplete, tentative, and revisable according to the contingencies of present life circumstances, the present from which we narrate (Gadamer, 1991; Ricoeur, 1984a). Narrative explanations of one's past do not stand still in a way that allows for certainty. Instead, we exist, however unconsciously or uncomfortably, with unsettled meanings. A case in point: Geist and Dreyer (1993), drawing on Bakhtin (1981, 1984b), argued for a dialogic perspective of medical encounters that recognizes the ever-changing dynamics that fuse and differentiate providers and patients in relationships of interdependence and independence across time and space.

The multiple and shifting nature of meanings should not, however, be perceived as an excuse for scholars to escape choice or dismiss evaluation (Cheney, 2000). Bakhtin (1981) celebrated the novel as an egalitarian site of multivocality—a cacophony of worldviews. Although his concept of *heteroglossia* encourages us to consider the range of voices and understandings present in any particular discourse, Bakhtin also emphasized plausible and defensible interpretations. In other words, our confrontation with *heteroglossia* operates within certain parameters. While the parameters themselves may be contingent and not absolute, they provide individuals with places to stand to consider viable and compelling meanings among which individuals must choose at that moment in time and space. There remains value in trying to identify intended, preferred, and dominant readings of narratives, as long as we recognize that "it's not a project we'll ever complete or get completely right" (Ellis & Bochner, 2000, p. 752).

Many authors in this volume capture the partial and indeterminate nature of narrative sense-making. Miller, Geist-Martin, and Cannon Beatty (chap. 14) share their work with the Tariq Khamisa Foundation, an organization that seeks through pedagogies of peace and forgiveness to alter patterns of violence among youth in the United States. As you read their chapter, you witness the transformation of teachers and students alike as they reframe learning, manage conflict in alternative ways, and shift, if even slightly, the stories of their lives and dominant societal emplotments of violence. Singhal, Chitnis, and Sengupta (chap. 8), in their discussion of how Indian viewers consume health-related Western media, draw our attention to narrative transparency— how texts are read through the lens of religion, ethnicity, culture, politics among other factors that produce diverse reading positions. Singhal and his colleagues aptly demonstrate how text, context, and audience intersect toward polysemic meaning formation. Individuals negotiate unique meanings about health and sexuality with mediated artifacts, in this case *Friends*, in the differentiated contexts in which they act in their everyday lives.

## CONCLUSION

This book features the work of scholars who embrace narrative inquiry as an interpretive, rhetorical, and/or critical framework from which to explore symbolic attempts to understand and enact illness and wellness. Drawing from an intriguing array of theoretical, existential and empirical orientations, these essays pursue the implications of health narratives for individuals engaged in personal and relational sense-making and the construction of multiple, simultaneous, yet perhaps incompatible, realities. As the chapters attest, knowing and being are narrative acts. Moreover, health narratives emerge as complex performances in the midst of enveloping life and social narratives that can enable or constrain, stigmatize or empower, confuse or enlighten individuals as they attempt to restore continuity when faced with the disruption of illness, suffering, or trauma. Embracing such persistent problematics, the authors in this volume do not search for a universal and fixed meaning in discourses. Rather, they attempt to present rich portraits that are life-like and ring true, and participate in richly contoured and nuanced discussions about narrative, health, and healing.

Collectively, the chapters illustrate the aspirations of narrative theory, research, and practice to comprehend key problematics of life: knowing and being, continuity and disruption, creativity and constraint, and the partial and indeterminate. We believe that the issues dramatized in these chapters provide theoretical resources for more complex and fruitful thinking about narrative and health. We hope they offer you the reader, as witness and co-creator of meaning, insights into the implications of narrative for health care participants as individuals, relational partners, agents in organizing processes, and members of society.

## NOTE

1. We thank Bill Rawlins for his thoughtful reflections on an earlier draft of this manuscript.

# 2

# Narrating Problems and Problematizing Narratives: Linking Problematic Integration and Narrative Theory in Telling Stories About Our Health

**Austin S. Babrow**[1]
*Purdue University*

**Kimberly N. Kline**
*Southern Illinois University*

**William K. Rawlins**
*Ohio University*

Unstable subjective estimates of the chances and value of survival make it difficult for the individual to interpret messages (e.g., judge the honesty of the physician's prognosis), sustain a particular outlook (e.g., maintain optimism), make decisions (e.g., choose between a lumpectomy and a mastectomy), and act consistently with prior choices (e.g., continue chemotherapy).... *(P)roblematic integration* is the difficulty we experience when probabilistic and evaluative orientations to a particular object (e.g., person, thing, event, idea) destabilize one another and unsettle such orientations to associated objects.

—(Babrow, 1995, p. 284, italics added)

Life can be regarded as a constant *effort*, even a struggle, to maintain or restore narrative coherence in the face of an ever-threatening, impending chaos at all levels.

—(Carr, 1986, p. 91)

*For almost two weeks, Kim had been teaching her health communication course to students from her university who were participating in a study-abroad course in England. A small class of seven women, this class had been a particularly exciting opportunity for her because she could concentrate on the women's health issues that had been the predominant focus of her scholarship for the past 7 years. With great zeal, she discussed one of her favorite topics—pregnancy and childbirth. As a staunch advocate of the midwifery[2] model of maternity care, she regaled her students with stories decrying the benefits of and need for medical interventions. Doctors, invested in an objective, scientific approach to health care, tend to spend little if any time with the expectant and/or delivering mother; they often do not attend to the woman's concerns or feelings. Moreover, the medical paradigm, one which pathologizes and medicalizes this very normal experience, typically necessitates technological interventions such as fetal monitoring, epidurals, labor inducement, episiotomies (if you're lucky enough to make it to a natural, vaginal birth), and Cesarean sections, known by medical professionals to be detrimental to mother and child. It's all so impersonal.*

*The midwifery paradigm, on the other hand, advocates attention to the subjective experience of the mother. And, during delivery, practitioners privilege patience, permitting the laboring mother to progress at her own pace so that interventions are needed less often than in the medical model. Birth, from a midwifery perspective, is a natural process that can be challenging but rewarding.*

*Then Kim found out she was pregnant with her second child. As she shared this good news with her students, she knew they would ask, "So, are you going to have this baby at home?" To everyone's surprise, including Kim's, her answer was, "Well, I'm not sure."*

Throughout our lives, experiences of our physical being call forth the construction of (and, in turn, challenge) basic understandings. For example, sexuality, pregnancy, childbirth, diet, exercise, aging, illness, and death elicit—and often call into question—bedrock understandings about body, mind, self, relationships, and the nature of our own life and of life in general. Under such circumstances, that is, when we no longer take for granted the well-being of our bodies and our worlds, communication with others is essential to ongoing meaning-making.

In the spirit of these ideas, this chapter discusses two approaches to the study of health communication that we believe complement each other in compelling ways: narrative and problematic integration (PI) theory and research. We first discuss three complementary suppositions of these two perspectives: meaning-making constitutes a basic characteristic of human being, meaning-making is fundamentally contextual, and meaning-making involves reckoning with time. We then examine in detail how these two approaches can be used together to comprehend the ongoing (co)construction of meaningful configurations of contingencies that emerge through telling and living stories about our health.

## SYNTHESIZING PI AND NARRATIVE THEORY: COMPLEMENTARY SUPPOSITIONS

Rather than offering an extensive review of PI and narrative theories, the following discussion focuses on central claims relevant to health communication that these perspectives share and develop in complementary, mutually elaborating ways. We begin with the argument that meaning-making is a basic characteristic of human being.

### Meaning-Making and Human Being

Fundamental to narrative approaches to sense-making is the assumption that meanings emerge from individual interpretation and rearticulation of the relationships among countless seemingly unconnected experiences, beliefs, attitudes, and understandings, and so on. That is, "meanings are found in interpretation of phenomena, not in objective observations" (Vanderford, Jenks, Sharf, 1997, p. 17). With regard to health and illness, the concern with meaning exemplified by a narrative approach is perhaps best understood in contrast to the concern with so-called facts associated with the logico-scientific approach to reasoning that has pervaded modern medical practice. Comparing narrative- and evidence-based medicine, Greenhalgh (1998) explained: "Conventional medical training teaches students to view medicine as a science and the doctor as an impartial investigator who builds differential diagnoses like scientific theories and excludes competing possibilities in a manner akin to the falsification of hypothesis" (p. 248). Thus, she continues, "the discovery of 'facts' about the patient's illness is exactly equivalent to the discovery of new scientific truths about the universe" (p. 248). In contrast, rather than making predictions or formulating general laws of human behavior, a narrative approach privileges the particularities of individuals' lives and attempts to understand how specific persons in particular times and places describe their experiences of living their lives. Continuing with the previous example (which we refer to throughout the chapter),

Kim's story reveals that the understandings she could glean from more objective articulations of available evidence about pregnancy and childbirth (whether the medical or midwifery versions) simply did not provide answers to the questions she faced. In short, a focus on the meanings that people attribute to their experiences as they construct narrative accounts shifts the focus from a search for universal truths about an objective reality to the subjective experiences of individuals.[3]

Acknowledging that a narrative approach emphasizes interpretation does not in and of itself account for the effects of narrative in sense-making, however, for narratives themselves concomitantly demonstrate and constitute the relationships between experiences and understandings. As Polkinghorne (1988) noted in discussing narrative meaning, "The question, 'What does that mean?,' asks how something is related or connected to something else" (p. 6). Narratives comprise the means by which individuals organize a host of random emotional, perceptual, physical, and social experiences into a meaningful account of their situation. In doing so, persons telling stories reveal the "time and space relations and cause–effect links they have made in their own understanding and management of illness and health" (Vanderford et al., 1997, p. 18). Although noting the definitional stipulation that the events in narratives typically must exhibit some "intrinsic, meaningful connection to one another" (L. P. Hinchman & S. K. Hinchman, 1997, p. xv), the actual significance of the experiences or events for the teller emerges through the narrative told to self and others that articulates the perceived relationships among those experiences (Polkinghorne, 1988; Vanderford & Smith, 1996).

This clarifying and dramatizing of connections that characterizes narrative sense-making is particularly important for persons interested in empathic understanding of another's health situation (especially health care professionals). As Greenhalgh and Hurwitz (1998) pointed out, "Since patients almost invariably place their most important experiences—birth, death, grief, and illness—within very different narrative streams than do doctors, it follows that doctors and patients often assign very different meanings (and different streams of causality) to the same sequence of events" (p. 11). Moreover, with each retelling of a narrative, different experiences and understandings may be invoked, relationships established, rejected, or reconfirmed, and in that process, meanings transformed.

Narrative theory and research, then, emphasize the meanings that persons assign to their lives as they orient to experience. Hence, narrative researchers ask, what interpretations do people construct for their lived experiences? What significance do they assign to the events and moments of their lives? For example, aging, illness, and death challenge a host of meanings—about the nature of life, bodily integrity, self and identity, relationships, and so on. Through narrative activity, people develop storied understandings about how they reached their current age and physical state of being, how they see themselves now, and how they think the processes of aging, illness, and death will play out in the future.

PI theory complements these ideas by illuminating key themes and dynamics in sense-making. The theory suggests that, at the heart of our efforts to make sense of experience, to make life meaningful, we must form two interdependent sorts of understandings. These two forms of understanding or orientations are suggested in stress and emotion researcher Richard Lazarus's (1991) assertion that "People are continually seeking *knowledge* (that is, beliefs about how things work in general and in the specific adaptational encounter) and *appraisals* of the significance of the person–environment relationship for personal well-being, whether about a specific encounter or life as a whole" (p. 127, italics in original).

> As Kim struggled with the question of whether to have a mid-wife attend a home birth or give birth in a hospital, she asked herself, "What happens if something goes wrong? Does it matter that my first child was born by Cesarean section (and could my uterus burst if I attempt a vaginal delivery)? Could the cervical surgery I had years ago cause complications? Will my family and friends think I'm nuts? Can I handle all of the details for preparation normally taken care of by hospital personal (who exactly cleans up after what we all know is a pretty messy process)?" Just as importantly, she wondered how to prioritize each of these concerns. Her and the baby's health were, of course, at the top of the list.
>
> However, in spite of the fears that she had about giving birth at home, she found as much evidence that a home birth would be safe and that a hospital birth had its own hazards. She weighed heavily the kind of experience she might expect from the two options. She recalled her daughter's birth 10 years before and the loss of control she had experienced. She remembered how the medical staff had whisked her daughter away within minutes of her birth. Kim had been left in a recovery room (snagging any passerby who'd listen to her talk about the few details she knew from the mere minutes she'd had with the 9 pound, red-headed baby girl), forced against her wishes to wear a nursing bra (which she subsequently hung on an IV stand since she couldn't remove it entirely), and then stuck in a room with another woman who shared none of Kim's enthusiasm for midnight calls to friends and family to revel in the exis-

*tence of this new person. She didn't hold her daughter, born at
10 p.m., until around 7 a.m. the next morning. Certainly, these
factors in conjunction with her knowledge of the health risks
associated with both birthing options made a home birth seem
much more preferable (though still a scary proposition).*

According to PI theory (and countless other perspectives), all
knowledge is associational, and all such associations are inherently
unverifiable in any ultimate sense . Hence, in his description of PI theory, Babrow labels this aspect of meaning construction or understanding of experience as *probabilistic orientation*. For example, we
construct probabilistic orientations when we answer questions such
as, "Was I vaccinated for smallpox in my youth?" "Are we pregnant?"
"Will you stop drinking and driving?" As these examples illustrate,
probabilistic orientations can be formulated for past, present, and
future experience. In each case, we may be absolutely certain, believe
but with some uncertainty, or conceive the understanding as the
slightest of possibilities.

Although probabilistic orientations remain foundational to human
understanding, they do not in themselves constitute the meaning of
experience. That is, human understanding involves more than beliefs
about what things are, what they are like, how they work, and so on.
According to PI theory, the meanings that we attach to experience also
entail appraisals or evaluations of whatever we think we know about
the world. In other words, human beings cannot orient to their world
based solely on probabilistic orientations (beliefs, assumptions, and
so on) no matter how well warranted. To orient ourselves thought-
fully, reasonably, meaningfully, we also must consider the evaluative
meanings that these associations hold for us (e.g., for our happiness,
well-being, survival; Babrow, in press). Extending the previous examples, to make sense of these experiences or potentialities, we must
evaluate having had a smallpox vaccination, being pregnant, and
stopping drunk driving. How good or bad was/is/will be each of these
potentialities?

As the discussion thus far indicates, PI theory is relevant to important dualisms common in everyday thought/talk and scholarly theory.
For instance, scholars and nonscholars commonly distinguish between belief and evaluation (or value judgment), expectation and desire, reality and wish, and other such formulations loosely related to
the modernist fact-value dualism (see J. Stewart, 1991). However, unlike much of the relevant discourse, although PI theory makes a distinction between probabilistic and evaluative orientations, it also
emphasizes their deep interdependence. Indeed, the central phenomenon addressed by PI theory is the communicative construction of the

(often problematic) integration of these two basic aspects of human meaning/being.

PI theory asserts that we forge meanings in the creation of probabilistic and evaluative orientations (i.e., understandings of "the way things are" and evaluations of the reality so constructed, respectively). However, these meanings are not simply co-occurring aspects of understanding, like planks laid side by side to form the deck of a ship. Rather, they interrelate more like the threads of a fabric; though distinct, they are intertwined, taking their shape, texture, and hue from one another in the pattern of weaving. Put less metaphorically, another basic claim in PI theory is that probabilistic and evaluative orientations, while distinguishable, must be integrated in experience. In part, this assertion means that what we think is so (or possible) is shaped by and also shapes what we think is good and bad, and vice versa (Babrow, 1992, 2001).

For example, the desire to become a vegan shapes the perceived possibility of becoming one. Desire impacts effort which, in turn, alters one's chances of success. However, desires also influence expectations directly, as in wishful thinking (Babrow, 1991; Weinstein, 1987). Alternatively, perceived probability (e.g., success in becoming a vegan) often influences evaluation. For example, Kim's concerns about the possible health risks of a home birth were most likely tempered by her desire to give birth at home and thereby avoid a hospital birth. This process has been called *self-protective rationalization* (McGurie, 1960). In addition, these interdependent orientations to any one issue (e.g., home birth or becoming a vegan) must be integrated with surrounding probabilistic and evaluative orientations, such as those related to our sense of self or identity, perceptions of our body and health, relationships with other people, spiritual considerations, and so on (see Babrow, 1992, 1995).

We believe that we accomplish much of the integrative meaning making illuminated by PI theory through narrative activity in the form of stories.[4] Reflexively, then, narrative activity largely involves the production of a coherent understanding of "the way things were/are/will be" and the meaning of this apparent arrangement or probabilistic construction for our happiness. To better appreciate these ideas and their relevance to health and illness narratives, we must consider another basic characteristic of the two perspectives.

## Meaning-Making and Context

Narrative and PI approaches share the idea that meaning-making is fundamentally contextual. Narratives become informed by and reveal the contexts within which their relevant understandings are formed and acted upon. Notably, a narrative perspective invokes two relevant contextual forms: the lived context of the events being retold and the living context of the telling itself. On one hand, narrative research concentrates on the context in which events of the narrative have transpired; that is, their setting. It probes what a person considers to be the enveloping circumstances that frame and give meaning to the events recounted in that person's stories about her or his life. What she or he selects for inclusion and exclusion is important. The setting for the story matters. Imagine, for example, two different narratives, one that recounts a childbirth that took place in a hospital and the other that recounts a childbirth that took place at home.

Even more broadly, we enact and express cultural values and worldviews in and through story telling. As Freeman (1997) observed, "Lives are lived in culture—in language, in social relations, in communities, in the web of quite specific rules, conventions, beliefs, discourses and so on" (p. 172). Notably, we derive individual goals, desires, and perceived (im)possibilities, expectations, and choices from surrounding culture, and these in turn, impinge on the elements chosen for inclusion in a narrative formulated to make sense of some circumstance. Again, consider the narratives of childbirth already mentioned: Given the United States' cultural commitment to medical intervention in birthing, the narrative describing a hospital birth most likely does not include/necessitate explanation for the choice to deliver in a hospital (unless told to a group of direct-entry midwives) whereas the home birth narrative (as a counter to the dominant medical narrative) incorporates substantial justification. So, narrative scholars ask, as seen through the eyes and expressed through the voice of the storyteller, what does a given story reveal about the assumptions, everyday activities, practices, and values of the culture in which it is authored? What moral issues are at stake in the community presupposed by the story? For instance, in their study of the silicone breast implant controversy, Vanderford and Smith (1996) found that some women experiencing difficulties did not blame the problem on inherent, predictable, and hence avoidable flaws in the implants because "their health issues fit within the larger narrative concerning the imperfection of medicine" (p. 18).

On the other hand, the context within which the story is told impinges on the meanings inherent—and possible—in the narrative. Geist-Martin, Ray, and Sharf (2003) suggested that narratives constructed by a 1-month pregnant, 15-year-old young woman might take on significantly different forms in the contexts of talking to parents who do not consider abortion to be an option, with a counselor in a private office at Planned Parenthood, and during a conversation with the 15-year-old young man who impregnated her and who favors an abortion. This case affirms the relevance of story context as well as the ways in which context can affect and constrain narrative possibilities. For instance, most of us have, at some point, commented that physicians are limited in their ability to spend enough time with their patients because of appointment scheduling; the pressing question is whether medical appointments are rigidly teleological, therefore demanding that the patient's narrative be emplotted in a specific way that drastically constrains or denies her or his voice. Additionally, whose values does this plot serve? In short, stories may be told about the contexts for telling stories in health care settings.

*Ten years after the birth of her first child, the world was a different place for Kim, allowing her to tell the story of her first birth in a way that supported a wider range of choices than might have been available to her 10 years earlier. Not only did she have the academic background to validate the claims she made with regard to childbirth practices, she could substantiate the strength of her convictions with her personal experiences and relationships (which included numerous women who had given birth at home as well as a direct-entry midwife who had, at that time, attended over 800 home births). Moreover, she was relatively successful in her chosen (dare we say, upper middle-class) profession, giving her the financial wherewithal to expand her range of options.*

*Given another place and time, Kim might not have been able to even consider the question posed by her student or to revise the story of her first birth to accommodate a socially, culturally, and politically unaccepted childbirth option. Notwithstanding the change in her circumstances, Kim still felt that she had to rationalize the choice she faced, which required the ability to reconcile the myriad of concerns about what might happen given either choice with the personal and political values with which she had come to be identified.*

Like narrative theory, PI theory and research illuminates the contextually accomplished construction of meanings in various ways. As noted, in its most basic conceptions, the theory holds that our sense of what was/is/will be and our evaluations of these elements of understanding (i.e., our probabilistic and evaluative orientations) must be integrated with one another. That is, each form of orientation provides the most fundamental context within which the other form of orientation is understood. Is it good news that you or your partner is pregnant? This judgment may depend on several considerations relevant to your probabilistic orientation toward being pregnant. Appraisal of the pregnancy will be influenced by the extent to which you believe that you can eat properly, avoid dangerous substances; the expectation that the pregnancy is likely to end in another miscarriage; the judgment that your partner supports childbirth, and so forth. Conversely, knowing that a baby is on the way may prompt reconsideration of one's evaluative orientations.[5] Moreover, integration is problematic when probabilities and values destabilize one another (see Babrow, in press, for a discussion on the various PI forms). Health communication, in general (and health-related narrative activity in particular) largely involves an ongoing matter of values forcing the rearticulation of (un)certainty and (un)certainty compelling the rearticulation of values (Babrow & Mattson, 2003).

Not only does PI theory assert that probabalistic and evaluative orientations must be integrated with one another, more to the point, this integration takes place in experience thereby implicating the social context of meaning-making. PI theory serves essentially as an inquiry into the "nature of the relationship—whether representational or constitutive—between communication and one's conception of or orientation to the world" (Babrow, 2001, p. 554). Communicative activities or our symbolic interaction (Burke, 1966) form the context within and through which we make sense of our lives. In other words, developing probabilistic and evaluative orientations to any one health-related issue and integrating them with one another and with surrounding beliefs and values entails not merely psychological but social processes (see Babrow, 1993, 1998).

In keeping with this attention to social processes, PI theory emphasizes the contextuality of meaning-making through its conception of the interpenetration of levels of experience. By implication, then, our probabilistic and evaluative orientations to any one event, such as reaching or leaving middle-age, intersect with a host of surrounding beliefs or expectations, values, and desires. For example, efforts to narrate some specific ailment or milestone in aging—to understand where we are, what's happening, what it means for our happiness— necessarily implicate surrounding stories about our general physical health, relationships, career, and other concerns. Extending the contexts or levels of experience, Babrow (2001) contends:

> Communication in families and friendships, impersonal relationships, and private and public contexts provides the categories for perceptions and the grist of cognitive and emotional processes. In so doing, communication content, structures, and processes create, shape, clarify, obscure, challenge, and transform probabilistic and evaluative orientations and the PI they so often occasion. (p. 555)

This interrelated accomplishment of our judgments and understandings transpires whether illness experiences are mundane and self-limiting or extraordinary. In the former case, socially given stories apply straightforwardly to experience. For example, think of the infinite storied instantiations of the folk belief that getting a chill causes a "cold." In short, understandings of mundane experiences take shape within and in turn reinforce available stories. However, the importance of context to narrative meaning construction is magnified when health issues are extraordinary. When readily available frames of understanding don't seem to fit, ongoing communication—with family and friends as well as the scientific–technological, literary, artistic, spiritual, and political resources of our culture—become the *sine qua non* of meaning-making activity (Babrow, 1992, 1993, 1995, 2001; Babrow & Dutta-Bergman, 2004).

## Meaning-Making and Temporality

The idea that the resources, processes, and fruits of meaning-making are embedded within multiple layers of context relates closely to a third shared characteristic of PI and narrative thinking: Both perspectives wrestle with meaning-making through time. Most basically, narrative constitutes a form of discourse by which individuals attempt to develop a coherent accounting of their experiences by placing events in a sequential order. Even so, Mishler (in press) cautions against relying solely upon linear, temporally ordered models when conceptualizing the influence of time in narrative sense-making. Rather, he directs us to Ricoeur's approach, which indicates that narrative time is composed of two dimensions, the episodic and the configurational. In proposing that narratives are made of events (i.e., episodic) and that these events are rendered as significant wholes by way of the plot (i.e., configurational), "Ricoeur's formulation ... gives the ending of a story the primary function in how a story is plotted or constructed" (Mishler, in press, p. 3). In this sense, articulated relationships between events not only give meaning to past events, they also give meaning to possible future events. That is, narrative "imaginatively reconstructs the past so that it has meaning or purpose for the present" (Williams, 1997, p. 189), but it also "retrieves previous experience and imaginatively creates alternate scenarios which anticipate the consequences of possible actions" (Polkinghorne, 1988, p. 16). Thus, the rearticulation of sequence in narratives contributes to the meaning of the events because, "if the sequence were changed, the meaning of the account would alter" (Gwyn, 2002b, p. 140).

Freeman (1997), in turn, explicated the temporality of narrative with the idea that the perspective is "historical in orientation" (p. 174). According to his analysis, this historicity is reflected in several ways: (a) Most stories are retrospective accounts of events that have already occurred and are now being recounted; (b) each person can select and relate events from his or her own life history stretching from the time he or she was born until the present telling, and we can only recount a completed life history of someone who has died (Holquist, 2002); (c) each life history contributes to a larger human history in the same way that our individual stories present snapshots of lives lived in the culture where they transpire. As Freeman (1997) stated, "In this sense, turning to narrative, to concrete human lives, is a way of becoming engaged with history—with memorializing or commemorating not only the life in question but its cultural–historical surround" (p. 174); (d) listening to stories thereby expands our historical and cultural consciousness because of the meaningful and textured ways in which stories dramatize the lives and choices of people who are different and similar to us in discussable ways (Gadamer, 1975).

Acknowledging the difference between clock/chronological and narrative/experiential models of time (Mishler, in press) is particularly important in health communication contexts. As Sharf (1990) observed, "The natural inclination of the patients is to present a sequence of events, rather than the chief complaint or problem list in which the doctor is interested" (p. 222). Accordingly, a narrative approach seeks to understand how events unfold in time according to the storyteller. Researchers ask: What do individuals select as the significant events that occurred before and set the stage for the story being told? What events are identified as pivotal in composing the story itself? What have been the consequences of the story's events and actions from the vantage point of the present moment of telling? How are these events arranged in the plot of the story as it is told? In Bruner's (1996) words, narratives thereby enact and reveal "a structure of committed time" (p. 133). Hence, narrative researchers ask: What do specific stories reveal about how persons understand their lives in time?

*With 10 years between pregnancies, Kim was poignantly aware of how time had altered her perspective on childbirth. Trying to make sense of her radically different concerns and desires during this pregnancy as compared to the last, Kim realized the difficulty of trying to tell someone 10 years younger (or 20 or 30 years younger) what a difference those years made in the way she understood the choices she made "back then." It didn't necessarily help her in making the choices she faced, but it did help explain the conundrum she confronted in justifying to herself and others the possibility of a home birth when her first child had been born using surgical procedures in a hospital.*

PI theory offers complementary ways of understanding the motivation for and character of sense-making through time. First, it recognizes that probabilistic understandings depend on time and temporal sequences for working out causality, both intentional and mechanistic. That is, to understand what causes what, what goes with what, we necessarily track and make sense of events through time. Similarly, evaluative understanding requires that we follow causes through time to their effects in order to determine whether these effects—and hence their causes—are good/bad, valuable/objectionable, and so on.

Moreover, we have already noted that the integration of expectations and desires (i.e., probabilistic and evaluative orientations) is often problematic. Regardless of the form that problematic integration takes—whether it extends from diverging expectations and desires (i.e., when hopes are slim or sorrow seems likely), uncertainty (about realizing hopes or avoiding sorrows), ambivalence (mixed blessings; similarly valued, mutually exclusive alternatives), and impossibility/certainty (hopelessness)—as PI experiences occur, we enter ongoing struggles that can be more or less protracted (see Babrow, 1992, in press, for more extended discussions of the various PI forms). As individuals and members of social groups, we attempt to make sense of experience, to formulate and synthesize expectations and desires in comfortable, workable, or at least meaningful ways. Hence, meaning-making inherently unfolds through time.

Finally, when we put this idea together with the previous discussion of the contextuality of meaning, both PI and narrative theory tell us that "context" is itself dynamic, ever-evolving, and that the subject/object and its context, the figure and its ground, interpenetrate in the process of constructing the meanings of experience through time. By conceptualizing meaning-making in this way, we challenge theories of knowledge (e.g., logo scientific) that regard meaning as the immutable product of organizing static events. Hence, we acknowledge Fink's (1970) assertion that "Theories of knowledge have unaccountably neglected the significance of the simple fact that experiences come to us *seriatum*, in a stream of transience, and yet must be held together in a single image of the manifold of events in order for us to be aware of the transience at all" (p. 547).

## NARRATING SEQUENCES AND PROBLEMATIC CONFIGURATIONS

Thus far, we have discussed the features of some corresponding aspects of PI and narrative theories (i.e., their emphasis on the centrality of meaning, its contexts, and temporal dimensions), suggesting the compatibility of these two approaches for explicating the challenges and strategies of human sense-making. In the following section, we extend this line of thinking by considering the complementarity of PI and narrative theories. Thus, as suggested by the title of this chapter, challenges to forming and integrating probabilistic and evaluative orientations can problematize narrative activity; concomitantly, by narrating these problems, we give structure to our orientations and their integration.

*How hard can it be to tell the story of the birth of your first child? Kim's experiences suggest that the difficulty lies in the relevance the story has for current choices. When she was asked whether she would have a home birth, Kim began to question the integrity of every story she had ever told about the birth of her first child. Shouldn't it always be as it was? she wondered. Then she reflected on the way life has a tendency to prod a person in different directions. "Yes," she said, "the story has taken a different turn." "But," she asked, "is that so surprising given the different directions my life has taken?"*

Echoing Fink's concerns, Ricoeur (1981a) called our attention to a fundamental quandary of narrative thinking that we find useful in characterizing the ways that narrative and PI perspectives can be brought together to understand more fully the presence and value of stories in health communication. As already mentioned, Ricoeur argues that all narratives involve two dimensions, a "chronological" one and a "nonchronological" one, that combine in varying ways to perform the narrative function. On one hand, in "following a story," the episodic "dimension is expressed in the expectation of contingencies which affect the story's development; hence it gives rise to questions such as: And so? And then? What happened next? What was the outcome?" (p. 278). This dimension describes the raw temporal succession of events embodied in stories.

However, because neither telling nor following stories can be reduced to the mere sequential addition of episodes, Ricoeur stipulates a second dimension, the "configurational" activity of constructing "meaningful totalities out of scattered events" (p. 278). Ricoeur (1981a) continues, "This aspect of the art of narrating is reflected, on the side of following a story, in the attempt to 'grasp together' successive events" (p. 278). These two dimensions work together to compose the plot of stories. Importantly for our purposes, Ricoeur concludes, "This complex structure implies that the most humble narrative is always more than a chronological series of events and, in turn, that the configurational dimension cannot eclipse the episodic dimension without abolishing the narrative structure itself" (p. 279).

Revisiting Ricoeur's explanation of narrative form, we envision the episodic dimension as suggesting that a story comprises sequenced events and PI orientations, and the configurational dimension identifies the plot as the static rendering of events and PI orientations as significant wholes. Thus, we believe the tension between arranging sequential events and meaningful configurations within narrative activity also lies at the heart of the animating tension connecting PI theory and narrative perspectives. Accordingly, we are led to ask: What intertwining perceptions of probability and evaluation inform and transform the expectation of contingencies in living and telling the stories of our lives? How are scattered events and feelings meaningfully clustered, connected, and addressed? What is the relationship between each perspective's way of figuring human predicaments and the forms of temporality composing and composed by them?

We have argued throughout this chapter that narrative provides a way to make sense of experience. Stories provide particularly important ways of understanding when unexpected, unpleasant, ambiguous, or uncertain bodily experiences challenge what had previously been taken for granted or when we experience our body in significant new ways. Much has been written about the imperatives of (re)creating meanings in illness (Frank, 1995; Greenhalgh & Hurwitz, 1998; Gwyn, 2002b; Kleinman, 1988; Sharf & Vanderford, 2003). As Kleinman (1988) put it, "Nothing so concentrates experience and clarifies the central conditions of living as serious illness" (p. xiii). More specifically, Gwyn (2002b) explains:

> ... in the area of illness experience telling stories of the self has particular importance, since the process of adjusting to illness, or remaking a life after a period of illness, necessitates a more intense degree of self-disclosure and of sense-making than might normally be encountered in other everyday activities. (p. 164)

However, even when we are well, changing experiences of the body, such as a significant new sexual discovery, becoming pregnant, altering diet substantially, and so on, can call forth quite substantial efforts to remake our understandings. Any change in health—whether physical or perceptual—can constitute what Bochner and Ellis (1995) referred to as an epiphany, "an event in which individuals are so powerfully absorbed that they are left without an interpretive framework to make sense of their experience immediately" (p. 205). Moreover, stories are demanded by family members, friends, co-workers and employers, and health care providers and agents of the industry that surrounds them, all of whom want to understand what happened, is happening, and will happen (see Frank, 1995).

The resulting stories provide assertions about the structure of the world, and hence provide the substance of our probabilistic orientations to experience. That is, they select out a coherent set of objects (e.g., people, places, issues), specify characteristics and relationships, connect causes and their effects, and even order chaos by the act of conceiving of experience as random and unpredictable. Stories also provide logics for working out the probabilistic relationships that make up experience. These logics become most apparent in stories related to human action, where character, motivation, conflict, and so on explain "what goes with what" (Burke, 1973, p. 2), why the world is arranged in this way, and what is probably true even if it is not depicted explicitly within the story. Explanations of physical (e.g., biological) processes also highlight narrative logic. Those in the know ("experts") construct stories to explain sexuality, conception and childbirth, the "life" of cells, bodily "battles" against disease, senescence, and death. In all such tales, storytelling structures a host of discrete features of the world, placing them into coherent interrelationship, and hence, they transform discrete probabilistic and evaluative orientations into coherent, extensive understandings.

From the perspectives of both PI and narrative theories, living, telling, and being told about one's life/bodily experiences involves the ongoing construction of meaningfully composed configurations of contingencies. Such narrative work responds to the question: To what am I or should I be paying attention and how does it or should it relate or lead to what might happen next? Fink (1970) offered an intriguing depiction of the narrative positioning of contingent configurations:

> ... a number of things may be comprehended as elements in a single and concrete complex of relationships. Thus a letter I burn may be understood not only as an oxidizable substance but as a link with an old friend. It may have relieved a misunderstanding, raised a question, or changed my plans at a crucial moment. As a letter, it belongs to a kind of story, a narrative of events which would be unintelligible without reference to it. (p. 551)

In short, both narrative and PI analyses try to comprehend our embodied stances toward the contingent features of our lives. How do we recognize, communicate, and (co)construct the contingencies patterning our vulnerable existence? In some cases, we appeal to available stories from trusted narrators. If they do not allay our concerns, express our hopes or despair, or allow for the alternatives we desire, sometimes we must (co)create our own.

PI theory emphasizes that, even as stories develop interrelated probabilistic orientations, they also formulate evaluative understandings. Evaluation is implicit as stories draw together characteristics, acts, and consequences to construct patently appealing and distasteful actors, lines of action and interaction, and consequences. However, evaluation is often explicit and perhaps the central theme in stories designed to construct a moral or pragmatic judgment. Hence, as narrative theorists have argued, stories are inherently or overtly moral; in Holquist's (2002) words, "Stories are the means by which values are made coherent in particular situations" (p. 37). PI theory adds and accentuates the idea that evaluation, and hence morality, frequently entails direct wrestling with the tension between expectation and desire, with the mutually conditioning construction of what is possible/likely and what is good/bad (Babrow, 1992, in press), and with ambivalence or conflicting evaluative orientation. We develop stories to formulate, analyze, resolve, and reconsider experiences of (im)possible ultimate desires, ambivalence and the like.

PI theory reminds us that narratives often serve as the vehicles through which we cope with the difficulties of formulating probabilistic and evaluative orientations and their problematic integration. Culture can be understood as artifacts of a people's efforts to deal with widely if not universally shared problematics of being: the nature of the world, existence of God, fertility, vagaries of weather, nutrition, human relationships and conflict, aging, sickness and death (e.g., think of the works of Joseph Campbell, Carl Jung). That is, we create stories— from "myths" to relatively context-specific narratives—to construct meanings when we face diverging expectation and desire, uncertainty about substantial values or interests, marked ambivalence, or impossible wants and wishes. For example, Vanderford and Smith (1996) identified a wide range of stories developed by women, doctors, and journalists caught up in the uncertainties surrounding silicone breast implants (e.g., stories of loss and confusion, diagnosis and direction, success and satisfaction, safety and risk, surgery and profit, and corporate downfall).

Bruner (1991) further emphasized the evaluative strain characterizing narrative activity when he stated, "because its 'tellability' as a form of discourse rests on a breach of conventional expectation, narrative is necessarily normative. A breach presupposes a norm" (p. 15). As we have mentioned, the expectations and thereby values breached and addressed by emerging health narratives include norms and taken-for-granted aspects of physical health and social well-being. Such breaches voiced by narratives in health care circumstances include the assumed normalcy of bodily functions and capabilities, appropriate relationships between patients and health care practitioners, the stricken or encouraged person's knowledge of him or herself and the heretofore "normal" unfolding of his or her life and possibilities for growing older. All are now breached in some way or another and demand/give rise to a story.

The necessary attention drawn to narrator(s) constitutes one of the most powerful and inherently moralizing features of a narrative perspective. We have already discussed how a story's plot selects features and aspects of circumstances, including characters and their actions, and (re)arranges temporal sequences to call attention to relations among occurrences (Leondar, 1977). But who gives rise to plots? Bruner (1996) is unequivocal: "Narrative construals of reality lead us to look for a 'voice' " (p. 138). The voice(s) of the teller, the narrator, even if it is that of a third person or multiple speakers, must be identified or owned, however implicitly. Of course, clear reasons exist for this palpable moral presence in storytelling. As Bochner (1994) cogently observed, "Every narrator has a stake in her story; she is never indifferent" (p. 29).

Hence, narrators work to construct probabilistic and evaluative understandings of their health or illness situations. The stories told represent and rebuild an individual's sense of her or his body and life (Gwyn, 2002a; Sharf & Vanderford, 2003). In general, "personal identity, the answer to the riddle of 'who' people are, takes shape in the stories we tell about ourselves" (L. P. Hinchman & S. K. Hinchman, 1997, p. xvii). With regard to health and illness, narratives function as the means by which individuals renegotiate a self-image altered by changes in their health and/or illness status. For instance, learning that one has little chance of recovering from an illness or injury can disrupt the expectation and evaluation of achieving the self-identity associated with the absence of that illness or injury.

Thus, "stories have to *repair* the damage that illness has done to the ill person's sense of where she is in life, and where she may be going. Stories are a way of redrawing maps and finding new destinations" (Frank, 1995, p. 53). In the case of one man suffering from debilitating rheumatoid arthritis, the damage done to his sense of self was poignantly revealed in his troubled query, " 'how the *hell* have I come to be like this?' ... 'because it isn't me' " (Williams, 1997, p. 185). Narratives are no less consequential in the experience of substantial, although fundamentally healthy bodily change. In either case, we construct for ourselves new understandings by authoring new stories. Hence, in addition to its moral demands, the calling card of narrative emphasizes individual and collective agency, hearing one's own voice, and ongoing self-formation. As L. P. Hinchman and S. K. Hinchman (1997) stated:

> Narrative theories of identity have the virtue of making the self seem a "work in progress" that can be "revised" as circumstances require. Such theories put the individual in the position of being author of his or her own story, an active shaper of outcomes rather than a passive object acted upon by external or internal forces. (p. xix)

As such, narratives also constitute justifications for choices made or avoided in the past and those that will be made in the future as individuals negotiate physical, emotional, ethical, and social challenges prompted by changes in health. In other words, narratives form a basis for decision making (Polkinghorne, 1988; Vanderford et al., 1997).

In its extensive analysis of specific forms of uncertainty, such as the distinction between ontological and epistemological uncertainties, and various subforms of each (Babrow, 2001; Babrow, Kasch, & Ford, 1998), PI theory offers a variety of sensitizing concepts for understanding the kinds of dramatic tensions that drive storytelling. For example, narratives either assume or forthrightly examine their authorial conceptions of the nature of reality, or their *lay ontology*.[6] As more concrete and specific examples, narratives might reflect the author or actors' efforts to live with a reality conceived of events related probabilistically to discrete causes ("biomedical" stories), or events caused by more complex though still understandable and "manageable" transactions among biological, social, psychological, and/or communicative processes ("biopsychosocial" or communicational stories), or they may conceive of reality as the incomprehensibly complex "interbeing" (Hanh, 1988, 1998) of all of its aspects.

Moreover, PI theory suggests that uncertainties produce considerable dramatic tension when they must be integrated with significant values, intentions, interests, or desires. This tension sparks a central (if not a substantial) motivation for authoring or attending to a story; to construct expectations or probabilities and values or desires, to construct ways of coping with PI (see Babrow, 1992). Further, when PI is particularly pronounced (e.g., when divergence of expectation and desire is great, ambivalence is profound, uncertainties about important values are irreducible, or we face tragic or terrifying certainties/impossibilities), actors likely struggle often unsuccessfully to maintain any one story (see Babrow, 1992). Accordingly, we develop multiple, competing, perhaps conflictual, stories through time.

Finally, by its very nature, PI is pliable, fragile, and for these reasons, often heavily reinforced and fundamentally unstable (see Babrow, 1992, 2001). As in fabric weaving, the stories we tell are not seamless goods. The very nature of narrative is to create something new out of disparate threads, and to do so in a way that both preserves some of the character of its components while combining them in ways that make their configured character supremely interdependent with each other. Hence, the weave of a story inevitably leaves seams, spaces, weaknesses, and hence possibilities for further adornment, reinforcement, and unraveling. Every probabilistic and evaluative thread, particularly when woven hastily, fitfully, in anguish or uncertainty, is both the substance of a given narrative as well as the material of its unraveling and the fiber out of which new stories are spun.

> *Kim will tell you that the conclusion to the story of her first birth is always the same—she brought into the world a wonderfull baby girl who has given her nothing but joy every day of her existence. And, she regrets nothing about her birthing experience. Even so, the narrative she tells now about that experience clearly articulates to the careful listener the concerned perception of potential occurrences and values that informed the choice she made for her second birth experience. Her son was born at home, attended by a midwife, her apprentice, and numerous friends and family members.*

## CONCLUSIONS AND IMPLICATIONS FOR THE MOMENT

"[T]he consoling plot" is not the comfort of a happy ending but the comprehension of plight, that by being made interpretable, becomes bearable.
                                                    —(Bruner, 1991, p. 16)

In this chapter, we have explored some complementary aspects of PI theory and narrative theory for experiencing and shaping, that is for coping with, our plights (and contingent good fortunes) as vulnerable, embodied beings.

In our view, PI theory provides a useful existential anatomy for understanding human situations that demand our attention, those situations where our responses compose and reveal our characters. Meanwhile, we hold that the insights provided by PI lend themselves to narrative exposition, application, fleshing out. PI's configurational probings invite the input, the choices and voices of actual characters for whom these problematic situations compose unfolding realities. In short, PI theory helps us to understand the murky, interdependent, and reflexively emergent nature of the contingencies we live with such poignancy in experiencing health and illness. Taken with narrative processes, those of PI allow human communicators to embrace the possibilities, address the contingencies (and in doing so, clarify precisely to whom the contingencies are addressed), and, when feasible, to make choices. In doing so as active speakers, listeners, and co-tellers, we narrativize our lives, and we perform our characters.

In complementary fashion, narrative theory teaches us that stories propose selves, identities, and communities—possible worlds for dwelling and co-dwelling. Narratives situate us in socially constructed time, space, and relationships. In doing so, we may say that narrative performance emplots the concerns and existential predicaments highlighted by PI theory; it embeds them in temporal and reflexive structures of activity that highlight the importance and potential consequences of our human choices, actions, and inactions. As a result, Callinicos (1995) observed, "Narratives ... allow us to recover the contingencies of the historical process, the junctures at which particular choices and chances tipped the balance between significantly different possible outcomes" (p. 54).

At the same time, the ambiguous, uncertain, and ambivalent understandings embodied in narratives may be teased out and understood using the theoretical concepts and displays of PI. To accomplish such insights in edifying ways as researchers, patients, health care professionals, friends and loved ones, we need to listen carefully to each storyteller's words. How is the plot's coherence constituted as a dynamic matrix of contingencies unfolding and transforming themselves over time? We need vigilantly to attend to narratives to learn the active interplay of perceived probabilities and experienced desires that are seeking to be integrated through this rendering.

We have identified reflexive links between PI and narrative activity in both living and telling stories of our lives. We find double meanings for the two gerunds in the previous sentence to be instructive. On one hand, "living stories" connotes the stories that actively unfold around and may or may not involve us at any moment. We believe the interaction of PI and narrative perspectives is useful in recognizing, analyzing, and seeking to understand such stories, whether it is from the third-person vantage point of a health care professional, communication researcher, or even the individual in the waiting room. On the other hand, we also acknowledge that "living stories" of our lives involves active participation and engagement in composing our possibilities as first person narrators, and here too, we see value in connecting PI and narrative perspectives.

"Telling stories" has at least two meanings for us as well. On one hand, it extends the active participation theme just mentioned in its own depiction of voicing our narratives—so that our concerns, joys, and possibilities can be heard and shaped by others as well as by ourselves. In these moments of utterance, we take responsibility for the place we occupy in our own accounts, our own stories, our own lives (Bakhtin, 1993). In a second sense, "telling stories" are those that are consequential for us, for what they reveal about our embodied circumstances as they unfold. If we have less say about the ultimate course of some of these stories, it is because, as physical beings, we dwell within the contingencies of the human condition. Even so, we would hope that narrative renderings and insights facilitated by PI theory might provide some comprehension and appreciation of and consolation for the profound sadness or celebration occasioned by these telling stories of our physically embodied and communicatively meaningful existence.

## NOTES

1. Authors are listed alphabetically. All three authors shared equally in the conception and writing of this chapter.
2. The midwife most people are familiar with is the Certified Nurse Midwife (CNM). These are typically nurses trained in established medical institutions who work as assistants to physicians and, thus, practice in accordance with state mandated restrictions that require them to supplement medical care given in hospitals. Our references to midwives are to Direct-Entry Midwives (DEM), who have learned their practice by apprenticing with other DEM experienced in attending pregnancy and childbirth. Notably, DEMs advocate and attend home births (even when, as in the case presented here, the law does not allow this choice).
3. Sharf (1990) demonstrated the manner in which these two approaches to sense-making can undermine shared understanding between doctors and patients whose narratives are "based on the dichotomy between disease and illness" (p. 223). In contrast, Bochner and Ellis (1995) illustrated the potential for achieving shared understanding when sense-making is approached by using individual stories to co-construct a narrative that "incorporates both partners' voices and subjectivities" (p. 205).
4. We do not mean to claim that narrative is the only way that people make sense of experience. In addition to narratives, people form understandings through a variety of processes and structures, such as metaphoric, dialectic, and what has been called paradigmatic thought (Bruner, 1986; Dennis, 2001; Zukier, 1986).
5. We are reminded of the scene in "The Rock" where the FBI chemical weapons expert played by Nicholas Cage who, having just neutralized a chemical bomb with only seconds to spare, laments to his girlfriend that "the world is being FedExed to hell in a handcart ... anyone's even thinking about having a child in this world is coldly considering an act of cruelty" only to be met with her revelation that she is pregnant. When she asks if he meant what he just said, he replies, "I meant it at the time." "At the time," she retorts, "you said it 7½ seconds ago"—to which he counters, "Well, gosh, kind of a lot's happened since then."
6. Previous discussions (Babrow, 2001; Babrow, Hines, & Kasch, 2000; Babrow et al., 1998; Babrow & Klein, 2000) of types of uncertainty have included *lay epistemology* (a nonphilosopher's view of the nature of knowing and knowledge) but have failed to notice its counterpart, here termed *lay ontology*. Following J. A. Anderson (1996), we understand lay ontology as relatively unschooled understanding of the nature of the phenomenal world and being(s) in that world.

# II

## Personal Narratives and Public Dialogues

༄

### INTRODUCTION

#### Phyllis M. Japp
*University of Nebraska-Lincoln*

*Benson Campbell, an attractive, physically fit, and successful young husband and father, was diagnosed with testicular cancer at age 27. After absorbing the shock of the diagnosis, the Campbells took charge. They found out what had to be done and immediately went at it. After several rounds of chemotherapy Benson was pronounced cancer free. Now as active as ever, Benson is working to raise money for research for testicular cancer, supporting a website and golf tournaments to raise awareness and solicit contribution.*
—McCafferty, 2004, pp. 14–15

*Briana Lane, age 22, an uninsured waitress, rolled her car and was thrown through the windshield. She was charged with DOI and driving with an expired license. Doctors saved her life by removing nearly half of her skull and placing it in a freezer, to be reattached a few weeks later when bleeding and swelling had diminished. Four months later, Briana was still missing her skull. Forced to wear a hockey helmet constantly, she experienced extreme pain when she moved, as her brain shifted from side to side. The wait for the replacement surgery was not due to her condition but to the hospital's unwillingness to proceed without assurance of payment from Medicaid. Finally her mother's insurance agreed to cover the cost of surgery as well as nearly $200,000 in other medical bills.*
—Sage, 2004, p. 2D

53

*David Mitchell, a 50 year old former salesman, is losing balance, peripheral vision, short-term memory and language capability. He has constant and severe headaches. The left side of his brain is shrinking and doctors—he has seen 15 different neurologists—have no idea why. The Mitchells were dropped from their insurance when they inadvertently missed a payment and now have over $100,000 in medical bills. David is scheduled for a brain biopsy at Mayo Clinic if they can raise enough money to pay for the procedure.*
                    —Man Being Robbed of Mind, 2004, p. 9A

Scarcely a day passes that I do not encounter stories like Benson's, Briana's and David's; in my morning newspaper, the magazine I pick up at the dentist's office, on the local and national evening news, in conversations with friends and colleagues. Recent years have brought what some (borrowing a medical metaphor) call an epidemic of personal narratives of all sorts, certainly of stories of illness, death, caregiving, health economics, and the multitude of issues surrounding health. Although I formerly might hear only stories of close friends and relatives (those who trusted me with their narrative), now stories of the physical, emotional, familial, and economic difficulties of those I do not know compete for my attention and sympathy, if not for my monitory contribution. Via public discourse, we become intimate with strangers in a way that we may not with our closest kin. Yet if some personal stories seem to be shared too glibly, with little regard for the occasion and the audience, other stories remain untold, to the loss of both the narrator and the audience. When bereaved parents of an accident victim tell their story, they can assume a sympathetic response. In contrast, the story of a child's suicide, although just as painful a loss, often remains untold; parents uncertain whether they will receive sympathy or blame. In the aforementioned stories, Benson and David are presented as worthy recipients of public sympathy and financial support; David's wife told his story to a public audience in part to solicit contributions for treatment. Briana's story suggests she is responsible for her accident, rendering her less worthy of public sympathy.

As I reflect on the ubiquity of personal health narratives, I raise a curious question for one who has made public narrative the focus of research: Is it possible to become so saturated with public variations of private stories that we become deaf to their appeal? At what point do we hear of so many needs, so much pain, that we become desensitized? When stories of illness and death are sandwiched between weather reports and baseball scores on television news, next to an ad for the grand opening of a new shopping center on the newspaper page, do they become so commonplace they are simply part of "another day, another ad, one more illness story?" Tester (1994) cautioned:

... the more the face of the other is communicated and reproduced ... the more it is denuded of any of the moral authority it might possess. Increased visibility to the gaze seems to go hand in hand with increased invisibility from the point of view of the responsibility of moral solidarity. Media significance means moral insignificance. The image of the other, and therefore the face of the other, which should be so compelling ... becomes commonplace and incapable of attracting a thoughtful or deliberate second glance. (p. 130)

Whether or not we agree with Tester, we must acknowledge that being inundated with stories has implications for personal narrators and their audiences, as well as for public dialogue about health and illness. The intersection of personal illness stories and public discourses of health and illness, creates "personal/public" narratives, personal stories shaped and constructed for public consumption, often to serve ends other than the needs of the individual narrator. These narratives are simultaneously personal and public, therefore open to contradictory expectations and assumptions. Personal stories are vital to healing across a spectrum of health and illness experiences, but as stories migrate into public dialogue, they can no longer be understood solely as personal expressions of experience.

Morris (1998) argued that the postmodern era is characterized not only by the plethora of narrative but by the blurring of boundaries between public and private. The blurring is age-old, of course; what is new is the recognition that life is not carved into separate and distinct domains. Personal identities have always been constructed within the language, images, and values of communal cultures; public discourse always dependant upon stories of personal experience. Personal stories are shaped by the narrative forms of a culture; they embody the familiar and pervasive patterns that shape ways of thinking and collective understandings. In sum, any personal story is constituted in dialogue with relevant public narratives, whether in confirmation, denial, or challenge. Benson's story is a story of triumph over adversity; David's of courage in the face of chronic pain; Briana's of need for support in spite of her own negligence.

Although personal narratives encompass an implied public and mediated public discourse (from legislative testimony to newscasts to public health promotion), these personal narratives rely on individual stories to illustrate problems, shape arguments and engage emotions, as well as to persuade, evaluate, reward and punish. Personal stories increasingly provide a focus for any issue, a convention of news, advertising, promotional campaigns, and entertainment. Thus, public narratives build on and connect to personal and institutional narratives, drawing from the experiences and understandings of those within their domain. David's story reminds us that there are still medical mysteries, conditions for which no diagnosis has been reached; Benson's of the miracles of modern medicine; Briana's of the power of economics to dictate treatment.

How do we engage this mix of personal and public narrative? H. L. Nelson (1997) suggested that there are five things to do with stories: we read or hear stories, we tell stories, we compare stories, we analyze stories, and we invoke stories. Across the continuum from intrapersonal to public communication, we do all of these things with the stories we live out and live among. But the last two responses, analyzing and invoking, are directly relevant to personal/public narratives.

When personal stories are shared interpersonally, the hoped-for response is acceptance of the narrative as a valid and unquestioned account of the narrator's lived experience. However, when such stories become part of public dialogue, framed in the purposes and assumptions of that broader arena, they cannot remain so privileged. In addition to their function as testimony to individual experience, they serve as public persuasive discourse, thus their selection, presentation, adequacy, and truth value are open to analysis. Auditors can and should raise such questions as: Whose story is this? Why this story (or version of events)? Why is it told here, for this audience? Why is it told now? What does it ask me to believe? Briana's and David's stories, for example, constitute an indictment of a heartless and mismanaged health care system as well as personal expressions of trauma. Benson's story, on the other hand, makes absolutely no mention of insurance or economic hardship, implying the cost of treatment as insignificant.

We must also ponder why a particular narrative deserves media time and space when others do not. I will be forever grateful to a very astute undergraduate student who, after watching a video of personal illness stories recorded from television news and documentaries, blurted out: "I'm glad I'm ugly, only good-looking people get sick and die." Certainly, media prefers attractive, articulate, educated, middle-class exemplars, the photogenic individual or family that can eloquently describe their health trauma. David and Benson fit this norm; White, well educated, successful businessmen with loving and supportive families. Audiences can comfortably identify with both. Briana is a less sympathetic character, although at 22, perhaps she can be forgiven her faults and learn from her experience.

H. L. Nelson (1997) suggests that when we invoke a story, we create an alternate use-value by employing it "to make or illustrate a moral point" (p. xii). With a larger narrative frame in place, communicators select stories to fit their purpose, subjecting the personal story to the structure of the broader discourse (just as I am doing here with Briana, David, and Benson). So placed, the personal/public story represents a category of stories and becomes a vehicle to educate or persuade, furthering the goals of the larger narrative. Frequently, a personal story becomes the "face" of a given illness, the case that illustrates the need for increased awareness or funding for the illness in question. Hardwig (1997) argued that "any story silences others" (p. 59); "when one individual becomes the 'face,' it renders other sufferers faceless. Moreover, every story is told from a point of view, a position that silences alternate versions of the story, and marginalizes others as mere characters in its emplotment" (p. 59). Thus, when a personal story is invoked for a public purpose, it is appropriate to ask: Who, or what group, does this story claim to represent? What stories are silenced by the choice of this particular story? Whose point of view is embodied? Who in the story is marginalized or relegated to supporting roles with little voice of their own? What is emphasized or deemphasized as the personal story is shaped to the purposes of the public narrative?

Benson, Briana, and David told their stories to reporters who selected and arranged elements to suit their purposes. I read these second-hand accounts, and summarized and extracted what I needed to support my arguments. Benson and David are constructed as the heroes of their stories, the former as a successful disease warrior, the latter as displaying courage in the face of great adversity. Briana is plotted as a victim of an unfeeling system, but also of her own stupidity. In all three stories, families play a supporting role whereas physicians enter only as marginal characters. Benson's story, a saga of endurance of hardship and pain with restitution at the end, casts his wife as caring but relatively inconsequential.

The chapters in this section all address the implications of personal/public narratives as they engage the tension between personal stories and public discourse, and the social, political and ideological issues invoked by that tension. Beck (chap. 3) deals sensitively with Cathy Hainer's personal/public narrative of life with, and death from, cancer. Her personal story employs familiar narrative forms, from the "battle metaphor" to the "adventure motif." She positions her story as a public dialogue with her readers; it comprises the final chapter in her public persona as a journalist. If we wipe tears away as we read, we cry not only for Cathy, but because she has borne public witness to a painful and commonly experienced sense of loss. Cathy's story becomes a volume in our public library of cancer narratives, a resource for others who will experience this horrible disease.

Harter, Kirby, Edwards, and McClanahan (chap. 4) reveal the powerful constraints public narratives exert on personal experience. For women dealing with issues of fertility, the language of ARI—the metaphors, equations, narrative constructions and visual images—constitutes the terrain on which they must articulate their needs and concerns. This public discourse is so constraining and ideologically powerful that it is difficult, if not impossible, for women to write their story outside its parameters. Even if a woman is able to construct a resistive personal narrative to explore her needs and explain her decisions, she realizes her experience will be evaluated within this set of powerful public narratives of ARI.

P. M. Japp and D. K. Japp explore the personal narratives of those whose lives are caught between illness and health. The ability to construct a coherent and meaningful personal illness narrative is constrained when the biomedical master narrative is unable to provide legitimacy. Those who claim to be ill when the biomedical narrative refuses to validate that experience are forced into the realm of alternate public narratives, those of imaginary illnesses, mental dysfunction, or malingering. Personal stories of BII attempt to counter the dictates of these public narratives, but so often have internalized their damaging orientations and values.

Workman (chap. 6) clearly demonstrates the tension between personal and public narrative in his analysis of how a dramatic personal story functions as a core component in public discourse of binge drinking. The generic death story, fired by the real-life death of MIT freshman, Scott Kruger, represents the scope of the campus drinking problem and serves as the centerpiece of prevention campaigns. The power of this personal story, reconfigured and reinforced by extensive media coverage, unfortunately, does not resonate with those most at risk. Yet, the dominance of this one personal story silences other stories that might be more realistic and appropriate.

Carabas and Harter (chap. 7) demonstrate how public and personal narratives—or lack thereof—are entwined in the politics of oppression. State-induced illness, from neglect to torture, silences stories of abuse and pain. Abusers and abused both must remain mute so that citizens can pretend to be ignorant and power structures can maintain their authority. When silence is broken, stories pour forth, stories of the abused and justifications of the abusers. These personal stories legitimate suffering and promote healing. Simultaneously personal, public, and political, they cumulatively will eventually rewrite the public narratives of history.

Singal, Chitnis, and Sengupta (chap. 8) provide a fascinating case of narrative "border crossing," from culture to culture, from public to private and private to public, as the mediated narratives of one culture are viewed within the frame of the public narratives of another culture. *Friends* is a mediated narrative that represents, to some degree at least, the values of its culture of origin, the United States. Although a public narrative, *Friends* is composed of a series of personal stories, in which fictional characters engage the issue of "safe sex." Indian audiences necessarily pull these fictional personal stories through the public narratives of their own culture and then into the realm of their personal lives as they examine the relevance of these fictional stories for their own experiences with sexual activity.

Each chapter, while providing closure for a specific focus on narrative, is also heuristically rich. Collectively, as these chapters address the interface of public and personal narrative in a variety of venues, they provide rich suggestions for "what to do with stories."

# 3

## Becoming the Story: Narratives as Collaborative, Social Enactments of Individual, Relational, and Public Identities[1]

**Christina S. Beck**
*Ohio University*

> ... I left work in the middle of the day and went to Georgetown University Medical Center to visit my friend and colleague Cathy Hainer. I knew it was the last time I would see her. So did she ... I offered up a stack of mail she has received—a mere handful of the hundreds of letters from USA Today readers who had been following her battle with cancer in the public diary she shared with them. Six of the letters on the top of the pile were from the same man, a prisoner somewhere who addressed each envelope the same: Cathy Hainer (reporter with cancer). "As opposed to Cathy Hainer, reporter who does not have cancer?" she asked. "Evidently," I replied. She chuckled.
>
> —Wilson, 1999, p. 1D

As a relatively regular reader of *USA Today* in the late 1990s, I routinely turned to the "Life" section. I searched for Hainer's name, hoping for another article about her experiences with breast cancer, dreading possible bad news. To be honest, before her first column in the series on March 10, 1998, I was unfamiliar with Hainer's work as a journalist. I didn't know anything about her as a person, an individual with friends, family, colleagues, and a family history of breast cancer. As a reader of a national news publication, I would not have perceived any of that information as my business.

From her articles in this special series, I learned that we were roughly the same age, both college grads in the same year with a journalism degree. Our similar age sparked my initial interest in Hainer's journey—but for the grace of God, Hainer's story could be my own.

I came to know much more about Hainer than I do about women in my own church who have battled cancer. Through her columns, she confided the challenges of enacting her complicated and, at times, conflicting, identities as a journalist, a girlfriend, a daughter, a colleague, given the physical, emotional and spiritual saga of living with (and dying from) cancer.

For some readers (unfortunately, myself included at times), Hainer became "the reporter with cancer," no longer merely a journalist yet, because her artful reflections about her journey got featured in USA Today, not just someone with cancer. In fact, Hainer even reflected on those particular identities (journalist and cancer patient) as she detailed medical procedures and encounters. During one surgical procedure in the later stages of her treatment, she passed gas. She bemoaned that "the truly embarrassing part was the intercom ... Would I forever be remembered as 'that flatulent woman from USA Today'?" (Hainer, September 27, 1999, p. 7D).

However, as her articles attest, she refused to accept the narrowing label of only "reporter with cancer." She positioned herself as a reporter from a national newspaper, still a viable colleague and contributor, even when her illness forced her to take extended leaves. She picked out an engagement ring and a house with her fiancé; she mourned the loss of potential children. She wrestled with emergent physical limitations while obtaining an inner peace about her illness, wellness, and mortality.

For personal and professional reasons, Hainer opted to write about her doctor visits, treatments, tough medical choices, interactions with friends and family, and ultimately, her peace with dying. She chose to share raw, riveting, deeply personal perspectives with thousands of readers (as opposed to a few close friends and family members). Consistent with Frank's (1995) notion of "quest narratives" (p. 115), Hainer did so not just as a breast cancer patient but as an investigative reporter with the goal of enlightening readers about the uncertainties of contemporary health care based on her first-hand experiences. As she closed that first column on March 10, 1998, Hainer explained:

> I prayed that I could find a way to turn my cancer into a transformational, healing experience. I asked God for help in showing me the path to make that happen. I believe that writing this article, sharing my experience with others, and possibly providing help to others who will get a similar diagnosis this year, is part of that path. (p. 1A)

As a health communication scholar who has written about her own health care sagas (Beck, 2001), I am drawn to narrative—voices of others and aspects of ourselves that intersect and intertwine throughout our complex and multifaceted existences. Much like Melanie Griffith's character in the movie, *Working Girl*, I clipped Hainer's articles and letters to the editor that were published in response from March, 1998, to December, 1999.[2] Indeed, Hainer's narrative struck me as valuable for scholarly reflection and discussion. I decided to explore Hainer's articles, focusing on the rhetorical constructions of this personal health narrative situated in such a public forum.

Yet, as I started to type this chapter, I wondered about my right to comment on Hainer's articles, her personal peek at living with (and dying from) breast cancer. Certainly, the installments of Hainer's narrative were published in "America's newspaper," *USA Today*, usually on the front page of the "Life" section. Clearly, their publication constitutes publicly available "data." However, I felt odd as I highlighted passages of the text in preparation for writing. Hainer bared herself for us, I thought, disclosing physical and emotional details that I would not even likely get from family members or one of my best friends. What authority do I have for analyzing such private perspectives without gaining her permission? What right do I have to advance my analytical insights about her lived reality without the opportunity to speak with her, given that she died in December of 1999?

As I wrestled with this ethical dilemma, I realized that my queries paralleled a point of this chapter—the ways in which such a "personal" story becomes co-constructed as "public" domain—"our story." As one *USA Today* reader responded in a letter to the editor, "I want to thank Cathy Hainer for her bravery and for telling the world of her cancer. But really, it's not just her cancer—it's everyone's" (Ciotti, 1998, p. 14A). Thus, in this chapter, I employ the public conversation surrounding Hainer's illness as a catalyst for contributing to scholarly conversations about communicative enactments of narrative (see, e.g., Harter, Japp, & Beck, chap. 1, this volume; Sharf & Vanderford, 2003) and the construction of personal narratives as part of public dialogues about health, wellness, and disease, such as breast cancer.

Notably, as I detail throughout this chapter, the blurring of public and private identities and space, the morphing of "my story" into "our narrative," powerfully illustrates the contemporary complexities of co-defining experiences with illness (see related arguments by Gergen, 1991). Not completely private, not entirely public, fluctuating and fragmented, this public conversation about life journeys detoured by cancer, prompted by Hainer's disclosures, provides a compelling example of negotiating "illness" (and concurrent, dynamic individual and relational identities) in the postmodern era. Indeed, this discourse underscores the temporal nature of narratives (see related works by Brockelman, 1985; Freeman, 1998; Ricoeur, 1981b, 1988). As Hainer articulates in her accounts, the passage of time and her own positioning within a "usual" lifespan flavored those complicated and continual negotiations. Moreover, the broader context of this narrative as situated in the late 1990s—with the ever-increasing proliferation of media and technology (and their expanding role in public dialogues), blurring boundaries between public and private, and loudening cries for breast cancer and women's health to be situated as politically and medically relevant—serves as an integral backdrop to Hainer's articles and the responses to them by readers.

In this chapter, I argue, first, that health care narratives are implicitly embodied rhetoric. Our bodies constitute a critical, co-constructed, co-negotiated, and perhaps contested, springboard for rhetorical enactments of individual and relational identities. Extending from that argument, I contend, second, that health care narratives are implicitly relational. Although health care narratives may stem from an individual's experience with disease or disability, that individual cannot construct the narrative in isolation; others inherently (even if inadvertently or unintentionally) contribute to the emergent, temporal enactment of health narratives, and as such, those narratives constitute relational constructions. In light of my assertions about narrative as implicitly embodied rhetoric and implicitly relational, I explore, third, the rhetorical implications of health narratives as public constructions.

## NARRATIVE AS IMPLICITLY EMBODIED RHETORIC

On July 19, 1999, Cathy Hainer called herself, "The chemistry experiment who wore tennis shoes." She clarified, "No, it's not the latest summer kid's movie; it's become the story of my life" (p. 7D).

Health narratives constitute complicated social accomplishments, expanding far beyond mere physical manifestations of disease or disability (see, e.g., Frank, 1995; Garro & Mattingly, 2000; Kleinmann, 1988; Langellier, 2001; Mattingly, 1998; Riessman, 2000; Sharf & Vanderford, 2003). Yet, as Frank (1995) contended, "... illness stories are not only *about* the body but *of* and through the body" (p. 140). Actions on and by the body reflexively and rhetorically contribute to health narratives, powerfully shaping critical aspects of the health care and wellness process. As embodied rhetoric, the ever-emergent health narratives impact the ways in which health care gets accomplished and the ways in which individual and relational identities develop.

## Implications of Emergent Health Narratives
## as Embodied Rhetoric for Health Care

In earlier works, I argued that health care participants collaboratively co-construct health care encounters (C. Beck, 2001; C. Beck, with Ragan & duPre, 1997). Through their verbal and nonverbal behaviors, including silence, health care participants coordinate their actions and affirm or negate preferences for identity, relational roles, and courses of health care treatment, and so on (see related classic works by Berger & Luckman, 1966; Garfinkel, 1967; Gergen, 1991, 1999; Goffman, 1959, 1963, 1967; Schutz, 1962). In particular, though, the co-definitions and orientations to the body work rhetorically to flavor ways in which health care gets co-accomplished by health care participants (and, reflexively, the emergent health narrative).

For example, on March 10, 1998, Hainer detailed:

> As he [the doctor] left the office so I could get dressed, he held up the specimen jar, proud of the good biopsy samples he'd gotten. "Want to see?" he asked. Not really. Once Dr. Petrucci had left, I turned to my boyfriend David and said, "This guy is crazy. I'm 36 and in love. How could I possibly have cancer?" (p. 1A)

Through the way in which Dr. Petrucci displayed those good biopsy samples that he harvested from Hainer's body, he communicated pride, a medical procedure well done. Although artifacts from Hainer's body, now separated for the purpose of disease diagnosis, Hainer did not return Dr. Petrucci's enthusiasm. How could she? For her, those snippets from herself symbolized the potential of a life-altering problem—her body had somehow produced tissue that could harm the rest of her. Further, the idea that cancer could be present in those bits of her body conflicted with the rest of her lived reality—as a well person, someone in love, someone relatively young. Borrowing from Fisher's (1984, 1985a, 1987) description of narrative rationality, Hainer struggled to juxtapose the diagnosis with her age (36) and chronologically consistent activities—being in love, feeling attractive, contemplating children. She hadn't penciled cancer into how she envisioned her life to unfold, instead privileging a predictable, linear ideal of time—consistent with Freeman's (1998) concept of *historical time*. Yet suddenly, the cancer occurred, vastly disrupting her ideal timeline (physically, personally, and professionally) and clashing with her perceptions of what should be and what can still happen in the future. Extending from Ricoeur (1981b), Freeman (1998) argued persuasively:

> ... in dealing with human time—that is *temporality*—the notion of historical time qua chronology and linearity is insufficient; for the act of in-

terpretation, via memory, brings with it a mode of time that is rather more like a circle or spiral, embodying a dialectical movement from present to past and past to present, at once. This movement is in turn conditioned by the future as well, in the form not only of hopes, expectations, and so on, but of the projected self that both emerges from and gives form to the landscape of one's history. (pp. 42–43)

Charmaz (1991), Kleinman (1988) and Frank (1995), among others, wrote eloquently about the ways in which individuals respond to and enact illness. For Hainer, the initial incompatibility between her diagnosis and her apparent health and appearance proved difficult to reconcile, exacerbated by the likely consequences of treatment for an illness that she could not yet fathom.

> I was having a hard time integrating the fact of my cancer into the reality of my life. I still felt fine, was going to work, looked the same as ever. David had been taken by surprise at the news of the extent of the spread and wasn't feeling optimistic. Worse yet, the doctors had said it was probable that the chemotherapy would leave me infertile. I was devastated ... we had hoped for a child of our own. The news left an icy pit in my stomach. (Hainer, March 10, 1998, p. 1A)

The body serves us as a vessel, a shell for our soul, an outward manifestation of who we are and who we want to be. As a woman, Hainer yearned for her body to enable her to produce a child, yet ironically, the prescribed treatment for preserving her own life would rob her of the chance to create one. She mourned the would-be child, the possibility of that type of family unit, and the missed relational opportunity to give birth and to nurture her own child.

S. Smith (1994) explained that bodies "... provide us, as individuals, the boundaries of our isolated beings" (pp. 267–268). However, Smith also contended that bodies "are obviously and critically communal and discursive bodies, and community creates a superfluity of 'body' that marks us in practices, discourses, and temporalities" (p. 268). Very much in keeping with other doctors who adhere to the biomedical model, Hainer's initial doctor oriented to her body as something to be diagnosed and treated. However, the responses of Hainer (and her loved ones, to some extent) contributed to the ensuing decisions about how her body (e.g., as the vessel for her self, the container of the disease, etc.) became symbolically constructed (and physically acted upon). After learning of her diagnosis with stage IV metastatic breast cancer, Hainer reflected on her pending choices about courses of action and orientations to her body, her self, and others who would play critical roles in co-constructing the emergent health narrative. Hainer wrote that "... it's undeniably comforting to feel you're in the hands of professionals. It's so tempting to say, 'OK, no more decisions for me. Doctor, take care of me now' " (Hainer, March 10, 1998, p. 1A).

Hainer's ultimate decision to resist that initial temptation by seeking information, alternative health care, and new medical advances reflected the way in which she wanted to position herself in relation to health care professionals. In so doing, she reflexively claimed ownership of her body and rhetorically positioned herself as active in the health care process. As Park-Fuller (1995) contended, though, a different orientation would also indicate, reflexively and rhetorically, a particular perspective of the body. In her writings about the performance of breast cancer, Park-Fuller (1995) noted that individuals who do not seek their own voice in health care experiences may well start to "... perceive themselves as 'victims' upon which the medical community may succeed or fail in working its miracles. With such a self-image, patients are 'docile bodies,' co-conspirators in their own victimization" (p. 62).

## Implications of Embodied Rhetoric for Individual and Relational Identities

In the introduction of her book on embodied theory, Davis (1997) suggested that bodies are "... the means for self-expression, for becoming who we would most like to be" (p. 2). In her critique of earlier feminist writings on body theory and embodiment, Davis (1997) contended that "bodies are not simply abstractions, however, but are embedded in the immediacies of everyday, lived experience" (p. 15). Moreover, especially for women, Smith (1994) maintained "... communities surrounding us normalize certain bodies and render abnormal or grotesque other bodies, thereby situating our body somewhere in the field of bodies" (p. 268).

Goffman argued in 1963 that society stigmatizes certain illnesses or conditions, impacting an individual's preferred identity, that is, labeling someone as not *normal* or not *complete*. Given the ramifications of treatment, not only do women with breast cancer face the potential of death; they may also fear and resent the loss of bodily markers of being a normal and complete woman (see Kleinman, 1988; Langellier, 2001; and a related argument by Nelson, 2001). Langellier (2001) explained "treatments for breast cancer, sometimes referred to as the Slash/Burn/Poison triology (surgery, radiation, chemotherapy) are traumatic and often mutilating, an additional source of stigma, often starkly visible and a challenge to body image and feminity" (pp. 145–146).

Hainer's reflections on March 26, 1998 illustrate Langellier's observations:

It's a subtle psychological process. With my hair in place, I felt like my healthy old self. Once my hair was gone, I felt like I might as well wear a sign saying, "I'm getting chemotherapy." I had already bought a wig, but I'd hidden it away in my closet, hating the very sight of it. Nevertheless, I decided to take the direct approach at work. So on Monday morning I walked in and announced to my colleagues, "Well, I'm going bald." Craig Wilson, a fellow reporter who has chronicled his own battle against a receding hairline for this paper, joked, "Oh cry me a river, honey, I've been fighting that battle for years." Laughter definitely helped ease the sting. (p. 6D)

Although cushioned by the reactions of her colleagues, the "sting" remained. Wilson's collegial comment offered a possible recasting of Hainer's hair loss, but for Hainer, the impending hair loss symbolized something far different than Wilson's. As Hainer noted, she "might as well wear a sign" that something was amiss, something was not normal, something was not right (see related work by Bell, 2000; Bury, 1982, 2000). Her body became that sign, exacerbated by the impact of additional treatment. After acknowledging that she felt like "my own life had become analogous to the Passover story," Hainer detailed her 10 personal "plagues" on April 15, 1998. She explained:

Next, tiny wrinkles showed up near my mouth, on my forehead, even on my chin. Overnight I became George Burns. My skin took on a sallow, waxy look. My fiancé, David, continued to tell me I looked beautiful, but I knew I looked different, like some pseudo-Cathy. Even the wig seemed suddenly to hang on me differently. (p. 9D)

Almost a month later, she scheduled her mastectomy. Hainer's comments on May 13, 1998, highlight turbulent temporal undercurrents regarding orientations to her body and the physical consequences of combating the cancer within it:

Months earlier, right after diagnosis, I had been very cavalier about the breast. "Just take it off," I remember thinking. But as the date approached, I felt differently. I was nervous about the surgery, but also sad. After all, that breast had served me well for 36 years, and I'd miss it. "There's always reconstruction," my friend Rachel said. And though I planned on having reconstructive surgery, that would be more than a year away. (p. 1D)

The physical transformation of her body contributed starkly and significantly to the emergent health narrative, especially in terms of perceived ability to enact preferred individual and relational identities (e.g., "complete" woman, attractive fiancé, productive colleague). Although perhaps taken for granted (and even initially dismissed during an early phase of her illness), Hainer's breast became more than just an expendable body part that could someday be "rebuilt." As time passed, she came to recognize her breast as an essential part of who she was and who she could be. Without it, she would be forever different than she had been for the prior 36 years. Her hair, her energy, her health could return one day, but at that moment just before the mastectomy, she paused, pondering what had been "just my breast" and what could be reconstructed after its removal.

Herzlich and Pierret (1987) observed "... the sick person also, indeed above all, appears to the world as an inactive and unproductive member of society" (p. 97). Through Hainer's decision to chronicle her battle with cancer, she overtly worked to reposition herself as ill yet also productive and professional. Although Hainer resisted casting herself as "sick," especially in early installments of the journal, Hainer's reflections after she went into remission indicate the ways in which her body hindered preferred individual and relational identities. Hainer wrote on June 22, 1998:

> ... I came to understand that it [quality of life] means much more. I had my life back again. Black peach fuzz covered my head as my hair started growing back. David and I had moved into our new home. My energy level was high, and I felt great. I had a life of quality again. I didn't want to go back to sick-person mode. (p. 1D)

On October 1, 1998, Hainer continued:

> Nine months is a symbolic chunk of time in a woman's life. In my case, it didn't represent a pregnancy, but a gestation period of renewal in body and spirit ... Except for the wig I still wear and the pill I pop each morning, life has pretty much returned to the way it was B.C.—before cancer. I'm traveling again for work, which is a good thing, since it's tough for a sometime travel writer not to travel ... My energy level has returned to normal, and I'm back to working out. (p. 1D)

As Freeman (1998) contended, "... as a general rule we don't live lines, moving inexorably through one thing after another; we live spirals of remembrance and return, repetition and reconfiguration ..." (p. 47). Interestingly, Hainer contrasted her 9-month experience with the time frame of a typical human pregnancy, a physical accomplishment that may not now be possible yet something that she considered "B.C. —before cancer." Although she cycled through disappointment about the impact of her cancer on her hoped-for pregnancy, in this passage, she emphasizes getting back to normal in terms of her energy and her work. With restored energy, she could work again. More than simply earning a livelihood, Hainer could once again really do her job by traveling, thus legitimately performing tasks and roles necessary to enact her identity (and job) as a journalist. Yet, she necessarily reconfigured "normal"—she still wore her wig and took her pill. She confessed that cancer never completely left her consciousness. However, in the "new normal," she could relegate her identity as "cancer patient" (which had been prioritized in the preceding 9 months) to the background, instead foregrounding how she wanted to be as partner and reporter (see related arguments by Beck, 2001; Gergen, 1991).

Unfortunately, in mid-March of 1999, Hainer's doctors discovered that the cancer had returned, spreading to her brain and into her bones. Hainer called the multiple lesions "a serious act of guerrilla warfare. Cancer 10, Cathy 0" (Hainer, April 20, 1999, p. 1D). As she battled overwhelming pain and pondered increasing physical limitations, she did so within the context of her preferred individual and relational identities.

> After five months of feeling well, was I finally failing? Would I soon be stuck in a hospital bed? Would I have to wake David up for bedpan duty in the middle of the night? Who would take the dog on her morning walk?... The three hours at the office totally depleted my energy ... For several nights in a row, I went to bed weeping. Afraid, exhausted and in pain, I was tired of fighting. This wasn't Cathy Hainer, but some other woman in a deteriorating body. Running my life has become such a burden. Not for the last time, I asked God to bring me a quick and painless death. David was a constant support, but I knew this downturn in my physical and emotional state was draining for him, too. How could it not be? (Hainer, September 27, 1999, p. 7D)

In subsequent published accounts of Hainer's health narrative, she reiterated the integral nature of her body's condition for her perception of self, individually and in relation to others. On November 4, 1999, she explained that "sometimes I felt like an old doll, once a beloved present, now forgotten in the back of the closet. My batteries were dying down, and parts of my body were wearing out ... To feel one's body fading away is a strange and scary thing" (p. 6D). In her final column, Hainer admitted:

> For months, I have dreaded this very moment. I remember when my mother was dying from breast cancer and was forced to wear diapers. The indignity seemed impossible to bear. Now I find myself "dropping trou" in front of anyone who happens to be in the room at the time. When you gotta go, you gotta go. I never thought I'd have to rely on my dad to wipe my bottom, but he lovingly does so with a warm washcloth ... I must rely on family and friends for virtually every movement of my body ... In effect, I am a virtual prisoner in my body. (December 6, 1999, p. 9D)

As Hainer's accounts attest, the body constitutes an integral, component of health care narratives. Individuals necessarily embody physical manifestations of disease or disability. Moreover, they also embody the emotional, spiritual, and relational meanings and messages of those impacts of disease or disability on the body. As social beings, our embodiments of "wellness," "illness," "fitness," "physical challenges," and so on. flavor our constructions of self in relation to others in powerful, persuasive ways. Thus, our health narratives constitute embodied rhetoric that contributes to our co-accomplishment of social selves.

## HEALTH NARRATIVES AS IMPLICITLY RELATIONAL

Reviewing the work of Mead (1934) and Goffman (1959, 1961), in particular, Holstein and Gubrium (2000) developed the notion of self as socially constructed. In their excellent analysis of the implications of Schutz (1962) and Garfinkel (1967) on the construction of self, Holstein and Gubrium (2000) depicted "self" as emergent and discursively accomplished. Importantly for the purposes of this chapter, Holstein and Gubrium argued that "narrative practice lies at the heart of self construction" (p. 104) and that "the selves that stories convey, as well as the identities of storytellers and listeners, are thus shaped and edited as storytelling proceeds" (p. 113). Indeed, McAdams and Bowman (2001) agreed "life stories are not imagined out of thin air. Instead, they are based on reality as both personally known and consensually validated" (p. 28).

Despite the emphasis on social selves and social constructionism in writings on narrative, the tendency has been to treat "a" narrative as primarily "a teller's story" with varying input from others (see, e.g., P. Atkinson, 1997; Bavelas, Coates, & Johnson, 2000; Capps, & Ochs, 1995; Frank, 1995; Garro, 1992, 1994; Holstein & Gubrium, 2000; Young, 1987). As P. Atkinson (1997) maintained, "Whether they stress the exotic or the ordinary, they celebrate the individual. The speaking voice, the subject of recorded or reported speech, is represented as a unique and privileged locus of character and experience" (pp. 326–327).

In this portion, I challenge a prioritizing of the individual in narrative research, contending instead that health narratives are implicitly relational in nature. P. Atkinson (1997) asserted that narrative research invites us to celebrate "some—but by no means all—narratives. These are stripped of social context and social consequences. They are understood in terms of an individualized view of the self" (p. 339). Although I agree with Atkinson's point about the privileging of certain narratives in private and public discourse (see related arguments in Beck, 2001), I take issue with the implication that narrative research, per se, must be so limited.

Indeed, extending from my earlier argument that health narratives constitute embodied rhetoric, I suggest, first, that we inherently experience life issues (including our physical selves) in relation to others, not as isolated individuals. Second, I contend that multiple, concurrent health narratives may spring from a single health episode as others become co-tellers from their own relational perspectives (i.e., significant others, family members, colleagues). Although participation by such others certainly fluctuates, depending on relational identities, personalities, situations, institutional contexts, and so on, those others (intentionally or unintentionally, overtly or subtly) collaborate in our co-construction of what health episodes mean to us and to others.

## Health Narratives as Collaborative Co-Accomplishments

In their classic ethnomethodological work, Wieder and Pratt (1990) detailed the enactment of positioning oneself as a "real Indian." Based on their research of one Native American community, Wieder and Pratt found that individuals cannot simply assert their identity as "real Indians." Instead, they necessarily engage in the interactional work of presenting themselves and receiving affirmation of their legitimacy/inadequacy as particular types of members of the community. Through their taken-for-granted treatment of specific behaviors and orientations as indicative of membership, the community collaboratively constructs cultural artifacts, norms, and preferences, including its definition of what counts as a "legitimate" member of the community (see Wieder & Pratt, 1990; and related work by Garfinkel, 1967).

As individuals engage in health care experiences, they do not do so in isolation. Gusdorf (1980) contended "no one is rightful possessor of his life or his death; lives are so thoroughly entangled that each of them has its center everywhere and its circumference nowhere" (p. 28). Much like the Native American participants in Wieder and Pratt's (1990) investigation, health care participants do not interpret or respond to diagnoses, physical conditions, or treatments in a vacuum. As Bateson (1972) and Goffman (1974) argued in their respective work on framing, individuals assert and affirm preferred and shared orientations to aspects of interaction, including the very ways in which individuals present themselves physically (see Goffman, 1959). For example, as noted earlier, Goffman's (1963) work on stigma clearly suggests that certain manifestations of disease or disability become socially constructed as problematic by interested others in society, not simply by an individual's personal perspectives on that condition.

With that said, individuals certainly do have their own viewpoints. Yet, the interplay of individuals in relation to others—health care providers, family members, colleagues, friends, and sometimes, perhaps even strangers—contributes to codefinitions of meaning in emergent health narratives. Hainer's narrative exemplifies that interplay.

Hainer struggled a great deal with reconciling her deteriorating body with her sense of self—who she really was and who she could still be in relation to others. Near the end of her illness, Hainer recounted a conversation that spoke to those questions.

> My college roommate came down for a reunion visit, and we spent lovely hours reminiscing and catching up. After a while, she told me how happy she was to still perceive "my essential Cathness." The true me was still very evident, she said, not buried under layers of fear, anger, or pain. I was especially glad to hear this since Mr. Pain had moved into Cathy's Cancerland. (November 4, 1999, p. 6D)

On March 26, 1998, Hainer shared a special moment during her journey, an occasion made significant through the ways in which Hainer and her boyfriend, David, framed it as relationally meaningful (not simply medically essential):

> My boyfriend, David, had learned to do the injections as well. So on Saturday morning, hands shaking, we loaded up the syringe, and he injected it into my thigh. To ease the anxiety, we made a couple of lame jokes about shooting up together. It was certainly one of the most intimate moments of our relationship. Although another was yet to come ... That morning, feeling that my health was in question, David and I got a fever to get the rest of our lives in order. We'd talked for several months about getting married ... we decided to spend the rest of the day looking for engagement rings and homes. (p. 6D)

Hainer's relationship with David was not just a backdrop to her health narrative; it shaped, to a large degree, what cancer meant to her and how she confronted symptoms and even the possibility of death. On April 20, 1999, Hainer admitted, "hearing that you have multiple lesions in your brain is not an easy thing" (p. 1D). She continued:

> But David and I took the news with an eerie calm. We spent a few minutes holding each other, crying. I have to laugh now, but my first words were: "Can you afford the mortgage by yourself?" A practical Capricorn rising, to the end ... it's giving up on life that's the tough part. I don't have too many regrets, but the thought of leaving David, leaving my family, leaving my routine—it's too soon. I suppose it's always too soon.

Especially because she enacted her health experience in an overtly discursive manner, Hainer invited others to contribute their voices to her emergent health narrative. In that April 20, 1999, column, she noted:

Whether I was accepting my possible demise or denying it, I wanted very much to talk about it. I wanted to be keenly aware of what was happening to me, what death might mean, how it would feel. I didn't want to be cheated out of the experience because the subject was taboo. Of course, it was nearly impossible to discuss such an unknowable subject in any rational way. But I demanded that my family and friends engage me on this matter. And I'm happy to report that, to the last one, they have risen to the occasion. (p. 1D)

Of course, not all individuals choose to engage others in such interaction about illness and impending death. However, even if a person does not opt to confide in a single other person, that person's health narrative still gets shaped and co-constructed by the orientation of health care professionals and by the tenor of texts that he or she may read. For example, early in her illness, Hainer visited a naturopath. She wrote, "I left the center refreshed and upbeat. These people had given me a great gift: They'd helped me to remember that I was Cathy Hainer, not some faceless cancer victim. Unlike hospitals, which are suffused with the culture of disease, they promoted the culture of wellness" (March 26, 1998, p. 6D).

## Health Narratives as Multiple, Concurrent Accomplishments

If health narratives are collaborative, not individual, accomplishments, they also become multiple, concurrent accomplishments because each participant in the narrative construction impacts (and reflexively gets impacted by) the process of illness and quest for wellness. On July 19, 1999, Hainer wrote:

Some in the cancer community talk about the "gift" of the disease ... A friend of David's helped me to see that. One day, feeling down, David e-mailed Bob, a wise former teacher and loyal friend. "Why is this happening to us? It's so unfair," David wrote, "Cathy and I are in love and she even eats her vegetables." Bob wrote back: "Isn't it great that you guys are in love and that Cathy eats her vegetables?" What a great response! And what a perfect reminder to see the extraordinary in each ordinary moment. To find the magic in every day. (p. 7D)

Interestingly, the friend's response resonated with Hainer, serving as a message to her as well as to David. She treated it as a powerful reframing of their situation and a motivational reminder of how to view the world.

Moreover, this exchange also offers insight into the multiplicity of health narratives. Although David did not undergo treatment for cancer, he suffered through the diagnosis, surgeries, and what must have been a tremendous sense of loss. Indeed, he did not position the health episode as "Cathy's situation"; he wrote, "Why is this happening to *us*?" In that same column, Cathy recalled David's interaction with a doctor, noting that David inquired, "Which would give *us* the best chance of stopping cancer's spread?" (July 19, 1999, p. 7D).

By viewing a health episode as prompting multiple possible health narratives, we can gain a deeper understanding of the broad-reaching impact of wellness and illness for communities of people, not just for one individual. In her letter to the editor of *USA Today* in response to one of Hainer's articles, Mary Lee Hahn wrote:

> Like Cathy Hainer, my life turned upside down in January with a diagnosis of breast cancer ... Also like Cathy, there is nothing, besides surviving, more important to me than sharing my experience with everyone my life touches. I teach fifth-graders—my girls are just beginning to grow breasts and my boys can't say the word without giggling. They have been part of my journey into the cancer universe from the beginning, from the disbelief of the diagnosis of their young, healthy fit, energetic teacher through the surgeries and on toward the chemotherapy and radiation. Their mothers are coming along on this journey as well ... Every woman with breast cancer touches the lives of friends, family, hometown acquaintances, colleagues, and students. (March 13, 1998, p. 14A)

## RHETORICAL IMPLICATIONS OF HEALTH NARRATIVES AS PUBLIC EXPERIENCES

Through this chapter, I have asserted that health narratives are necessarily and implicitly social and relational constructions. As Hahn affirms, individuals who experience illness do impact (and are impacted by) the lives and lived realities of others.

Hainer's choice to chronicle her journey for an international readership vastly broadened her "community" of confidants, thus contributing to conversations between readers and the text and, potentially, between readers and their loved ones. In this portion of the chapter, I explore, first, the emergence of Hainer's story as "our story" and, second, the legitimacy of this shared interpretive experience for public conversations about lived experiences with illness and the process of dying.

### "Our Story"

In her theory of Communication Privacy Management (CPM), Sandra Petronio (2002) discussed the communicative accomplishment of boundaries as individuals choose which information to reveal to others and, indeed, to which specific others. As part of CPM, Petronio argues that individuals weigh the benefits and risks of disclosing versus privacy. Especially with potentially stigmatizing conditions, Petronio contends, individuals may avoid risk by guarding information carefully, disclosing in a limited, restrictive manner.

By opting to disclose information to others, we expand our personal boundaries to those others with regard to that particular issue. According to Petronio (2002), confidants become co-owners of that information, sharing what has been confided with the confider and implicitly gaining "insider" status as someone who now knows what had previously been unknown.

Hainer's decision to include her readers in her emergent health narrative inherently expanded the boundaries around her cancer journey to include strangers, not just friends, colleagues, family members, and health care professionals. As I have detailed throughout this chapter, Hainer wrote about harsh indignities and consequences of cancer treatment. Her journals included vivid accounts of implications of cancer for her relationship with her fiancé, her reflections on her body and her emergent self. To borrow from Petronio (2002), Hainer's articles necessarily worked to involve readers, even if reluctantly, as confidants of intimate information.

Notably, Hainer's disclosure of "her" narrative in *USA Today* reflexively, relationally, and rhetorically invoked co-construction of Hainer's medical situation as "our story," contributing to (and being impacted by) multiple, concurrent life (and health) narratives of her readers. Her colleague, Karen Peterson, affirmed, "Cathy Hainer did not walk alone. As she shared her journey, she touched readers who e-mailed and wrote from around the world" (Peterson, December 16, 1999, p. 1D). Hainer (June 22, 1998) noted, "Six months ago, I opened my life up to the readers of *USA Today*. The response has been overwhelmingly supportive, uplifting, and rewarding. Readers have added me to prayer lists, written words of support and sent chemo-coping tips ..." (p. 1D).

However, reader response surpassed mere messages of encouragement. Meyrowitz (1985) explained that readers of mediated texts blur boundaries between public domain and private space, diminishing perceived separation between selves and strangers. As she confided in her readership, Hainer facilitated dwindling distinctions between private and public domains. One reader, Jennifer Mitchell, commented:

> Cathy Hainer is a beautiful and brave woman who has chosen to be vulnerable and transparent and to share with so many the emotional story of her struggle with breast cancer. How can we read her account without feeling as if we know her, ultimately recognizing our own humanity and

asking ourselves how we will face up to these kinds of trials when our time comes? (September 30, 1999, p. 18A)

Consistent with Meyrowitz, readers of Hainer's articles responded with expressions of kinship and companionship in their respective health narratives. Anne J. Rislove (March 30, 1998) wrote, "Thanks again for your heartfelt article. It is a lonely battle, this fight against cancer, but it really makes us each feel much better to read that others have been through it, so we are not really alone" (p. 14A). Bruce Shorts agreed, noting that:

I have followed every printed article of Cathy's poignant and emotional "guerrilla warfare" with cancer. I almost feel as if I know her personally ... [after sharing about his own cancer experience] cancer changes one's entire perspective on life and living. I strongly feel a bond or kinship with people I don't even know who suffer from the pernicious cancer disease. (April 23, 1999, p. 14A)

Notably, individuals who opted to write messages to Hainer reflected on the intersections between Hainer's journey and their own experiences. Michelle Murphy (April 30, 1999) recounted that "reading Cathy's articles, I saw many parallels between the two women [Hainer and Murphy's mother-in-law] and what they were feeling. Cathy helped me understand a little better just how the cancer patient feels" (p. 12A). Sharon Collins (October 8, 1998) linked Hainer's illness with her mother's battle with breast cancer, claiming that "my mom's death and Cathy's illness have made me very committed to doing everything I can to support the fight for a cure" (p. 18A). Russell Shaw shared:

A little more than 11 years ago, I lost a very special woman in my life to uterine cancer ... My friend, Anicia, worked with words too. She also shared Cathy's heritage. Cathy had spoken so eloquently and beautifully—not only for those who have or have had cancer, but also as a teacher for those who love someone with cancer ... There are many who have learned from Cathy's words. The world is a better place because she lived and wrote. Because her words live on, she will, too. (December 17, 1999, p. 30A)

Through their mediated interactions with each other and, indeed, with readers who did not opt to submit letters to the editor, Hainer and her confidants collaboratively and reflexively co-authored to their respective health narratives. At the same time, they co-constructed an active, fluid, public text about the lived reality of cancer—"our story." On November 8, 1999, Michael Wilson stressed:

But what I want Hainer to realize is that she has given me and other readers insight into the life process of death ... Hainer, in her writings, has
portrayed herself very much as an Everyman. For all of our sakes, I wish
it were so. Nevertheless, I will try to keep the lessons she has taught me
with me until I die. (p. 26A)

## Legitimacy of Narrative in Public Dialogues about Health

As her illness started to take its toll on her body, Hainer pondered what
might remain after her body ceased to function.

I especially read that [an obituary] where the person has died young or
died from cancer. And I can't help imagining what my own obituary will
say: "Cathy Hainer graduated from college and went to work for a newspaper." Will I be disappointed that it doesn't describe me as "Pulitzer
Prize winner and author of best-selling novels"? A little. But I hope I'm
more concerned with my legacy than my obituary. Will people remember
me fondly? Have I brought a smile to anyone's face, helped anyone out of
a difficult time? Have I made someone laugh when they were down, done
anything for the common good of mankind? (July 19, 1999, p. 7D)

Hainer's awareness of the embodied nature of her experience, the
complexity and temporality of her experience, and the intimately relational nature of her experience enhanced the uniqueness and social
value of her last work as a journalist. According to her readers,
Hainer's health narrative sparked insights, validated perspectives,
and facilitated meaning-making of situations that defy easy understanding or reconciliation. Antoinette Cleveland observed:

I've followed Hainer's journey through this devastating disease since the
beginning. She is, without a doubt, one of the bravest and most honest individuals I've ever had the pleasure of knowing through her extraordinary writing ... Most of us know someone—a relative, a friend, a
neighbor—who has suffered from terminal cancer. I doubt if many of us
know someone like Hainer who has the courage not only to face the disease but also to share her most intimate thoughts and feelings about its
affect on her life—everything from whether to buy a house, get married,
renew her driver's license or any other of the daily decisions we make
without staring our mortality in the face. She is awesome. (December 9,
1999, p. 18A)

In the spirit of Fisher (1984, 1985, 1987, 1989), I argue that the public conversation prompted by Hainer's articles constitutes an exemplary
example of narrative as an integral component of human understanding
and, ultimately, public decision-making. In his description of the narra-

tive paradigm, Fisher (1985a) maintained "... a significant feature of compelling stories is that they provide a rationale for decision and action. As such, they not only constrain behavior, they may also determine it" (p. 364).

Although public sphere scholars continue to debate the value of personal experiences from the private domain (see, e.g., Barnett, 2003; Calhoun, 1999; W. Clark, 2000; Deem, 2002; DeLuca & Peeples, 2002; Habermas, 1987; Sitton, 2003; Warner, 2002; Wittenberg, 2002), I contend that Hainer's work offers a concrete illustration of text as a postmodern conversation in a public forum. By implicitly inviting her readers to become confidants in her emergent health narrative, Hainer exemplified the relational nature of narratives, drawing them into the community of individuals who live with (and die from) cancer. Through such a positioning of narrative as relational (i.e, it impacts "us," not just "me"), the call for concern (about others and self) gets underscored. As Mike Sturgeon (December 17, 1999) asserted, "She had remarkable courage to share her ordeal with the world, and one can only hope that perhaps maybe another life was saved through early cancer detection" (p. 30A).

## CONCLUSION

Through the exploration of Cathy Hainer's published articles about her journey with breast cancer, I began with the notion that bodies constitute active, dynamic, social texts. Because illness and injury gets located in the physical body, I argued that health narratives are necessarily embodied rhetoric—powerful, persuasive, deeply personal yet inherently social.

As actors in the social world, health care participants necessarily engage with others, to varying degrees, as they experience illness or injury. Even to the extent that individuals attempt to mask symptoms or conditions from others, they do so in the relational context of what others might think or how they want to construct individual or relational identities in light of such others.

In Hainer's case, her wig marked a special symbol for herself and also for her colleagues. When Craig Wilson wrote about that final visit to Cathy Hainer, he observed that "the hope-filled days of the perky black wig were long over" (December 16, 1999, p. 1D). Hainer bemoaned "having" to wear the wig. Yet, it marked an effort to resemble "normal"—just a temporary phase between instances of her real hair. She chose not to wear it anymore when hope of restoring "normal" (in terms of her self presentation and her emergent relational identities) faded. Although an individual decision, the absence of the wig quietly communicated volumes to her loved ones about Cathy's current psychological and physical condition, thus contributing reflexively to emergent relational and interactional framing. As Hainer's writings illustrate, health narratives emerge as temporally bound, implicitly relational (not individual) constructions.

Hainer's choice to share her story with an international readership enabled her to engage thousands of others in a discourse about their respective journeys. By blurring the boundaries between personal health experience and public conversation, Hainer invited readers to join her journey as she "spoke" to them in the context of their own. In so doing, her articles constitute a compelling example of a postmodern public dialogue about health, wellness, illness, and dying.

This analysis and theoretical reflections advance our narrative understanding of health experiences in three key ways. First, extending from Atkinson's (1997) critique of published health narratives, this study illustrates not only that narratives can be more than individual; it provides evidence about the ways in which they are implicitly relational, social constructions. By treating narratives as relational, we move forward in understanding how family members, health care providers, social support system members, and in this case, newspaper readers, participate in the co-telling (and the co-experiencing) of health narratives.

Second, this examination of an emergent health narrative offers insight into narratives as temporal, emergent co-constructions. Hainer and her readers' reflections on the spirals and cycles of understandings throughout their respective and shared health experiences supports assertions by Ricoeur and others about the nature of time. As Hainer's articles exemplify, Western conceptions of time and the biomedical model project a linear framework—diagnosis, treatment plan, health outcome—that clashes with lived realities. Yet, as Hainer's articles indicate, the "interruption" of a life due to illness, the "one step forward, ten steps back" frustration of struggling through treatments, resembles a maze more than a straight line (see related arguments by Beck, 2001)—contributing to confusion and recurrent reshapings of the emergent health narrative.

Third, this examination of the public conversation that stemmed from Hainer's articles highlights postmodern blurring of boundaries between public and private spheres. As such, this analysis indicates the dialogic potential of narratives in public forums. In response to Hainer's articles, readers offered support by sharing their own stories and perspectives. Moreover, they participated in the ongoing co-construction of meanings about breast cancer, illness, and even the process of dying. I encourage future researchers to pursue the implications of these published conversations for those who contribute overtly and for those who lurk—participating through reading and reflecting on public interactions about otherwise private health issues.

## NOTES

1. The author would like to thank Lynn Harter and Phyllis Japp for their most insightful suggestions on a previous draft of this chapter.
2. The primary data for this investigation emerged from Hainer's articles, published in *USA Today* (as well as in a tribute book, *The Cathy Hainer Journals: A Story of Courage*). In all, 13 installments of her journal were published. The original publication dates include: March 10, 1998; March 26, 1998; April 15, 1998; May 13, 1998; May 26, 1998; June 22, 1998; October 1, 1998; January 11, 1999; April 20, 1999; July 19, 1999; September 27, 1999; November 4, 1999; December 6, 1999. Additional data stemmed from three *USA Today* articles in tribute to Hainer after her death. All three were published on December 16, 1999. A search of the *USA Today* Web site revealed 29 letters to the editor; however, the publication indicates that "thousands" of letters were received. Consistent with the newspaper's policy, a select few were published. Due to confidentiality, my request to obtain the unpublished letters was denied.

# 4

## Time, Technology, and Meritocracy: The Disciplining of Women's Bodies in Narrative Constructions of Age-Related Infertility

∞

**Lynn M. Harter**
*Ohio University*

**Erika L. Kirby**
*Creighton University*

**Autumn Edwards**
*Ohio University*

**Andrea McClanahan**
*East Stroudsburg University of Pennsylvania*

The public preoccupation with age-related infertility (ARI) focuses sharp attention on the salience of reproductive control and shifting boundaries between public and private. Since the 2001 "Protect your Fertility" campaign sponsored by the American Society for Reproductive Medicine (ASRM) and the publication of Sylvia Hewlett's (2002) *Creating a Life: Professional Women and the Quest for Children*, procreation once again resounds as the subject of talk shows, autobiographical accounts, and the evening news. Widespread interest with ARI was generated in April of 2002 when the cover of *Time* magazine posed a naked baby on a piled-high inbox and asked "Babies vs. Careers—Which Should Come First for Women Who Want Both?" The accompanying article (Gibbs, 2002) chronicled Hewlett's "creeping

83

nonchoice" narrative—women who focus on their careers and wait until it is too late to conceive often experience the despair of ARI.

Infertility, however, is not a recent phenomenon; it existed long before the gendered separation of public and private spheres and advent of assisted reproductive technologies (see May, 1995 for an historical overview). Moreover, infertility does not plague primarily career-oriented women who delay childbearing. Consumers of the popular media might be surprised to know that the highest rate of infertility has been among poor Blacks, not prosperous Whites, throughout the 20th century (Centers for Disease Control and Prevention, 1997; United States Census Bureau, 2001). Furthermore, far from witnessing an "infertility epidemic" in our culture, the overall incidence of diagnosed infertility in the United States has decreased since the mid-1960s. The renewed sense of urgency about ARI can be located in the convergence of several factors: (a) the medicalization of infertility and growth of reproductive endocrinology consumed primarily by affluent women, (b) evolution of a social milieu conducive to public discussion about reproductive issues, (c) women and men's ability to "control" (and delay) reproduction, and (d) the increasing foray of women into the public realms of work, politics, and higher education. Embedded in these discourses is a renewed concern about women's autonomy, with ARI often positioned as the bedfellow of reproductive freedom—the price women pay for prioritizing careers, consumerism, and sexual pleasure.

Despite complex social changes that have altered gender roles, biological reproduction remains central to women's identities in pronatalist societies such as the United States (see Becker, 1994, Becker & Nachtigall, 1994, and Britt, 2001, for discussions of pronatalism as a powerful gender narrative that assumes women are naturally fit for parenthood and should bear children).Yet, we argue against locating the compelling character of ARI exclusively in pronatalist or patriarchal agendas. Middle-class Americans' faith in hard work, justice, consumerism and medicine illuminate the class-related and time- bound nature of the discourses. The media coverage given to new or improved biomedical techniques that provide hope of biological children for those of financial means contributes to the renewed interest in infertility. From surgical interventions that eradicate dysfunctions impeding conception to drug therapies stimulating or controlling the timing of reproductive events, contemporary couples are situated in a time and place characterized by ever-evolving technologies to cure or circumvent infertility.

We position the discourses of ARI as an occasion to explore narrative as a rhetorical resource in the social construction of healing and health. The story of ARI offers a unique opportunity to foreground shifting intersections between the most private aspects of our lives (i.e., relations with partners and kin, sexuality, and procreation) and the public domain around us. The discourses are easily narrativized, with aesthetically compelling life stories of White, middle-class, heterosexual couples. By putting a personal face on a now medicalized issue, the narratives invite audiences to share in the private lives and problems of "likable characters" (Condit, 1994). Throughout this chapter, we argue that the discourses of ARI privilege certain narratives of women's identities/bodies as society disciplines them through discourses about time, technology and middle-class values. We include ourselves as figures in narrative constructions of ARI, as audience for its performance, drawing on contemporary concepts of *gender, class, narrative* and *critical theory*. We do not present a "universal" or "fixed" meaning in these discourses. Meanings take shape—for different critics in different ways and to different degrees—in the symbolic space between reader, text, and context. We present one reading of the discourses, and in so doing invite you to enter, as witness and co-constructor of meaning, the public dialogues about ARI.

## NARRATIVE THEORIZING

Increasingly, scholars draw attention to the storied nature of our lives. We adopt an interpretive–critical perspective toward understanding narratives as constellations of relationships embedded in time and space and constituted by causal emplotment (see also Mumby, 1987). Indeed, a chief characteristic of narrative is its ability to render understanding by connecting (however unstably) parts to a constructed configuration or a social network of relationships composed of symbolic, institutional, and material practices. We focus attention on the ideological nature of health and healing, assuming that healthcare activities perpetuate hierarchies, structure identities, and construct identifications or divisions among those that practice the rituals and consume the related commodities. Yet, as argued by Boje (2001), narratives are not always the self-contained and structured linguistic events (i.e., beginning, climax, end) conveyed in most scholarly writing. Rather, stories constitute dynamic, interruptable, fragments frequently challenged and changed to meet institutional and individual needs.

Narrative theorizing provides a particularly fruitful framework from which to address the discursive understandings through which subjectivities are constructed (Somers, 1994). In today's world of proliferating sites and scenes of identity work, the self comprises an increasingly institutional project "disciplined" by diverse social circumstances and practices (Gergen, 1991). These settings, as Lyotard (1984) informed us, present the self with "a fabric of relations that is now more complex and mobile than ever before" (p. 15). If we set aside the notion of an integrated self, the multiple self-constructions that emerge in various settings become the identity-bearing subjectivities that serve complex social environments. We agree with Holstein and Gubrium (2000) who argued that Lyotard's (1984) obituary for master narratives and the paramount self does not obviate an empirical self so much as it redeploys it into varied contexts of everyday life.

Self-construction is not merely extemporaneous. It is profoundly conditioned by its circumstances and available resources. Goffman (1959) foreshadowed this by highlighting the situatedness of self-presentation. People construct identities by locating themselves or being located within a repertoire of emplotted stories. "Human conduct must to a significant extent," suggests Maines (2001), "be talked into existence through the strategic deployment of master symbols such as ideographs and through taken-for-granted ordinary symbols such as those contained in myth and local tradition" (p. 174). People act according to how they understand their place in any number of given narratives, however fragmented or contingent. Focusing attention on narrative as an ontological condition of social life affords the opportunity to explore how stories of the self are continually mediated by the increasingly institutionalized circumstances of contemporary life (Somers, 1994). Individuals orient their life worlds by way of diverse stocks of knowledge that are social in origin. Paralleling what Wittgenstein (1953) and Burke (1969) taught us about language, stocks of knowledge are part and parcel of everyday life, not separate and distinct from it.

Foucault (1975) illustrated how discourses of particular sites establish conceptual limits for storytelling; yet, narrative scholars rarely explore how stories are imbued with political, social, and aesthetic undertones (Atkinson, 1997; Clair, 2001). Tellers economically produce narratives for consumption, although the degree to which the audience buys the stories varies. Politically, narrative choice, structure, plot, and audience fluctuate, depending on aspects of privilege. The narrator and audience are aesthetically consumed by the emotional and artistic elements of the story. In sum, theorizing can be advanced by exploring how narratives, as one mode of symbolic structuring, are material instantiations of ideology (Clair, 2001; Mumby, 1987). We approach narratives as ideological forces that articulate meanings privileging some interests over others. Although narratives can function to legitimate meaning systems of dominant groups, narratives can also function as counterstories that resist oppression (Lindemann-Nelson, 1996, 1997, 2001). From this perspective, power is more than a phenomenon imposed on subordinate groups; power involves a dialectic of control (Giddens, 1979, 1984). As such, we take particular interest in how a narrative, or cluster of narratives, functions to enable and/or constrain behavior within the context of certain ideological meaning formations.

Our analysis explores ARI from the perspective of cultural drama, drawing on narrative to emphasize how lived experiences emerge through the complex interactions of agents who occupy different social positions, with differential access to power and space in the public sphere to articulate their story. Narrative enables individuals to recreate a sense of continuity and reconnect to the social and cultural order after the disruption of ARI. At the same time, narrative functions as an agent of social control and change.

Adopting a critical-interpretive lens, we explore how the discourses of ARI (see Appendix for sources of discourse)[1] support and sustain various structures of power and privilege, reflecting the imprint of institutionalized practices and ideology. We approach discourse from an explicitly broad vantage point, casting a wide net that incorporates research, social commentary, and personal experiences that surround a particular issue over time and across genres of communication. As Lupton (1994) explained:

> Discourse, in this usage, can be described as a pattern of words, figures of speech, concepts, values, and symbols. A discourse is a coherent way of describing and categorizing the social and physical worlds. Discourses gather around an object, person, social group or event of interest, providing a means of "making sense" of that object, person ... all discourses are textual, or expressed in texts, inter-textual, drawing upon other texts and their discourses to achieve meaning, and contextual, embedded in historical, political and cultural settings. (p. 20)

We move between *stories* of ARI, as experienced by women and shared in public dialogues and popular culture, and the dominant *narrative script* of ARI—the master narrative which is both medium and outcome of personal narratives. We argue that the discourses of ARI constitute narratives of women's identities/bodies, which discipline women through rhetoric about time, technology and middle-class values. We draw particular attention to (a) how the texts of ARI serve as points of struggle or tension over meaning, and (b) how the discourses both enable and constrain the human spirit, health communication, and health care decision-making.

## DIALECTICS OF CONTROL IN THE DISCOURSES OF ARI

In his writings, Giddens' (1979, 1984) vision of reciprocity of power within social systems is manifest in his concept of the *dialectic of con-*

*trol.* Giddens (1984) defined the dialectic of control as "the two-way character of the distributive aspect of power (power as control); how the less powerful manage resources in such a way as to exert control over the more powerful in established power relationships" (p. 374). Although social structures represent hegemonic interests of dominant groups, people in subordinated positions can and do strategically use resources to influence those in dominant positions and reach individual goals. Through dialectics of control, individuals engage in interplays of dialogue representative of shifting balances of power.

Mumby (1987) argued dialectics of control are present in narratives as well. According to Mumby, "All discourse, while often functioning as … a constraint on thought and action can also function simultaneously as a means of enablement" (p. 124). For example, the metaphor of the "birth-control generation" in the discourse of ARI illustrates how ritualized practices both enable and constrain. As members of the first birth-control generation, many Americans of childbearing age understand fertility as something that can be controlled. As argued by Condit (1994), the pill made the social demand for control appear as a biological and physical possibility. Yet, individuals do not solely exercise reproductive control. A host of biological (e.g., low-sperm counts), material (e.g., insurance coverage) and discursive forces (e.g., pronatalism) also impact the likelihood of reproduction.

Pamela Madsen, executive director of the American Infertility Association, captures these tensions, explaining: "It's great that we have birth control and that women have a choice. But we've … fed women this myth that they are in complete control of their reproductive lives" (Kalb, Springen, Scelfo, & Pierce, 2001, p. 40). Hewlett herself exclaims, "we've gone from fearing our fertility to squandering it—and very unwittingly" (Gibbs, 2002, p. 54). Hewlett (2001) and the ASRM justify their health campaigns because women harbor wildly unrealistic expectations of their bodies, reproductive control, and modern medicine. Subsequently, doctors and experts[2] frame the distribution of information about ARI as a means of empowering women. They are simply giving women information about the "fragility of fertility" so that women can then make their own choices about whether and when to have children. An exemplar of this discourse comes from Dr. David Adamson who notes, "It's important for women to be empowered with accurate information. We're all trying to get the facts out. The reality is reproductive capability does go down with age, and it's important for women to understand that so they can make intelligent decisions" (Hall, 2002, p. A1). Dr. Allison Rosen agrees, contending that, "This is not a case of male doctors' wanting to keep women barefoot and pregnant. You lay out the facts, and any particular individual woman can then make her choice" (Gibbs, 2002, p. 53).

Yet, a few commentators present a counterinterpretation by arguing the dominant discourses of ARI constrain rather than enable. At least one expert highlights how statistics continue to be selectively presented. David Dunson, a biostatistician explains "Although we noted a decline in female fertility in the late 20s, what we found was a decrease in the probability of becoming pregnant per menstrual cycle, not in the probability of eventually achieving a pregnancy" (Hall, 2002, p. A1). Echoing this concern, Hjul (2002) stated:

> Buried in the fertility report is the fact that the older women were not less able to conceive—it just took them longer. But that detracts from a good, alarmist story, which implies that all ambitious, successful females must be aching inside, clutching their barren bellies and regretting the day they chose boardroom over labor rooms. (p. 14)

Critics claim the dominant discourses simplify and exaggerate complex scientific findings, and, using visual images of women nursing briefcases instead of babies (Gibbs, 2002), trigger emotional responses to the discursively constructed "infertility epidemic" (p. 49). Kim Gandy, president of NOW (National Organization of Women), suggests that "the age issue is wildly overblown. The implication is 'I have to hurry up and have kids now or give up on ever having them' " (Gibbs, 2002, p. 53). Indeed, the implication has hit a nerve with many women. Cottle (2002) editorialized "I gotta admit, all this focus on aging ova has, among me and my kid-free girlfriends of various ages, provoked emotional reactions ranging from defensiveness 'Why are they always trying to keep us barefoot and pregnant?' to flat-out panic 'Oh God, what if it's already too late!' " (p. E-1).

Overall, then, discursive representations of the causes and consequences of ARI are both enabling and constraining. We further examine dialectics of control in narratives of time, technology, and middle-class values.

## Time as Enabling and Constraining

The discourses of ARI can be read as a narrative of women's bodies as they are disciplined through discourses about time. Especially in our professional lives, where time is money, we are encouraged to control time. Yet, time is often discursively positioned and materially experienced as an aspect of life that eludes our attempts at control, and, in fact, one that exerts control over us. Modernity's conception of time as a hegemonic structure whose essences include precision, control and discipline is epitomized in the key machine of the industrial age—the clock (Hassard, 1996). The clock has emerged not only as a disciplining force and key metaphor of public working life, but of women's bodies as well.

In explaining the vernacular of the "biological clock" that received widespread attention during the 1980s, Faludi (1991) revisited the 1982 *New England Journal of Medicine* article that first reported that women's chances of conceiving suddenly dropped after age 30. As she explained, the journal also contained a "paternalistic three-page editorial, exhorting women to 'reevaluate their goals' and have their babies before they started careers" (p. 27). *The New York Times* and other newspapers, magazines and television news programs also picked up on the story, and "by the following year, the statistic had found its way into alarmist books about the 'biological clock' " (p. 27). Indeed, references to the biological clock are now firmly reified as material actuality and permeate the contemporary discourse of ARI.

The metaphor of the biological clock serves to reconfigure women's relationship with time by highlighting the constraints of time and timing on women's reproductive successes and failures. Shortly after the publication of a study claiming that women's fertility rates begin to dip after age 27 (Dunson, Columbo & Baird, 2002), article titles like, "Study Speeds of Biological Clocks; Fertility Rates Dip After Women Hit 27" (Hall, 2002), and "Women's Fertility in Decline by Late 20s: Biological Clock Starts Earlier" (Boseley, 2002) appeared in numerous newspapers around the country. Much public dialogue centered on questions of whether the biological clock can be "reset," how fast the clock is "ticking," if biological clocks have "snooze buttons," and whether or not women are as aware as they should be of the incessant "ticking." Throughout the discourse, the biological clock is positioned as a fact of medical science, a predetermined given whose workings can be sped up, but never slowed down. "You can do things to shorten that clock, like with cigarette smoking," explained Dr. Cedars on a 2002 *Oprah* episode, "but there isn't yet anything we can do to extend the clock" (p. 7).

Women speaking publicly about their own reproductive experiences and choices often include references to the biological clock. Childress explains, "if I'm going to do it, I feel like the 'right time' to start is now. My biological clock is starting to come into effect" (Yarbrough, 2002, p. 60). Fertility doctors, too, rely on clock images, most notably in their very public attempts "to warn women that science can't always beat the biological clock" (Kalb et al., 2001, p. 40). For example, the metaphor has been visually instantiated in a controversial ad published by the ASRM (the American Society for Reproductive Medicine), which depicts milk dripping from an upside–down hourglass shaped baby bottle. Kim Gandy asserts "What it says visually is time is running out" (*60*

*Minutes* Transcript, 2002). Indeed, a number of critics argue that the focus on the biological clock may be unnecessarily alarming (if not oppressive) to many young women.

Prominent voices in ARI discourses maintain that the focus on women's biological clocks is justified and empowering. Pamela Madsen (2002) explained "Until women have the education about their true biological clock, we won't have reproductive choice. It's no more a pressure to offer women education about having babies as it is to offer women education about birth control" (*Oprah* Transcript, 2002, p. 4). Notably, though, "educators" primarily deploy the clock metaphor to describe the female body. The discourses of ARI highlight few (if any) medical science findings or narratives describing men as having biological clocks. Concomitantly, the texts portray ARI chiefly as a problem endemic to women. Although about 20% of infertility can be attributed to exclusively male factors, and more than one third of infertility cases can be attributed to both partners (Ehrenfeld, 2002), our discursive practices socially construct infertility as primarily a female condition.

The metaphor of the biological clock intersects with the master narrative of age as decline to discipline women's bodies. Such narrativizing encourages women to experience and express aging in terms of loss, isolation, and diminished material resources (Trethewey, 2001). This emplotment suggests that our peak experience is lived in youth and as we enter middle age, we begin the inevitable descent into "declineoldageanddeath" (Gullete, 1997, p. 8). Within ARI discourses, commentators frequently describe women's eggs in terms of their age, young and vital or old and decrepit. They couch such explanations in terms of medical science. "Biology," according to Kalb et al. (2001) "has always made fertility a delicate proposition. A woman is born with a finite number of eggs, which gradually get ovulated or die off as she ages. And older eggs, which are less energetic than younger ones, have a harder time making it through the fertilization process" (p. 40). Pamela Madsen has gone so far as to say that "women's eggs are like milk; they have a freshness date" (Liddane, 2002, p. L6). Similar notions are woven into the fabric of narratives told by everyday actors. Eisenhardt encounters other youthful women in their 40s, contemplates the unseen, and notes "I'm like, 'Your eggs are about to need a walker. Your eggs are going to need a respirator soon' " (Fergus, 2002, p. 1).

As Emily Martin (2001) argued, it is common for women's reproductive systems to be described and theorized primarily in their capacity to yield a product and seldom in their capacity to regulate other functions or as part of an ongoing cycle of maintenance whose goodness can be judged by its own continuity. For those experiencing ARI, age gets fingered as the primary culprit in the failed production of women's bodies. The discourses encourage women to experience and narrativize the inability to have desired biological children as yet another instantiation of the inevitable decline associated with aging. Because it positions women as individually responsible for managing the aging process, the accusation of a "failure" to act in time can be a painful reminder of aging and negatively impact their embodied identities. As Renee Borfreund shares, "I didn't want to admit my body had failed me and I had waited too long," (Fergus, 2002, p. 1).

Kim Gandy cautions that "the idea that you can choose what age you'll be to have your children is a ludicrous proposition for most women" (Kalb et al., 2001, p. 40). Yet, dominant discourses highlight time (and timing of personal and professional decisions) as something to be considered and controlled with regard to major life choices. In modern industrial societies, users of time are obliged to display good stewardship because time is a scarce commodity and must be used rationally (Hassard, 1996). Likewise, in ARI discourses, doctors, public health officials, and individual men and women promote (and resist) the notion that women must discipline their lives by implementing more effective time management. Thus, these discourses commonly encourage women to have children early, and to "catch up" professionally by reinventing themselves in careers later down the road. Hewlett (2002b) recommends that women start at age 45 and work backwards to determine when they should begin pursuit of each major life goal (especially childbirth). Indeed, many ARI texts center on the question "When is the 'right time' to have a baby?" They position age and the biological clock as key factors governing family planning decisions. Susan Dear Uhley suggested "The biological clock should play a role in the decision not only when to start a family but also when to complete ... Regardless of whether the baby you are dreaming of will be your first, second, or even third, keep your eye on the biological clock" (Mail Call, 2002, p. 14). Yet, in the same response in *Newsweek*'s Mail Call (2002), we are reminded that "in our carefully scheduled lives, some things do not happen according to day planners and palm pilots" (p. 14).

Like Frank (1995), we believe that the women who have courageously shared their personal stories in the public sphere do so, in large part, by adapting and combining narrative types that our culture makes available. Although these stories weave unique threads, the discourses collectively play out our cultural conflicts with time. However, ideologies of time coalesce with consumer reliance on modern medicine as a savior (i.e., technology can buy back "time") to enable and/or constrain those experiencing ARI in networks of relationships.

## Technology as Enabling and Constraining

As reproductive endocrinology progresses from drug therapy to freezing of eggs for future use, public hope and fear of technology comingle. The stories of ARI represent at once both disillusionment and faith in the restitution narrative. Frank (1995) argued that the restitution narrative (i.e., the journey from sickness to health, usually with help of institutionalized medicine) is the preferred narrative of Western medicine and continues to characterize most personal stories of illness and healing (see also Kleinmann, 1988; Morris, 1998). In the restitution narrative, technical expertise overtakes lay experience, including complex organizations of treatment. Although illness certainly becomes a circulation of stories (e.g., patient, family members, physician), not all stories are equal. The story that trumps all others is one of technology (Frank, 1995; Harter & Japp, 2001; Morris, 1998). In modern institutions of medicine, technology embraces more than mechanical tools of the trade. Rather, technology is epistemological—a way of thinking, talking, and acting that incorporates instruction, hierarchies, practices, and patterns as well as instruments developed within that paradigm (Harter & Japp, 2001).

At first glance, the personal stories of infertile women, doctors, and commentators woven throughout ARI discourses reflect distrust and disillusionment with the restitution "myth"—the grand narrative of progress told by Western culture about its journey through time. During a *60 Minutes* interview with Leslie Stahl, Melanie Curtright shared, "I just assumed that science would keep up with—keep up that pace, and that it wouldn't be a problem at 40. It never occurred to me that I wouldn't be able to have a child." Another 40-something woman, Nancy, shared with Oprah and millions of viewers (2002), "I was angry with my body for letting me down. I was angry with the doctors for not being able to help me" (p. 3) while Karen shared, "I always assumed that with the technology that they've advertised and promised us, that I would be able to have children now with no problem or even into my 40s" (p. 5). Dr. Sarah Berga suggested, "Even among fertility specialists, it was shocking to us that IVF didn't work so well after age 42 ... the early 90s, to my mind, was all about how shocked we were that we couldn't get past this barrier" (Gibbs, 2002, p. 51).

Hewlett (2002b) offered a sharp critique of the empty promise of high-tech reproduction and argued that young women are lulled into a false sense of security that assisted reproductive technologies (ART) will come to the rescue. Similarly, Pamela Madsen alleged, "We've fed women this fairy tale, they could have it all whenever they want ... these women could have had the children that they wanted if someone had told them the reality. Instead, these women had been blindsided by nature" (*Oprah* Transcript, 2002, p. 2). The devastating potential of a false sense of security about what science can accomplish is hauntingly evident in the discourses. Wendy Wasserman shared, "I've gone through so many—and been injected with so many drugs—I can't even keep track of them all. What did I get out of all this? All I've proved is that I can't get pregnant, that I'm really not a girl" (Hewlett, 2002b, p. 39). Stella also shared with Hewlett, "We took out a second mortgage on our house and signed up for IVF [in-vitro fertilization]. Twelve months and three cycles later I got pregnant again, only to miscarry in week five.... I needed to build some kind of wall between me and my co-lossal, cumulative grief" (p. 49).

Yet, technology inspires both fear and faith; it is both destroyer and savior of human life. The discourses of ARI comprise a microcosm of a broader cultural complex of acceptance and rejection of technology. Although disappointment with science is evident in women's narratives, at the same time they express hope that a scientific cure for ARI lies just around the corner. Yarbough (2002) suggested "Women didn't have the choices that we have now. Reproductive health and the technology that has come with it has given us a lot more opportunities to plan" (p. 60), whereas Kalb et al., (2001) reported "Scientists say they hope to figure out a way to determine each woman's reproductive age: she could take a test at 23 to predict how fertile she'll be at 40. Or science will unravel the mysterious molecular process that makes eggs age, then slow down the process" (p. 40). A team of doctors at Cornell University's Weill Medical college, *Newsweek* reports, are working on a "sci-fi" solution to aging eggs:

> Already, researchers have experimented with a procedure called "nuclear transfer," in which they suck the nucleus (which contains a person's DNA) out of an older woman's egg, then transfer it into the cytoplasm (which houses the cell's energy source) of a younger egg. VOILA! A 45-year-old woman, the theory goes, can have her own genetic child with the boost of a 25-year-old's eggs. (Kalb et al., 2001, p. 40)

Most news reports about ARI contain evidence of ever-evolving scientific advances that hold out the promise of hope for women experiencing ARI.

The restitution narrative is a modernist narrative of social control, and is encapsulated in the metaphor of the body as machine and the ongoing "war" saga between nature and science. As indicated earlier, Martin (2001) critiques the ways in which biological sciences depict woman's body as a factory whose primary purpose is to reproduce the species. Subsequently, science positions processes of menstruation and menopause, and in this case infertility, as forms of breakdown or failure. The role of science, drawing on the language of warfare, is to "attack" the enemy of nature:

> There's more going on in the lab, where scientists have been looking for new ways to *attack* the most frustrating problem in infertility today: the older women's eggs. Freezing eggs on college graduation day might seem like an ideal solution ... now researchers are experimenting with a variation on the theme: freezing slices of ovarian tissue, which contain thousands of eggs in an immature state. (Kalb et al., 2001, p. 40)

In the military drama, nature serves as the enemy, a threat to the victory of technology. "The top enemies can be described in two words," says one doctor in relation to male ARI: "heat and blockage" (Ehrenfeld, 2002, p. 60). The narrative consists of the struggle between technology and nature, as technology seeks to overcome nature and "win."

The restitution narrative is seductive. For middle and upper class Americans experiencing ARI, modern medicine offers a way to regain control. Comfortable with scientific solutions and medical authority, many Americans look to medicine for interpreting problems and enacting solutions. Ill individuals' own desires for restitution are compounded by the expectation that other people want to hear restitution stories. Yet, as with cancer and AIDS treatments chronicled by Sontag (1977, 1988), the military metaphors that undergird the discourses of ARI can contribute to the stigmatizing of those who are infertile. To use Erving Goffman's (1959) term, the experience of ARI is one of *spoiled identity*—identities that, for women, continue to be fused with biological reproduction. Thus, technologies both enable and constrain. Medical treatment provides routines and rituals that supply comfort and control in the face of chaos; yet, individuals may encounter a loss of control as regimens externally discipline micropractices of the body (e.g., ovulation monitoring, daily injections of hormones and blood testing, sexual encounters) and normalize women's notions of self. The loss of control is no longer just about the inability to control reproduction, technologies can constrain people's time, relationships, and bodies.

## Moral Imagination of the Middle Class

An unmistakable element of the discourse that reproduces (and resists) the restitution myth (i.e., technology will defeat the elusive temporal element of nature) is class; in fact, the compelling character of the discourse rests on its ability to draw on and reinforce the veneer of the middle-class work ethic. Through this perspective, women can control their choices and destinies, and children (read: biological/"natural" children) are part of the "American dream." This is due in large part to how the "face" of ARI has been portrayed—as the highly professional woman with regrets. Although Hewlett's (2002b) book has served as a catalyst for the renewed attention to ARI, she only selectively interviewed "high-achieving women"—those who are employed full-time or self-employed and earn an income that places them in the top 10% of their age group.[3] This rather homogeneous group of women narrativizes ARI; consequently, interwoven in stories of physicians, women, couples, and reporters are middle-class *meritocratic values* (where individual hard work is rewarded with individual merit and rewards) and faith in efforts, justice, technology and control.

Many women (and men?) now want to wait until the time is right to have children, and so numerous women spoke of ways they are trying to "protect" their fertility—to later receive the reward of a child. In their research on the (classist) discourses of popular success literature, Nadesan and Trethewey (2000) documented its suggestion "that the [White, middle-class, professional] body can be *successfully managed* by cultivating bodily regimes such as ... diet and exercise" (pp. 234–235). This mindset of "doing the right thing" to successfully manage the body—and thus deserving the merit of fertility—was echoed in ARI discourses. Suzanne was frustrated with her age-related infertility. During the *Oprah* (2002) episode, she shared, "I have always taken good care of myself. I've always had regular paps. I've never had an abortion. I exercise. I eat healthy" (p. 5), and Diana said:

> I've always been one to take care of myself. I love to exercise. It's—It's a hobby. I began taking prenatal vitamins before I even got married ... I can't tell you the loss that you feel and how you wonder where you go from here and that you thought you were taking 10 steps forward just to find out you have to start over again. (p. 6)

Britt (2001) argued that women's desire for biological children and their pursuit of pregnancy can be understood within the more overarching desire for "normalcy" (i.e., fertility) in American culture. In our pronatalist society, if women neglect their expected role of mother in their life paths, then they are, in many ways, stripped of one very important aspect of female identity. The identity of women as mother is overdetermined in our society, and as such, Giese (2002) charged that ARI discourses "implicitly suggest that an infertile life is not worth living" (p. A27). Hart (2003) served as an exemplar. She notes, "No matter what our feminist foremothers told us—'home and family be banned, pursue a career, that's what will make you happy'—no matter how much they tried to socially reengineer us, the truth remains that most women want children most of all" (p. A8).

Women compare themselves to others in the hopes that they are not "abnormal" in both their life choices and experiences with fertility. Intersecting with a desire for normalcy are narratives of success and failure. The narratives of success and failure, embedded in a tradition of individualism, encourage women to believe in the possibility of achieving success through hard work, determination and persistence. Especially for middle-class women, these cultural stories are pervasive and persuasive. Indeed, metaphors of success and failure saturate the personal narratives of women experiencing ARI. "Our generation takes it for granted," said Jodi Eisenhardt. "You think it's going to happen on a dime when you decide.... It's characteristic of women our age—we're used to getting what we want, we're assertive, and we take care of our business" (Fergus, 2002, p. 1). For those accustomed to success, the inability to have a child can represent the first major "failure" in their lives. Gala Verrangia, a mother who spoke about egg donation on the *Today* show, commented "I've always wanted kids, and when I found out I couldn't have them naturally, it was the hardest thing I ever had to—to accept. It was like someone struck me with lightning" (Couric, 2003).

The terms of any narrative are negotiated within dominant discourses. In the case of ARI, the rules and resources upon which narrators draw reproduce the moral imagination of the middle class where hard work should pay off. Subsequently, solutions to the problem of ARI reproduce values of productivity, efficiency, and control in that they are positioned as distinctly individualized, apolitical, and entrepreneurial (i.e., women are responsible for their own personal, professional and economic successes). Similar to broader societal discourses that position rejuvenation through consumption as the primary means of staving off eventual decline through aging, ARI stubbornly remains an individual problem for women that can be overcome through better strategic choices.

In the case of ARI, the only choices for women who want to pursue having a child cost money—and a lot of it. An article in the *Dayton Daily News* utilized the well-known MasterCard commercial to represent one couples' experience: "One round Clomid injections: $900. One round insemination injections: $1,600. One round-in vitro fertilization: $7,500. Holding your baby in your arms: Priceless" (Dempsey, 2002, p. E1). Thus, the "enterprising" way for women to confront this problem, if indeed they have "waited too long," comes with much financial hardship—money that women of lower socioeconomic class probably do not possess. We assert the consumerist framing of the issue is interrelated with the absence of male narratives in this public discussion. Because women are more likely than men to feel "abnormal" if and when they experience infertility in a pronatalist culture, they are more likely to seek health-related information and pursue medical treatment for ARI. Further, because there is at least potential success in these treatments to achieve biological or "natural" children, additional emplotments to the narrative—such as adoption or surrogacy—often linger unexamined.

In addition to notions of meritocracy, ARI discourses also reproduce a distinctly middle-class concept of (*White*) *privilege*. To begin, the discourses often criticize women for choosing to prioritize work first and family second. Middle-class White women can "choose" to work, yet women of lower socio-economic status have never usually had—and do not have—the option to choose whether to work for pay (Frankenberg, 1993; hooks 2000; J. Williams, 2000). Consequently, ARI discourses are not derogative of the "choices" of these women—in fact, popularized discourses omit them, as if they do not experience fertility issues.

Trethewey (2001) suspected women of color and women of lower socioeconomic status are even more vulnerable to decline and entrepreneurial discourses. We see this happening in ARI discourses; even though these discourses may induce guilt among middle-class White women, at least they have options—they (potentially) have the economic resources and support to choose to confront ARI. Poor minority women actually experience higher rates of infertility, but they are not the targets of these discourses—they are not typical beneficiaries of the meritocratic system, nor do they have insurance companies that pay for expensive treatments.

## CONCLUSION

"Whatever happened to Cinderalla?" is one [question] that is asked only when the taken-for-granted layers of culture are punctured and thus exposed. It is asked when gender narratives don't come true.

—Maines, 2001, p. 179

In examining the narrative construction of ARI, we sympathize with the women who cope with ARI and who provide a personal face and public voice for this now medicalized issue. Lynn and Erika were immediately drawn to these discourses because they were angry upon viewing the 2002 *Oprah* episode about ARI. On a daily basis, Lynn experiences "pressure from friends, family, and even colleagues, to have a second child because it is the right time." Erika finds the discourses very upsetting because "at 32, I have two children but probably want one more and my husband is not ready. What if it becomes too late?" Autumn is "particularly interested in the discourses of age-related infertility, in part, because of the relative youth (19) at which I entered parenthood.

Perhaps because of that aspect of my background, the issues of age and 'right timing' are particularly provocative (and personal)." Finally, when Andi encounters the narratives of ARI, she "as a never-married (still single) woman, closely approaching the doomed age of 27 when my fertility will plummet, I feel as though I am being attacked for making the 'wrong' decisions in my life thus far."

We witness, as women from diverse standpoints, the narratives of other women and co-construct meaning in the process. We recognize that our own personal reactions influence our interpretations—interpretations that we position as both partial and indeterminate (see Harter, Japp, & Beck, chap. 1, this volume). We identify with a woman's need to gain public recognition for her private anguish to validate her womanhood despite being childless (read: barren)—and perhaps prevent other women from "making the same mistake." Yet we are struck by the ways that "expert" voices in the discourses (i.e., physicians, ASRM representatives, AIA representatives) overshadow the voices of those experiencing ARI (age-related infertility). Concomitantly, the technical rationality of expert voices potentially shapes the ways in which women narrate their experiences—what women include (time, technology, career) and exclude (husband's influence, possibility for adoption) in their storytelling.

Personal narrative has always been the material of feminist theory and practice. Yet, we find the absence of particular narrators, characters, and emplotments in the ARI discourses to be problematic. Noticeably absent are the voices of men. ARI is cast as a problem predominately affecting women, with the discussion neglecting to recognize that men delay childbirth, experience infertility, and have vested interests and meaningful parts to play in the struggle to balance work and family. These messages serve both to illuminate and reinscribe the dominant cultural assumption that the choices of women bear the brunt of the responsibility for delayed parenthood.

We hope our analysis refocuses attention on the socially constructed nature of ARI. Giddens (1984) argued that structure may be said to bind time and space through the routine reproduction of social practices, "making it possible for discernibly similar social practices to exist across varying spans of time and space" (p. 17). The discourses of ARI illustrate the stubborn persistence of pronatalist ideologies, notions of meritocracy, and modernist faith in science and technology as historical features of Western culture. The rules and resources upon which narrators draw are embedded in wider reaches across time and space (i.e., institutionalized practices). Yet, we agree with Giddens that actors and structure exist simultaneously and are equally responsible for the production of social practices. In the public specter of ARI, we find glimpses of hope and human agency in the concept of *counter stories*.

Lindemann-Nelson (1996, 1997, 2001) described a counter story as aiming to resist and undermine a story of domination. "Its teller uses her standpoint as Other to feature certain details and moral ideas the dominant story ignores or underplays," argues Lindemann-Nelson (1996), "retelling the story in such a way as to invite interpretations and conclusions that are at odds with the ones the dominant story invites" (pp. 94–95). By deconstructing master narratives that create damaged identities and replacing them with alternative, less morally degrading narratives, counter stories function to reidentify persons. In the case of ARI, we need alternative stock plots that capture the systemic nature of how reproduction (and ARI) is enacted symbolically, biologically, materially and in networks of relationships.

Our discursive rules and resources should recognize how parenthood and its timing often rely on the existence and readiness of a suitable life partner, as well as material and biological imperatives. Interestingly, "emotional readiness" to parent often takes a backseat to physical readiness in ARI discourses. Time is used primarily to refer to factors such as the age of ovaries, but rarely invoked to point out the benefits of time in giving women and men perspective, life experience, and emotional stability toward successfully parenting a child. For this reason, Yarbrough (2002) attributes the modern delay of parenthood to the fact that "having a child at a time when you're just old enough to experience life isn't a decision that a lot of women want to make these days" (p. 60). She editorializes that far too much emphasis is placed on physical preparation to the neglect of reaching a proper mental state. We agree, and find encouragement in the few counter stories that position childbearing as a multifaceted decision usually involving multiple parties—including scenarios in which men are infertile (e.g., Mundy, 2002).

The standard linear thesis on time is regularly used to overstate the rationality of production practices and understate the qualitative construction of temporal meanings (Hassard, 1996). For this reason, the question of the "right time for a woman to have a baby" has a dual meaning. There is a medical–scientific answer to this question based on normative study data. But, there is a more difficult and less valued way of answering the question as well; one that places emphasis on experience and sense-making. In other words, an alternative way to conceptualize *time* (as in *right time*) requires careful scrutiny of the subjective life circumstances (including physical, financial, mental, and emotional) of each woman and man contemplating parenthood.

Finally, our discussion begs the question of the materiality of our linguistic practices and labeling choices. For example, the label *infertility* is only one of many possible labels that can be used to give meaning to the experiences and identities of those who cannot give birth to desired children. Britt (2001), for instance, distinguished between the labels *involuntary childlessness* and *infertility* as a means of problematizing infertility as part of a distinctively medicalized discursive account of experience. Because naming practices have the potential to both diminish and enrich our lives, they are deeply consequential. Although the medical label infertility affords us the possibilities of exploring technology, science, and entrepreneurialism in consuming, authoring, and embodying narratives to remedy our problems, we must remember that it is part of medicalized discourses. Subsequently, ARI "naturally" lends itself to the restitution narrative wherein technology comes to the rescue.

Yet, as we have argued, this restitution narrative can be constraining. One such constraint is that medicalized solutions rarely provide space in the narrative fabric of our lives for social answers to our pressing problems. Notably, there is little to no discussion of adoption in public discourses surrounding ARI. Though it is arguably an option exercised by many people who have experienced ARI, its absence from public narratives is a powerful reminder of the appeal and prominence of the restitution narrative and its emphasis on technology as cure. Although adoption does not "cure" the biomedical condition of ARI, it certainly eradicates "involuntary childlessness." Thus, the types of stories we tell heavily implicate and are implicated by the labels upon which we build our collective understanding and to which we assign meaning.

A different name for the central problematic in ARI narratives may well provide the material and space for the emergence of different plots, the forging of different identities, and the engineering of different endings. Those who reject a medicalized interpretation of their difficulties (infertility) and adopt in its place an alternative explanation (involuntary childlessness) may have radically different stories to tell. Not only would such stories differ from ARI narratives in their conception of the *role of technology*, but also the *role of time* in relation to parenthood.

We do not argue that our reading of ARI discourses is the only, or even best, reading of these texts. We present our arguments as tentative, and open to revision by others. Interpretations of stories can always be otherwise, or "unfinalizable" as argued by Bakhtin (1981). Critics operating from an alternative perspective or with a different focus may read the discourses quite differently. Future inquiry is needed to investigate how various audiences negotiate unique readings with the texts in the differentiated contexts in which they act in their everyday lives.

Any analysis is always left gazing at what remains in excess of the analyzable.

—(Frank, 1995, p. 138)

# NOTES

1.  We collected sources of data to analyze by performing a search for ARI in newspapers and magazines/journals archived in Lexis-Nexis Academic Universe. The search was limited to the years 2000–2003 to restrict the data to articles relevant to the public discussion regarding ARI involving Hewlett's work, the ASRM campaign, and the much-publicized recent medical studies focusing on ARI. Three articles including terms similar to ARI were excluded from analysis because the terms were not used in the spirit of the public discussion regarding ARI of interest for the current study (e.g., the words "age" and "fertility" appeared in an article documenting population statistics in another nation). In addition, the authors gathered sources of data form a variety of media outlets, including network television, organizational Web sites, and online news sources. The Appendix includes the references of all books, articles, and programs comprising the database of public voices of ARI analyzed in this study. When citing these sources within our analysis, we have included the name of narrator, author of published source, year, and page numbers when available.
2.  These referenced doctors and experts include Dr. Sandra Carson (reproductive endocrinologist at Baylor College of Medicine); Dr. Allison Rosen (New York City clinical psychologist); Dr. Ann Davis (reproductive endocrinologist); Dr. Connie Moreland, (obstetrician at Northwestern Memorial Hospital in Chicago); Michael Soules (American Society for Reproductive Medicine); Pamela Madsen (American Infertility Association); Dr. Robert Gunby (obstetrician at Baylor University Medical Center in Dallas); and Dr. David Adamson (director of Fertility Physicians of Northern California).
3.  Hewlett's (2002) research began as a celebration of achievements of the breakthrough generation (i.e., women who broke through the barriers and became powerful figures in fields previously dominated by men). Unexpectedly, Hewlett discovered many of those she labeled as *high-achieving women* were without children as a result of the "creeping nonchoice." In identifying high-achieving women, Hewlett focused on highly educated/ higher-earning women. Hewlett targeted the top 10% of women in corporate American (companies with more than 5,000 employees) measured in terms of earning power. High-achievers were defined as those women earning over $55,000 or $65,000 or who have a doctoral or professional degree in medicine, law, or dentistry.

## APPENDIX: SOURCES OF AGE-RELATED INFERTILITY DISCOURSE

American Society for Reproductive Medicine. (2002). *Protect our fertility.* Retrieved from http://www.protectyourfertility.org

Appleyard, D. (2002, Oct. 3). Are IVF mothers better parents? *Daily Mail* (London), pp. 52, 53.

Are women waiting too late to have children? (2002, April 16). *CNN.com.* Retrieved from http://www.com/POLL/results/107911.contents.html

Arnst, C. (2002, April 29). The loneliness of the high-powered woman. *Business Week*, 23.

Ashley, J. (2002, April 24). We really can have it all—with a little bit of help. *The Guardian* (London), p. 16.

Bachu, A., & O'Connell, M. (2001, October). Fertility of American women: June 2000. *U.S. Census Bureau [on-line]*. Retrieved August 15, 2002, from http://www.census.gov/prod/2001pubs/p20-543rv.pdf

Bosely, S. (2002, April 30). Women's fertility in decline by late 20s: Biological clock starts earlier, say scientists after surprise survey. *The Guardian (London)*, p. 3

Carpenter, E. (2002, August 26). Trying for baby fails, for now. *The Post and Courier* (Charleston, SC), p. 1D.

Clocking male fertility. (2000, November). *Essence*, 96.

Cohen, E. (2002, April 17). Career vs. baby book sparks controversy. *CNN.com* Retrieved from http://www.cnn.com/2002/HEALTH/parenting/04/16/waiting.for.baby

Coping with Infertility. (2002, October 9). *CBSNews.com* . Retrieved from http://www.cbsnews.com/stories/2002/10/08/earlyshowleisure/books/main524822.shtml

Cooke, R. (2002, May 27). Fertility fears. *New Statesman*, n.p.

Cottle, M. (2002, April 28). Dads are parents, too. *Pittsburgh Post-Gazette*, p. E-1.

Couric, K. (2003, May 20). Using egg donors for infertile couples. *Today*, NBC.

Dempsey, L. (2002, Dec. 12). Infertility: Dashed hopes ... empty arms. *Dayton Daily News*, p. E1.

Douglas, S. J. (2002, May 27). Manufacturing post-feminism. *In These Times*, 9.

Dunson, D. B., Columbo, B., & Baird, D. D. (2002). Changes with age in the level and duration of fertility in the menstrual cycle. *Human Reproduction*, *17*, 1399–1403.

Ehrenfeld, T. (2002, March 25). Infertility: A guy thing. *Newsweek*, 60.

Fergus, M. A. (2002, June 30). In the struggle to balance career and motherhood, many women are left wondering if they waited too long; Is time running out? *The Houston Chronicle*, L-1.

Fields, J. (2001, June 29). U.S. adults postponing marriage, Census Bureau reports. *United States Department of Commerce News [on-line]*. Retrieved August 15, 2002, from http://www.census.gov/Press-Release/www/2001/cb01-113.html

Fields, J., & Casper, L. (2001, June). America's families and living arrangements. *U.S. Census Bureau [on-line]*. Retrieved August 15, 2002, from http://www.census.gov/prod/2001pubs/p20-537.pdf

Franke-Ruta, _. (2002, July 1). Creating a lie; Sylvia Ann Hewlett and the myth of the baby bust. *American Prospect*, 30.

Frase-Blunt, M. (2001, November 6). Misconceptions and missed conceptions. The *Washington Post*. F02.

Frean, A. (2002, May 17). Birthrate at record low as women opt for jobs. *The Times (London)*, Home.

Gibbs, N. (2002, April 15). Making time for a baby. *Time, 159*, 48–54.

Giese, R. (2002, May 30). Flawed logic obscures messages on having kids. *Toronto Star*, p. A27.

Hall, C. T. (2002, April 30). Study speeds up biological clocks; Fertility rates dip after women hit 27. *The San Francisco Chronicle*, p. A1.

Hart. B. (2002, April 14). Delaying motherhood ignores hard realities. *Chicago Sun-Times*. 33.

Hatcher, T. (2002, May 2). Careers and babies: Fertility decline underscores dilemma. *CNN.com*. Retrieved from http://www.cnn.com/2002/HEALTH/04/30/fertility.women/

Hewett, C. (2001, August 7). Ad plays up biological clock. *Chicago Sun-Times*, n.p.

Hewlett, S. A. (2002a, October 21). Baby hunger. *New Stateman*, n.p.

Hewlett, S. A. (2002b). *Creating a life: Professional women and the quest for children*. New York: Talk Miramax Books.

Hjul, J. (2002, May 2). Is there any hope for single career women? *The Scotsman*, p. 14.

Infertility press coverage may be worrying some women needlessly. (2002, June 25). *Canada News Wire*, n.p.

Kalb, C., Springen, K., Scelfo, J., & Pierce, E. (2001, August 13). Should you have your baby now? *Newsweek*, 40.

Liddane, S. (2002, May 26). Fertile at 40? Maybe not. Conceiving a mid-life baby is harder than many women think. *The Seattle Times*, p. L6.

Mail call. (2001, September 3). *Newsweek*, 14.

Mask, T. (2003, January 26). Waiting to be called mom. *Chicago Daily Herald*, p. 1.

Mundy, L. (2002, March 17). The late shift. *The Washington Post*, p. W21.

Pickett, D. (2002, April 25). Little room at top for women who want to be moms. *Chicago Sun-Times*, p. 38.

Poniewozik, J. (2002, April 15). The cost of starting families first. *Time*, 56–58.

Psychologist: How to balance career, children. (2002, April 30). *CNN.com* Retrieved from http://www.cnn.com/2002/HEALTH/ parenting/04/26/zappert.q.a.cnna/

Raising the issue of the biological clock. (2001, September 2). *CBSNews.com* Retrieved from http://www.cbsnews.com/stories/2001/01/31/health/ main327350.shtml

Rivers, C. (2001, August 15). Women are delaying childbirth for good reasons. *National Organization for Women*. Retrieved from http://www.now.org/enews/aug2001/081501childbirth.html

Rogers, K. C. (2002, May 12). True feminism. *The Times-Picayune (New Orleans)*, p. 6.

Rowe-Finkbeiner, K. (2002, Summer). Oops, I forgot to have kids. *Bust*, 44–49.

Seeman, N. (2002, June 5). Mothers, babies, and that book. *National Review*, n.p.

Thompson, M. (2002, August 5). Pregnant pauses. *The Daily News* (Los Angeles, CA), p. U4.

Weiss, R. (2002, August 28). Infertility campaign can't get ad space. *The Washington Post*, p. A02.

Wen, P. (2002, September 21). Infertility ads not appearing at a theater, mall, near you. *The Boston Globe*, p. A1.

Winfrey, O. (2002, May 1). When should you have a baby? *Oprah*. Harpo Productions, Inc., Burrell. Retrieved from http://www.oprah.com

Yarbrough, M. (2002, May 20). Is there a 'right time' for a woman to have baby? *Jet*, 60.

Zappert, L. T. (2002, April 30). Psychologist: How to balance career, children. *CNN.com*. www.cnn.com/2002/HEALTH/parenting/04/26/zappert.q.a.cnna/

# 5

# Desperately Seeking Legitimacy: Narratives of a Biomedically Invisible Disease

ॐ

**Phyllis M. Japp**
*University of Nebraska-Lincoln*

**Debra K. Japp**
*St. Cloud State University*

The shelves of libraries and book stores, newspapers and magazines, television, film, and Internet Web sites all give evidence of the popularity of illness narratives. Some stories are autobiographical book or film-length accounts; others are shorter and more informally told. Illness narratives serve varied purposes for authors and auditors, from personal to political. Stories constructed by ill persons reveal not only their physical and emotional concerns but also their communication with caretakers and families, with health providers and organizations, and with public acceptance or rejection of their illness status. They provide catharsis, testimony, identity restructuring, and the ability to connect to others. Such stories are an integral part of the process of constructing new identities in the face of life changes or physical and mental dysfunctions (Frank, 1995).

For the reader or listener, narratives forge connections to another person and his or her world and reflexively provide insight into one's own world. If readers share the illness, they find reinforcement and community. If not, they learn how others experience the world of illness, and prepare for the day when they too will need to adjust to an illness of their own or one they love. For physicians and health providers, illness stories can provide insight into the emotions of patients and the social support or lack thereof that impacts their ability to cope with their illness. For scholars, illness narratives illuminate the complex process of constructing health and illness. Illness stories also serve political ends as they raise awareness, destigmatize various illnesses, influence legislation, and/or lobby for increased medical research.

In this chapter, we focus on a specific variety of illness narrative, the stories told by those who suffer from symptoms the medical community does not recognize as indicative of a legitimate disease. These conditions, termed *biologically invisible illnesses* (BII) or *medically unexplained physical symptoms* (MUPS), include those for which medical science can produce no empirical evidence of physical change or deterioration and thus can provide no definitive diagnosis (Barker, 2002; Zavestoski et al., 2004). In the dominant biomedical model, only illnesses that are "objectively measurable" can be legitimated as a disease (Aronwitz, 1998, p. 12).

Such illnesses, although dramatically increasing in incidence, do not fit comfortably within the extant framework of biomedicine. Structured toward providing heroic measures to combat clear cases of physical injury or dysfunction, biomedicine rejects or marginalizes conditions that do not fit into its models of causation. Currently, bio-medicine classifies many illnesses from which increasing numbers of people suffer (and which large numbers of physicians are expected to treat) as BII, among them Chronic Fatigue Syndrome (CFS), Fibromyalgia Syndrome (FM), Gulf War Syndrome (GWS), Chronic Pain Syndrome (CP) and Multiple Chemical Sensitivity (MCS; Zavestoski et al., 2004). The collision of a rigid bio-medical model of disease and the growing number of illnesses that fall outside the parameters of that model constitute a experiential crisis for many ill persons. Biomedicine's inability to amend the model, unwillingness to take seriously symptoms without a definitive cause, and discomfort with ambiguity, means that often the only possible explanation for these conditions is to explicitly or implicitly blame the patient. Without medical acceptance of the validity of the illnesses, social, legal, and economic acceptance is difficult if not impossible, leading sufferers to experience social stigma, devaluation, and economic hardships. The fact that the women (with the exception of GWS) make up the bulk of sufferers from BII infuses the crisis with gender issues, as a masculinist-oriented institution collides with the needs of women patients (Richmond & Jason, 2001).

Although research debates the validity of the illnesses and activists work for public understanding, ordinary individuals attempt to cope with debilitating symptoms and the changes these inflict on their lives and livelihoods. Their personal stories reside in and are connected to a broader network of narratives, to master narratives of biomedicine and institutional and public narratives of reinforcement or challenge, as well as to other personal stories that reveal the complexities of being caught in the web of confusion surrounding these illnesses. These personal narratives, therefore, not only provide accounts of individual sufferer's experiences but serve as windows on the world of cultural values, norms, and expectations that comprise our understandings of these illnesses and those who suffer from them.

## LEGITIMACY NARRATIVES

The force and extent of the medical and moral ambiguities that surround such illness, we believe, require construction of a particular genre of illness narrative. Although sharing many features with typical illness narratives, such as those discovered by Frank (1995), legitimacy narratives present distinct differences as well.[1] We find that legitimacy narratives, personal accounts of experiencing BII, contain a core of four interconnected elements: the need to establish the legitimacy of suffering, the search for moral legitimacy, the search for medical legitimacy, and the search for public legitimacy. Although scholars have identified these concerns relative to BII (Barker, 2002; Garro, 1992), here we look specifically at how these elements are constructed and represented in personal narratives of these illnesses and, further, what those narratives reveal about the broader culture within which patients must live and give account of themselves.

This chapter represents our initial inquiry into legitimacy narratives, thus our conclusions are tentative. Our engagement is personal as well as scholarly. One of us, struggling to adjust to a BII, has read widely on the topic for some years, from medical journals to self-help literature. The other has listened, supported, and helped to co-construct a personal legitimacy narrative. Although we find these four features present in our own experience and in most stories we have read and heard, we hold them open to modification as we continue our work. After describing these features in more depth, we look closely at a prototypical published legitimacy narrative, supplementing that account with supporting evidence from other legitimacy narratives. We then engage the issues we find both revealed and concealed, accepted and challenged, in this limited selection of legitimacy narratives.

## FEATURES OF THE LEGITIMACY NARRATIVE

As noted, four interrelated elements comprise stories of BII: the need to legitimate the author's suffering, assertions of moral legitimacy, the search for medical legitimacy, and the desire for public legitimacy. These overlapping and integrated concerns drive the structure and functions of legitimacy narratives.

## Legitimating Suffering

Certainly, legitimacy narratives are not alone in chronicling the suffering associated with illness. Giving voice to pain and its effects on one's life is a major feature of any illness narrative. Persons with BII, however, have special and compelling reasons to document their suffering. Unable to begin the story with "I learned I had cancer" or some other recognized disease, the legitimacy narrative must persuade the reader of the validity of the author's illness. In typical illness narratives, naming the disease is central to the story, as the author describes coming to terms with the diagnosis and how she is able to recover from, learn from, or adjust to the illness in question. The diagnosis, thus, constitutes a critical moment. It brings uncertainty as the narrator wonders how she will experience her altered state of identity but also allows certainty and closure; the mysterious symptoms now have a name, one recognized and legitimated by the medical community. In the midst of physical discomfort and mental anguish, a diagnosis provides the comfort of validation—this suffering is real, it is recognized and deserves to be recognized, by family, friends, co-workers, employers, and insurance providers. Especially for some who may have been weeks or months in the limbo of uncertainty, the diagnosis provides an anchor, a turning point from which they can begin to redefine their lives, reassess their priorities and relationships, and map out their futures—however short they may be.

For sufferers of BII, however, uncertainty remains. They remain unable to function normally, troubled by persistent symptoms for which physicians cannot find a cause, compelled to chronicle their symptoms severity and continuation as evidence that they constitute a bona fide disease (Barker, 2002). The intensity of these often lengthy descriptions is driven by the need to prove, in the face of medical and public skepticism, that they are really ill. The narrative of the cancer patient, by contrast, may detail the pain and fatigue associated with the disease, but does not have the burden of proving that the cancer exists. As one sympathetic physician notes, BII patients often have to expend so much energy proving that they are ill that little is left to direct toward either getting well or coping with the disease (Zavestoski et al., 2004).

BII authors face a double bind: they must detail their symptoms intensity and severity in hope of being believed, yet if they appear to be exaggerating, they will only reinforce disbelief. As Werner and Malterud (2003) reported, patients who complained too much "risked being perceived as quarrelsome, whining, or mentally disturbed, getting no further help. Presenting with only minor complaints did not facilitate interest on the part of doctors" (p. 1415). Barker (2002) noted that such patients experience "a deeply felt contradiction between their subjective certainty of their symptoms and the inability of biomedical science to demonstrate their objective existence" (p. 280). In the absence of visible physical impairment, they continue to detail their symptoms to support their claim that they are ill; the symptoms constituting evidence of a bodily rather than an imaginative disorder. Unfortunately, chronicles of symptoms do not constitute evidence of a legitimate disease. Biomedicine turns on the demand for clinical evidence (Aronowitz, 1998), and self-reporting of symptoms, however detailed, cannot provide that evidence. As Frank (1995) noted, "The story told by the physician becomes the one against which others are ultimately judged true or false, useful or not" (p. 5).

Even if a chronicle of symptoms fails to convince physicians, family and others, however, it can certainly benefit its author by providing a record of pain, stigma, and other experiences that describe her life as it now is lived. When the patient finds some confirmation of the reality of her symptoms, even if only from stories of other sufferers, she can begin to address the question: "How shall I live with this mysterious, controversial, but life-altering situation?" As she reads and listens to other's stories of similar symptoms, she may be able to convince herself that what she experiences is real, even if it does not have a name recognized by biomedicine.

## Moral Legitimacy

Authors of legitimacy narratives relate and attempt to refute challenges to their moral credibility. When clinical evidence is nonexistent, physicians tend to believe the origin of symptoms must be in the patient's mind (Barker, 2002). Such encounters result in "self-doubt and alienation" for the patient. The victims of such illnesses "endure the additional burden of experiencing their symptoms in the context of public (including medical doubt)" (p. 280).

In the face of suspicion by the medical profession, family, friends and others that a person's suffering is self-imposed, legitimacy narratives must defend the author's moral character. A central feature of the legitimacy narrative, thus, is its need to mount a defense against the charge—implied or stated—that the sufferer imagines or exaggerates her physical problems. When medical professionals and others question the authenticity of the illness, such suspicions become an "ontological challenge to the integrity of the self" (Garro, 1992, p. 104). Suffers must deal with the assault on their moral integrity as well as with the mental and physical challenges wrought by the symptoms they are experiencing. As Ware (1992) reported:

> The reality for sufferers of CFS through de-legitimating experiences is that their illness is not "real" at all but rather a fabrication based either

on the needless exaggeration of everyday complaint (in which case they are malingerers) or on the perception of imaginary symptoms (in which case they are "crazy"). (p. 355)

The resulting dissonance, shame, and self doubt can be extremely debilitating, as suffers ask themselves: "Do I have the right to consider myself ill? Am I lying or deceiving myself and others? Am I using my health status to avoid responsibilities legitimately mine? Am I taking advantage of others' generosity and good will?" As Ware (1992) noted, shame "stems not from the fact of having an illness but from being told they do not. Their shame is the shame of being wrong about the nature of reality" (p. 354). Sufferers realize that, in the medical and social worlds, for an illness to be "not physical" equates to it being "not real," that is, imagined or imposed by the mind. Mahoney (2001) concurred, "In our culture, the existence of a disease as a specific entity is a fundamental aspect of its intellectual and moral legitimacy. If it is not specific, it is not a disease, the sufferer is not entitled to sympathy" (p. 577). Thus narrators have a great investment in refuting the charge of mental causation, for "attributing the pain to a malfunction of the mind rather than the body implies that it is the sufferer who is to blame for both the pain and for the failure of the practitioner to achieve a cure" (Garro, 1992, p. 104). As one sufferer remarked, "It's so frustrating to be legitimately ill and have people treating you as though you're faking it or you're just another crazy female. Or, you could be well if you wanted to be ..." (Garro, 1992, p. 128).

The quest for moral legitimacy can also be aided by access to the stories of others who verify the reality of the illness and affirm the moral credibility of the sufferer. Via self-help and other informal support groups, as sufferers began to believe in the validity of their illness and tell their stories to each other, they often seek a wider audience. Frank (1995) observed that the goal of authors is not just "to work out their own changing identities, but also to guide others who will follow them" (p. 17). As a sufferer finds a legitimate place in the community of the ill, she regains the moral and thus the narrative credibility necessary to author her story. Through her story and other's stories, she is reconstituted as a moral self, one whose story deserves to be told and holds truth value for others.

## Medical Legitimacy

Legitimacy narratives typically detail the continual and often futile search for a medical explanation of symptoms, one that exonerates sufferers from the moral culpability already described. Medical science, as noted, seeks to locate observable origins of bodily symptoms.

Only then, the biomedical saga goes, can those symptoms be defined as a legitimate disease. Diagnosis not only names the disease but also determines its value and locates responsibility for causation and treatment (Mahoney, 2001).

Legitimacy narratives testify to frustrating and often shameful encounters with the medical profession. Typically, they describe consultations in which the physician cheerfully announces: "You are perfectly healthy," meaning, of course, that she or he could find no clinical evidence of disease. If a patient insists that they are not healthy, physicians unable to locate a physical cause of symptoms often turn to mental origins as an explanation. If a patient answers truthfully that, of course, she is depressed by persistent pain that seems to have no legitimate cause and, of course, living with such pain affects her relationships and work performance, then physicians frequently invert the explanation and announce her mental state as the cause, not the result, of her physical symptoms. One patient remarked, "The biggest problem I had was not my disease, but getting any doctor to even believe I was sick. I know they all thought I was fat and lazy" (Fibromyalgia, Chronic Fatigue, 2001, p. 130). Another tells of a doctor who asked, "Have you considered that you may have a problem in your marriage? Perhaps you are afraid of sex" (Rosen, 2003, p. 101). "So am I really crazy?" the patient wonders as she limps out of yet another demeaning medical encounter. Certainly, she dreads telling family once more that "they didn't find anything specific wrong with me." After several such reports, she sees suspicion grow in the eyes of those closest to her, echoing the physician's assessment that "it is all in her head."

In this dilemma as well, the narrative process can aid sufferers of BII. Narrators describe their anger at the indifference, condescension, even verbal abuse they have endured from physicians. As they engage each others' stories of how they have been branded as depressed, mentally unstable, lazy, or hysterical and relate how the absence of medical legitimacy has exacerbated charges of moral failure, they can gain the agency and purpose needed to live with the illness and the attendant social and medical disapproval.

## Public Legitimacy

Finally, many authors of legitimacy narratives search for public visibility and acceptance. Arguments for public legitimacy draw on all three of the prior needs, as a cumulative voice emerges and insists that suffering is real, that sufferers are morally credible and that they deserve medical legitimacy and social acceptance. As many voices, over time, insist that attention be paid to their suffering, as they resist the trivialization and stigmatization of their conditions, a discourse grows that attracts medical and even political attention. For many, the push for medical legitimacy becomes not only a personal quest but a social responsibility, as they "make demands for public awareness, fight for public and private funds" (Barker, 2002, p. 295).

Often a breakthrough occurs when well-known persons publicly tell their stories of struggling with the illness, the moral stigma, and the medical community. Just as celebrities bring attention to legitimate diseases, for example, Christopher Reeve for spinal cord injuries and Michael J. Fox for Parkinson's disease, they also can bring awareness of BII. The testimonies of people who have attained public attention or respect in other fields, for example, actors, writers, athletes, politicians, musicians, not only publicize the illness and proclaim it to be authentic, they provide a powerful form of credibility for ordinary people whose stories have not been believed.

Clearly, these four dimensions of legitimacy narratives are overlapping and mutually reinforcing elements that constitute a narrative argument for legitimacy of the illness in question. Although stories may differ in the attention given to one or more of the elements, in most we have read they are all present, intertwined and articulated in greater or lesser degree. Before discussing these dimensions in more detail, we consider a compelling example of a legitimacy narrative. Although this is one story, by one person, about one BII, it echoes and resonates with the voices of numbers of sufferers of this and other illnesses. As we work through this narrative, we provide what we term *echoes* from other narratives that reinforce the words and emotions portrayed in this one extended story. The story is that of Laura Hillenbrand, the author of a best-selling novel, *Seabiscuit*. Hillenbrand suffers from CFS, a prototypical BII. Following publication of that book, which she wrote while ill, Hillenbrand began to write about her struggle with CFS. *A Sudden Illness* is the most complete and compelling of her illness narratives. The echoes come from other published or public narratives in books, articles and Internet communications.[2]

## CFS AND THE SEARCH FOR LEGITIMACY

Hillenbrand's illness, CFS, is one of the most ambiguous and misunderstood of recent illnesses. Symptoms are varied and range in intensity. Sufferers—those documented at least—are mostly adult women, although men and children are also afflicted. The onset and duration of the illness varies from person to person. Some fall suddenly ill and remain chronically impaired; others gradually experience the onset of fatigue, muscle pain, digestive problems, sleep disorder, headaches and the myriad of other symptoms associated with the syndrome. For some, the illness becomes totally disabling; for most, it results in a diminishment of activity and certainly of the quality of life. For nearly all, it brings a challenge to their moral credibility.

Because no clear cause of the symptoms can be located, the disease is usually diagnosed, if at all, by the elimination of other possible diseases. Even after the Center for Disease Control's (CDC) recognition of CFS as a "syndrome" (the designation denotes the invisibility of causal agents), questions continue about whether symptoms are physical or mental in origin; whether the illness is social or psychological rather than somatic (Aronowitz, 1998). Physicians, faced with patients who declare that their symptoms are real but for which clinical evidence is nonexistent, vary in their responses. As noted, the easy explanation is psychological, that is, the sufferer is constructing an illness in her mind and projecting it onto her body. Accordingly, physicians often advocate counseling and therapy in the hope that the patient will adjust her mental attitude so that she need not define herself as ill. Initial media attention to the syndrome, first called "yuppie flu," echoes the skepticism of the medical profession, a skepticism that remains lodged in public consciousness, in spite of recent efforts toward legitimation, including increased medical research.

## A SUDDEN ILLNESS

Hillenbrand (2003) wrote *Seabiscuit* while often unable to leave her bed or even raise her head, due to the fatigue, muscle weakness, and vertigo associated with severe cases of CFS. *A Sudden Illness* tells of her struggle to find a diagnosis for her debilitating symptoms and her quest for moral and medical legitimacy. Although she is still ill and has limited strength, she has granted interviews and made personal appearances to bring CFS to public attention.

### Legitimizing Suffering

Hillenbrand's story, like most CFS narratives, begins with a prolonged description of her suffering. Following what she believed was a case of food poisoning, her symptoms continued and increased in severity. She was unable to eat, unable to concentrate, and hardly able to walk but continued to try and attend college classes. However, after a few days:

> One morning I woke to find my limbs leaden, I tried to sit up but couldn't .... It was two hours before I could stand. On the walk to the bathroom, I had to drag my shoulder along the wall to stay upright.... After three weeks of being stranded in my room, I had no choice but to drop out of college. (Hillenbrand, 2003, p. 56)

*Echo: I had trouble breathing, walking up the stairs and to the car.*
*Waves of heat poured over my body, leaving me dizzy and weak.*
*(Goranson, 1996)*

Leaving the campus, unable to care for herself, Hillenbrand moved back to her childhood home. After several more weeks of lying in bed, hoping for recovery, Hillenbrand (2003) described continuing pain and dysfunction:

> ... I stepped on a scale. I had lost twenty pounds. The lymph nodes on my neck and under my arms and collarbones were painfully swollen. During the day, I rattled with chills, but at night I soaked my clothes in sweat. I felt unsteady, as if the ground were swaying. My throat was inflamed and raw. A walk to the mailbox on the corner left me so tired that I had to lie down. (p. 58)

> *Echo: At my worst ... I was barely able to function. It was an extreme effort even to do laundry or prepare a meal. Many times after doing these small chores I was barely able to get out of bed.... I've experienced blurred vision, muscle weakness, lightheadedness, shakiness, stomach upset, night sweats, lack of concentration, heart palpitations, shortness of breath, mind-splitting migraines....* (Akers, as quoted in Struck, 2000, p. 38)

> Sometimes I'd look at words or pictures but see only meaningless shapes. I'd stare at clocks and not understand what the positions of the hands meant.... I couldn't hang on to a thought long enough to carry it through to a sentence. (Hillenbrand, 2003, p. 58)

> *Echo: I have two post-graduate degrees and have had two careers. Now the spell checker does not even know what I am trying to spell and I cannot help it find the right word. I cannot even remember how to spell my last name consistently.* (Moonsage, 1998)

The graphic discussion of symptoms continues as Hillenbrand describes weeks extending into months and then into years of inability to find a diagnosis or any means of recovery:

> My world narrowed down to my bed and my window. I could no longer walk the length of my street. My hair was starting to fall out. I hadn't had a period in four months. My mouth and throat were pocked with dozens of bleeding sores and my temperature was spiking to a hundred and one every twelve hours. (p. 59)

Such detailed accounts of suffering are necessary to document the reality of the illness and the life restructuring that it has caused. Hillenbrand's focus on her physical symptoms forces the reader to enter into and verify her world of suffering, albeit at this point in the story, neither the narrator nor the reader know the name of the disease.

## Moral Legitimacy

Throughout this ordeal, Hillenbrand consulted physicians, seeking diagnosis and treatment. She describes a series of medical encounters that fail to take her symptoms seriously. Told her problem was mental, she is referred to a psychiatrist who refers her back to physicians. She chronicles her increasing physical and social isolation as friends stopped calling. She hears rumors that she has AIDS. She describes moving from frustration, to shame, to depression and finally to suicidal despair. Although she has some familial support, she experiences growing loneliness amid charges of moral weakness:

> Without my physicians' support, it was almost impossible to find support from others. People told me I was lazy and selfish. Someone lamented how unfortunate Borden was to have a girl-friend who demanded coddling. Some of Borden's friends suggested that he was foolish and weak to stand by me.... I was ashamed and angry and indescribably lonely. (Hillenbrand, 2003, p. 60)

> *Echoes: I felt overwhelming guilt. It was bad enough to be unable to work at my job, which had given me an identity.... Now I couldn't even take care of my home, my children were confused and scared, my husband was run ragged.* (Goranson, 1996)

> *With vacillating levels of self-confidence, I am compelled to justify myself to strangers. I possess a need for those I don't even know to understand that I am not lazy.* (Hahn, 1996)

> *No one would make up this illness and put themselves in this position.* (Shave, 2003, p. 4)

> *"... Some thought surely this was a mental health problem. Some thought it a convenient excuse to escape the rat race.... Some told me I was lucky to get it and be able to be at home ..."* (Goranson, 1996)

## Medical Legitimacy

After years of dealing with the stigma of moral failing, the story turns when Hillenbrand (2003) finds a physician who not only empathizes with her suffering but legitimates it by providing a diagnosis. He is unable to offer her a cure, but her shame and stigma begin to be removed as her suffering is authenticated and her moral legitimacy re-established, at least in her own eyes. Finally, she writes, she has obtained necessary diagnosis, "My internists, he said, were wrong. My disease was real." She has CFS, "one of the most frustrating illnesses he had encountered in his practice; presented with severely incapacitated patients, he could do little to help them" (p. 60).

*Echoes: Rest, that is all you can do. There is no treatment for it. Eat a good diet, get some exercise, as much as you can without pushing, and rest. You'll probably get better in a couple of months. call me every once in a while or if your symptoms get worse.* (Shaderowfsky, 1996, quoting her physician)

*I'm just trying to get you, no begging you, to think about the patient as you begin to practice medicine. That's why you are there. That's who pays your salary and who pays off your student loans. We patients are human, and we can be hurt by you and your medical position/power. We can also be abused by it.* (Pollman, 1997, to a medical student)

From this point on, for Hillenbrand, redefinition of self and reorientation to life can begin. She still must adjust to a life of uncertain physical abilities, learn to trust herself and accommodate her needs, and work to repair or redefine relationships. She still moves from specialist to specialist seeking treatment, now armed with the CDC's description of CFS, although many physicians were still unaware of an official recognition of the condition. She stops hoping for a cure and begins, with medical help, to cope with the up and down cycles of the illness. As she explains,

Whenever I over extended myself my health deteriorated. One mistake could land me in bed for weeks, so the cost of even the most trivial activities, from showering to walking to the mailbox, had to be painstakingly considered. Sometimes I relapsed for no reason at all. (p. 61)

*Echo: I have really good weeks and I have really bad weeks.... It is definitely a daily struggle. I hope I find more highs than lows.* (Amy Peterson, in Freedman, 2001, p. K6383)

Finally, Hillenbrand finds a specialist who "listened for the better part of an hour.... He couldn't cure me, he said, but he would do everything he could to help me cope with the illness" (p. 63). There is no "happily ever after" to Hillenbrand's story, or to those of other CFS sufferers. In her case, however, she was finally granted the legitimacy of a diagnosis and was thus able to begin to adjust as much as possible to a life dictated by her illness.

## Public Legitimacy

Although *A Sudden Illness* does not chronicle Hillenbrand's public activism, the story itself provides a public appeal for the legitimacy of the disease, a record of mistreatment at the hands of physicians, suspicion on the part of friends and relatives, and a chronicle of a painful journey from self-doubt to self-affirmation. In short, the story confirms in a public forum the experience and legitimacy of the disease for other CFS sufferers. As *USA Today* headlines an article about Hillenbrand, she "puts a face on chronic fatigue syndrome" (Fackelmann, 2003, p. 8D).

> *Echoes: I've grown tired of doctors, co-workers, the media and the public not paying attention to this disease. We need to change the perception that CFS is a trivial little illness that doesn't deserve notice.* (Holderman in Giuliucci, 2002)

> *Jay Leno told a national TV audience that CFS people did not show up for a CFIDS [The Chronic Fatigue and Immune Dysfunction Syndrome Association of America] rally because they were too tired. Bryant Gumble told TODAY Show viewers that CFS does not exist.... That's why CFIDS Advocacy is needed.* (Karasik, 1998)

Hillenbrand's willingness to talk about her struggles attests to her desire to help others. She bears testimony so that others who suffer from the disease can be encouraged to believe in themselves and their continued worth, despite their physical incapacities.

## LEGITIMACY NARRATIVES AS RESISTANCE NARRATIVES

Unquestionably, stories such as Hillenbrand's are of immense value to fellow sufferers, their families, and the medical community. Equally important, they provide a window on cultural attitudes and practices that surround an illness experience. Legitimacy narratives, like other illness stories, illustrate the master narratives of medicine, as well as public and medical attitudes and assumptions that circulate in our culture and that serve as conscious and unconscious frames for interpreting experience.

The agonistic tone of legitimacy narratives suggest that they may function as what H. L. Nelson (2001) labeled "counterstories." Counterstories "constitute a revised understanding of a person or a social group. They are stories that define people morally and are developed for the express purpose of resisting and undermining an oppressive master narrative" (p. 8). Legitimacy narratives certainly attempt to resist the trivialization of the author's suffering, the moral stigma imputed to sufferers, medical indifference to their problems, and public ignorance of their illness. To do so, however, they must challenge master narratives, those taken-for-granted explanations and assumptions that drive public and political action and infiltrate individual consciousness, such that people define themselves within their parameters (Somers, 1994).

When the identity imposed by a master narrative is an oppressive one, and those oppressed realize it to be so, H. L. Nelson (2001) argued that those marginalized can develop stories that resist the power of the master narrative to define their identity and limit their agency. These counterstories seek an opening, gap, or inconsistency in a master narrative and attempt to exploit that opening as they construct narratives that oppose the power of the master narrative. As H. L. Nelson (2001) noted, counterstories can resist oppression at three levels: refusal, repudiation, and contestation. At the most private level, counterstories can refuse to internalize the damaging identity. This strategy does not direct its efforts toward changing master narratives but toward limiting the damage done by those narratives. As she explains, "The point of counterstories that refuse is not to change the dominant perception of the group—it's to shift how individuals within the group themselves understand who they are" (p. 170). As a strategy of refusal, for example, one may say to oneself: I will not define myself as mentally deficient, even though I know others insist that is the case.

Counterstories that repudiate are a stronger but still private response to the oppressive identity of a master narrative. In this strategy, those marginalized not only refuse to internalize the damaging identity but challenge other's attempts to apply unacceptable and degrading labels (H. L. Nelson, 2001). A repudiating response, for example, might be: I don't define myself as *mentally deficient* and if you apply that label to me I will tell you that you are wrong and your judgment unacceptable.

The final strategy of counterstories—contestation—moves from the private to the public, as the marginalized join in a vocal and persistent challenge; contestation works systematically not only to repair the damage inflicted by master narratives but to undermine, revise, and/or replace that master narrative (H. L. Nelson). Contestation, for example, might respond to a label of mental deficiency by developing a public campaign of denial, one that insists such labels are inaccurate, unethical, and unacceptable to the group in question and demanding that they be changed. We now consider the type of challenges legitimacy narratives mount toward master narratives of biomedicine and assess the degree to which those narratives are effective in their efforts to resist the oppression of master narratives.

## RESISTING THE MASTER NARRATIVES OF BIOMEDICINE

Legitimacy narratives engage master narratives of biomedicine whenever they call into question the definitions and practices that are taken for granted in that realm. We locate three major areas of challenge: First, legitimacy narratives struggle against the master narrative's separation of body and mind and the attending stigma of mentally induced illness. Second, legitimacy narratives question the master narrative's ontological paradigm, the insistence on locating biological markers as the criteria for legitimacy. Third, they engage the gender biases of the biomedical master narrative.

## Body, Mind, and Stigma

The biomedical division of mind and body as separate and discrete realms permeates legitimacy narratives. Although most well-trained clinicians now agree that the mind and the body are interconnected aspects of human health, in practice, most clearly situate disease in one or the other. As Aronowitz (1998) noted, medicine's interest in more holistic models of disease is undermined by the reductionist practices of medical research and clinical diagnoses. Nowhere is medical resistance to interconnected mental and physical causation more evident than in the treatment of BII.

The resistance to psychosocial explanations by physicians and patients alike is rooted in the dualism described. This dualism also assumes that people can control their mind (thus are morally responsible for their thought processes), but are at the mercy of the body (thus innocent of responsibility for bodily dysfunctions). As Garro (1992) noted, "Attributing the pain to a malfunction of the mind rather than the body implies that it is the sufferer who is to blame for both the pain and for the failure of the practitioner to achieve a cure" (p. 104). Aronowitz (1998) concurs:

> For many medical practitioners and lay people today, to the degree that individuals suffer from a prototypically specific disease, they are held to be victims rather than in some measure just recipients of disease. As a corollary, patients whose suffering cannot be understood in ontological terms are more responsible for their illnesses. (p. 177)

If biomedicine grants medical legitimacy only to illnesses of somatic origin and withholds moral legitimacy if an illness is attributed to mental origins, patients have as much investment as physicians in the dualistic paradigm. The unwillingness of many legitimacy narratives to consider mental connections supports rather than challenges the stigma attached to so-called mental illnesses in our culture. If biomedicine were to acknowledge the complex interaction of mental, emotional, social, cultural and physiological dimensions of human health, it would mean that physicians might have to admit to ignorance of specific causes and cures. Neither physicians nor patients seem willing to accept such uncertainty.

CFS legitimacy narratives are characterized by assertions of refusal to accept the diagnosis of mental illness: "I am not depressed. My aunt and sister have clinical depression. I know the symptoms and I do not have them" (Pollman, 1997) and repudiation of that label when applied by others: "No one would make up this illness and put themselves in this position" (Shave, 2003, p. 4). However in the narratives we read, we did not find the move to contestation, that is, the overt challenge to the biomedical separation of mind and body as an inappropriate and damaging paradigm. It would take a great deal of courage for a sufferer to assert: Who cares what causes the pain, it is experienced in my body and I've come to you [the physician] for help in alleviating that pain. So put away your moral judgments, forget your need to decide who or what caused this problem, and get to work helping me deal with it.

## Ontology and Medicalization

The pervasive hegemony of the biomedical model of disease limits the stories patients tell as much as it does physician's practices. Authors of legitimacy narratives struggle to identify a specific physical cause, thus supporting, rather than challenging biomedicine's focus on origins and causes. When patient–physician interaction is predicated on the search for a specific diagnosis and cure, both parties believe their time is wasted and their relative expertise devalued if there is no progress toward that goal (Aronowitz, 1998). The search for ontological causation denies the role of experience, essentially all the patient has to offer. Thus, although the patient attempts to insist that his or her illness is legitimate based on his or her suffering, the focus on ontology prevents the physician from accepting that experience as evidence.

Unfortunately, the ontological paradigm, as it demands definitive clinical evidence of cellular or organic deterioration, delegitimates the illnesses of a large percentage of the population. Many people now suffer from illnesses such as CFS, FMS, and various other conditions that defy inquiries into causation. Estimates vary widely, because few patients have received a "legitimate" diagnosis, but recent accounts suggest that between 14 and 22 million people suffer from autoimmune disorders (Hales, 2003). Such patients find little help or support for their problems and continue to experience frustration in medical encounters. Many endure, as the authors of legitimacy narratives attest, what amounts to psychological abuse as they are treated with skepticism, accused of malingering, and shuttled from physician to psychiatrist and back again.

Understandably, the need for medicalization of their illness drives authors of legitimacy narratives. The process by which illnesses become medicalized is important for its social and political implications as well as for the impact on individual lives. In practice, medicalization remains far from a purely scientific enterprise. Rather, it is decidedly discursive and moralistic, as much a process of social redefinition as of clinical evidence. Aronowitz (1998) suggests a number of "nonbiological" factors that are part of the legitimacy process, including extant attitudes, the strength of advocates for medicalization, media coverage, and economic considerations (p. 27). Media attention, especially in the form of stories that tap into public emotions, functions as a significant factor in garnering both political and public support for medicalizing a given condition (Mahoney, 2001).

Public pressure has often overcome the lack of biological evidence and resulted in the classification of an illness as a legitimate disease. Certainly, the medicalizing of an illness instigates the mobilization of resources, and provides opportunities for employment, economic gain, and even political power (R. Smith, 2002). For the medical profession, medicalization means that personnel, services and research can be gathered to treat those with the condition in question. For the pharmaceutical industry, medicalization legitimates the search for drugs to alleviate the condition and advertising campaigns to sell such drugs.[3]

In addressing medicalization, CFS legitimacy narratives abound in statements of refusal and repudiation but seldom in contestation. The need to vindicate their suffering by acquiring validity within the biomedical master narrative leads them generally to insist that biomedicine find the cause of their illness rather than to question the need for causation. Patients as well as physicians await the discovery of "biological markers for CFS" in order to lay to rest the suspicion and misunderstanding regarding the illness (Richman & Jason, 2001, p. 25).

## Gendered Medicine

The lack of power and respect accorded to patients' voices and experiences in the biomedical master narrative echoes throughout legitimacy narratives. The fact that many CFS sufferers are women has, over the years, played into extant cultural assumptions about women's tendencies toward mental instability, hysteria, and all the other demeaning stereotypes that have survived 200 years of feminist challenge. Implicitly, if not explicitly, legitimacy narratives testify to the feminization of such illnesses, as they demonstrate how logic trumps experience, objectivity stifles emotion, and patriarchal power structures sanction those who challenge their authority. Social historians and other academics who speak with the surety of the medically ignorant about gender-related illnesses, because of the popular attention given their work, help to create and perpetuate a social pathology of the female experience (Shorter, 1992; Showalter, 1997). Research that addresses the gender gap in such illnesses often seems unable to discover in that gap anything but a social pathology of gender. Even respected researchers such as Ware and Kleinman (1992) connected their conclusions about CFS sufferers to social stereotypes of gender and the demands of feminist ideology:

> Liberated by feminism to enter previously all-male occupations, women in the 1970s found themselves exhorted to "have it all" by combining a demanding career with a rich and fulfilling family life.... "do it all, and do it now," became the watchword of the corporate and professional worlds.... They [these demands] are the cultural underpinnings of the exhausting lifestyles described by sufferers of CFS. In this sense the fatigue these individuals experience is emblematic of their social experience, a metaphor for the overcommitted life. (p. 554)

The stresses of contemporary life and the excessive demands on the human body and mind can well be contributing factors to illness, across gender, economic, and racial differences. However, linking any specific illness to the history of a gendered social pathology unnecessarily damages women's credibility and feeds into medical assumptions about women patients as chronic complainers.

As Richman, Jason, Taylor, and Jahn (2000) noted, feminist critiques of medicine question four major characteristics of practice:

> ... the "medicalization" of otherwise normal bodily occurrences, the "psychologization" of legitimate medical illnesses, the inequitable allocation of medical resources, and highly asymmetric medical power relations.... U.S. health policy, health care legislation, health-related research, and influential medical positions are all dominated by male-centered thinking. (p. 4)

These issues are clearly problems for CFS sufferers, who are predominately women. The psychologization of this illness reinforces associations with female mental instability. Unlike acute illnesses, chronic illnesses in general fail to garner extensive public attention; those, like CFS, that are experienced mostly by women, are even less likely to be noticed. Further, an institutional power structure that reflects male-centrism is unlikely to provide respect for an illness experienced by women but not validated by medical research.

CFS legitimacy narratives respond to gender pathologies, if at all, via refusal and repudiation arguments, assertions that the author is not a neurotic woman. As Shaderowfsky (1996) reported a conversation with her physician, "Are you depressed? [his question] ... I suppose I could always find a reason be," I said. (A rush of rage, how many times would a man tell me I'm depressed, that I have some sort of vague women's problem?) Few contest the gendered nature of the encounters of mostly female patients with mostly male physicians. Fewer yet raise an overt challenge to the gender pathology so evident in medical and social thought.

## LEVELS OF RESISTANCE

All legitimacy narratives, by their very nature, stand as testaments of resistance to the master narrative of biomedicine. Virtually all engage in some degree of refusal, as the author attempts to resist incorporating into her identity the charges of mental dysfunction, deceit, and malingering that are part of the medical and social discourse of CFS. Most stories demonstrate some degree of repudiation as well, as they not only resist the internalization of the moral pathology, but challenge the right of others to describe them using such labels. Implicitly, if not explicitly, they charge physicians, family, and others with lack of accuracy, empathy, respect and other qualities the sufferer feels she deserves in her interactions with others. Some CFS legitimacy narratives engage in contestation, openly drawing attention to the oppression of CFS sufferers and challenging the oppressive power of the master narratives. Few explicitly argue for remoralization of the biomedical paradigm. Yet all, by their very nature as stories, demand "recognition that the moral order itself requires reevaluation. The story joins these two levels of remoralization; the personal is political" (Frank, 2000a, p. 330).

CFS sufferers find it difficult to challenge biomedical master narratives because they remain trapped within them; medically, morally, economically, and politically defined within their parameters. However vocal they become, they are restricted in their ability to define their own conditions, create their own vocabulary or face down the entrenched power of the medical establishment. Dependent on physicians, insurance providers and others for treatment and support, they remain under the domain of biomedicine and its power to define their legal and medical status. Individual resistance may be difficult; cumulative strength can result in a public voice of contestation. In the case of CFS, some activists have drawn individual stories into a collective voice that seeks to rename the illness, redefine its meanings, and reshape social and political attitudes toward it. Sensitive to the power of language, among other issues, CFIDS activists address the need for a name change, arguing that the three words—"chronic," "fatigue," and "syndrome"—make the condition seem trivial in comparison to diseases that are exotic, fatal or contagious, and thus deserving of public and medical attention.[4]

## CONCLUDING REFLECTIONS

Our initial inquiry into legitimacy narratives as well as into the master narratives within which in they are embedded has raised more questions than it has answered. At this point, we offer reflections rather than conclusions, because the story of our engagement with these stories continues. Several topics remain of interest for further inquiry: the internal dissonance or ironies embedded in the narratives that weaken their power as counterstories, gender differences in legitimacy narratives, and the middle-class orientation of most published narratives.

### Internal Ironies and Tensions

The juxtaposition of personal experiences with biomedical and other master narratives creates unresolvable and often unnoticed tensions. We noted several such tensions in the narratives we read. The first involves the conflict between ability and disability. To be sick means to be unable to perform social roles and responsibilities; to be well is to be able to perform those responsibilities. CFS sufferers must engage in daily renegotiations about what they can and cannot do and this tension permeates their narratives.

Stories, as rhetorical critics realize, are often constructed according to appealing and successful cultural scripts; these scripts become the structure around which the narrator organizes the details of his or her experience. As Frank (1995) noted of illness stories, people learn from social models how such stories should be successfully constructed. Yet, these familiar formulas, so necessary to communicating and understanding, may serve to undermine a narrator's apparent purposes. For example, the "overcoming adversity," "good out of evil" or "quest" scripts are ubiquitous in our culture, probably a necessary form for a successful public narrative. Legitimacy narratives that stress success in spite of illness certainly provide inspiration for others dealing with that illness and satisfy the public's need for a satisfactory story. They can also implicitly trivialize the debilitating effects of the disease. Inspiring narratives attest that one can write a best seller, produce an award-winning documentary, play on a national soccer team, or produce academy award-winning films while ill; all extraordinary accomplishments well beyond the abilities of most healthy people. So although the public can praise the achievements of the narrator, those very achievements may sustain doubt about the severity of the suffering and undermine the moral legitimacy of illness claims. Michelle Akers embodies this tension when she notes "Some people are angry because they think that I belittle the illness by what I can do on the soccer field. They think that I am just not sick enough" (Stolting, 1998, p. 69). The nature of such illnesses—good days and bad days, remissions followed by recurring symptoms—means that ability and inability remain relative, always being negotiated, frequently on an hourly or daily basis. Few can speak definitively about their ability to perform any task on demand or to conform to social expectations on any given occasion.

A second tension occurs between validation and invalidation, as evinced in narrator's struggles to legitimate experience as an ontological reality. Patients believe their experience of symptoms should be taken as grounds for defining the disease, and respond with shame and outrage when that experience is devalued. As already noted, they often become more persistent in detailing symptoms in a futile quest for legitimacy, as if the degree and intensity of suffering ought to confer both moral and medical legitimacy. In the master narrative of medical science, however, suffering is not acceptable as proof, nor are patients willing to live with symptoms that are not linked to a definitive cause and validated with a diagnosis. To quote Frank (1995) again, "The story told by the physician becomes the one against which others are ultimately judged true or false, useful or not" (p. 5). Insisting that symptoms count as valid evidence in an attempt to resist the invalidation of their experience, legitimacy narratives are caught in the tension of reinforcing invalidation while seeking validation and confirmation.

We found a third tension in the simultaneous independence and dependence displayed toward the medical profession, evinced in narrator's language of desire for approval and betrayal when it was not extended. For these sufferers, the drive to reclaim moral agency remains dependent upon the definitional power of medical authority. The strong push for medical legitimacy that drives these narratives, although certainly necessary and understandable, reinforces the power of medical science to grant or withhold legitimacy on the narrow criteria of clinical evidence and plays into dualistic thinking and insistence on the search for ontological causation. Ultimately, many legitimacy narratives are as resistant to biosocial causes as the medical establishment, equally unwilling to admit the interconnection of mind and body, supporting rather than challenging the biomedical model and thus implicitly reinforcing the stigma of mental dysfunctions. By depending on medical approval to confer moral legitimacy, the stories grant science the power to determine moral worth. Thus they essentially seek their place within the master narratives of medical authority rather than declaring independence from their power.

Finally, we found a tension between association and dissociation as the authors sought to reconstruct their identities in the face of chronic illness. Embracing who one is by claiming identification with a community of sufferers can certainly empower individuals and solidify identity. Shared stories provide confirmation of one's pain and the realization that one is not alone. Yet stories also seek to dissociate the sufferer's identity from the social pathologies inherent in the illness, from charges of mental weakness and moral deficit as well as the stigma of a body that is often out of control. Thus suffers struggle with the dialectic of distance and engagement, an avowal that "this illness is me, I am one of a group defined by its parameters" often accompanied by an implicit denial, "this illness is not me, I am not to be evaluated by its parameters" (Frank, 1995, pp. 126–127).

## Gendered Voices

Do men and women tell different legitimacy stories? This is a fascinating question that cannot be addressed without more research. Women authored most of the stories we read. As noted, recent estimates indicate that between 14 and 22 million people suffer from autoimmune disorders similar to CFS and FMS, and that at least two thirds of these are women (Hales, 2003). Thus, the "face" of the illness is female (as well as White and middle-class). As we read and listened to the stories of female CFS sufferers, we found ourselves both saddened and outraged at the potentially damaging experiences of women being marginalized and delegitimized as they struggled to stay active in spite of often overwhelming pain, shame, and guilt.

Contrary to the popular stereotype of the whining, complaining female hypochondriac, in the stories we read, women narrators were possessed of great courage and resolve, willingness to help others, strong in their ability to think past their pain and look for the value it might have for their lives and others. They were amazingly articulate and compassionate. Even in their frustration and anger with the medical profession, they tried to be fair and just in their assessments. They were honest about the self-doubt, shame, and guilt they felt, even as they struggled against it. Of course, we seldom hear or read "chaos" stories, the stories of those whose experiences are too fragmented and confusing to order into an understandable narrative (Frank, 1995).

Men do suffer from CFS, although in lesser numbers than women. As Berne (1992) noted, "men who are no longer able to work suffer the stigma of no longer being the breadwinner, wage earner, achiever—in short, an inability to fulfill the traditional male role" (p. 121). A few men speak clearly of the stigma of being unable to fulfill cultural expectations of males. As one CFS sufferer comments:

> I'm the kind of guy who never falls apart. I'm always fair and honest and was always a good problem solver and a hard worker. I can't do that now;

I can't do the kind of job I can feel good about, so I don't work at all. It's a big hurdle for a Type A, workaholic, hard-driving, very successful, polyphasic thinker who loves what he does to change the rules.... Nothing like this has ever happened to me before. (Berne, 1992, p. 123)

In the few stories we found, male authors appeared either less troubled by the guilt and shame of moral illegitimacy or less willing to admit to those emotions; they appeared more assertive, or wanting to appear so, in insisting on respect and attention from physicians. Their personal relationships seemed less threatened by their chronic illness, or they were unable to articulate the pain of relational ruptures. However in others, we noticed the same guilt and shame evinced by women, perhaps exacerbated by the social stigma attached to men who are not strong and able to overcome weakness. Obviously gender differences remain a fruitful area for further research in legitimacy narratives.

## Class Differences

Finally, as Hawkins (1999) noted, most book-length illness narratives—and this claim would hold true for those accounts published in magazines and other sources—are by middle-class authors with some sophistication in writing and reading narratives and with some sense of the ultimate value of their experience for others. If educated and articulate sufferers find themselves almost silenced and morally devalued by their experience, what must be the case for those who have little sense of personal worth or a more tenuous position in society? As H. L. Nelson (2001) noted, when master narratives successfully instill self-doubt about one's mental incapacity, they systematically destroy a person's trust in her own judgments about her life and erode her sense of agency. Sufferers who internalize the values of the master narrative and feel little sense of agency to begin with either "cannot see through the medical ideology" or cannot free themselves from it (pp. 56–57). If educated, insured, middle-class women are driven to despair, self-doubt, and even suicide by the assault on their moral credibility, what must be the case with those who lack voice and resources that give them at least social credibility? Perhaps such women find alternate means of restoring moral credibility, for example, religious faith. Perhaps they experience less trauma from social disapproval and medical invalidation because they already endure stigma in many other areas of their lives. Until we can access their stories, we cannot know.

In conclusion, we believe that legitimacy narratives demonstrate how cultural constructions of health and illness are both resistant to and open to change. Legitimacy narratives situate an illness in the context of an individual life and simultaneously in a sociocultural and political context of meanings within which those lives are lived. As communicative messages, legitimacy narratives provide insight into the intrapersonal process of reconstructing identity, into interpersonal interactions with family, friends, medical personnel, and into how personal lives both reflect and resist the master narratives and ideologies of health and illness. Equally important, they serve as reflections on biomedical assumptions and practices. In these narratives, we see medicine in the mirror, framed by the experiences and emotions of those who most need its attention. The narratives provide poignant arguments for change in the assumptions of what constitutes illness, how experiences of pain and suffering should be respectfully addressed, and how medical, social, and moral attitudes are intertwined and can serve to silence and isolate rather than support and treat those who are ill.

## NOTES

1. We do not address here how legitimacy narratives fit with Frank's typology of restitution, chaos, and quest narratives. We see elements of all three but need time and space to reflect on the relationships involved.
2. An exceptional set of public narratives that we did not include because of the need to address visual as well as verbal dimensions of narrative is found in the documentary film, *I Remember Me*, written and directed by Kim A. Snyder. Snyder is an independent film producer and CFS sufferer. She chronicles the effects of the disease on her own life, interwoven with interviews with a number of sufferers, including among them Michelle Akers, women's U.S. soccer star, and Blake Edwards, film producer. Thus the film is composed of stories within a story, as the sagas of individual lives unfold within the narrative script of the film.
3. The debate surrounding GWS was characterized as much by socioeconomic and political concerns as it was for clinical evidence of the condition. The moral dimension was strongly evident as well; some believed sufferers to be faking, others questioned their mental stability. The subtext of the debate, of course, was that with legitimacy would come attribution of causation and implicate responsibility for compensation and treatment, even beyond the present generation of sufferers if the condition was determined to cause birth defects (Mahoney, 2001).
4. The Chronic Fatigue and Immune Dysfunction Syndrome Association of America (CFIDS) is an activist group that maintains a Web site, a newsletter, and outreach activities aimed at educating the public and the medical profession about the illness. See the Web site at www.cfids.org

# Death as the Representative Anecdote in the Construction of the Collegiate "Binge-Drinking" Problem

$\infty$

**Thomas Workman**
*University of Nebraska*

On Friday, September 26th, 1997, the brothers of Phi Gamma Delta (Fiji) fraternity at the Massachusetts Institute of Technology (MIT) engaged in a common ritual found throughout collegiate "Greek" organizations; freshmen pledges were paired with their "big brother" who would, among other things, guide the new member as a special mentor and friend. The occasion was celebrated, as are most events in fraternity life, with the consumption of alcohol. It was "Animal House Night," where the freshmen initiates were brought to a room with a large quantity of alcohol and told to have all of it consumed before the film was over (Herper, 1999; Watt & Schuermann, 2002). The festivity was a tradition in the house; drinking beyond personal capacity proved the new member's willingness to be a part of the brotherhood while yielding plenty of humorous stories of drunken stupidity.

That night, however, something had gone terribly wrong. At 12:12 a.m., Boston police, fire, and emergency medical officers swarmed the room of freshman, Scott Krueger, who lay unconscious and unresponsive amid fresh vomit and empty alcohol bottles in his basement room of the fraternity house. Scott's blood alcohol concentration, or BAC, was .410—more than four times the legal limit for drivers in most states. Krueger remained in a coma until he died late Monday, September 29th. He was 18 years old.

The local fraternity chapter, charged with manslaughter, disbanded in order to avoid criminal prosecution. MIT settled with Krueger's parents for $6 million dollars to avoid a wrongful death lawsuit for a much higher amount. A second lawsuit against the International Fraternity of Phi Gamma Delta was settled for more than $3 million dollars, and the promise to produce an educational video using Scott's story as a warning against binge drinking. New policies and programs were instituted at the prestigious university on nearly every aspect of student life, which for all students entering the gates of MIT or the staff hired to care for them would never be the same.

No active member of the fraternity could have imagined the impact of the stories that would be told not by half-drunken brothers in late-night recollections with their friends, but by the media and by health officials who shared the story of the MIT student from Orchard Park, New York, often and with a clear agenda in mind. Krueger's death would be retold for another 4 years in the national media and in popular books, used as an example whenever the subject of college drinking emerged.

The use of the "death story" to build the case for a public health problem, however, is nothing new. Tragic stories are often used to illustrate the personal impact of social problems or to assist in the adoption of policy solutions to problems (Carstairs, 1998; Joseph & Kearns, 1999). Ibarra and Kitsuse (1993) contend that the claims-making process—a critical element in the construction of social problems—accepts "as given and beginning with the participants' descriptions of the putative conditions and their assertions about their problematic character" (p. 24). Such stories assist in the construction of the "victims" and "villains" of problems (Loseke, 1999, p. 75), yet most theorists contend that in order for a social problem to be institutionalized, it must be perceived as "widespread" (p. 6), forcing claims to be grounded in statistically significant trends of a entire population and not necessarily on the personal experiences of those who have actually lived the problem firsthand (Best, 1995; Gusfield, 1996; Holstein & Miller, 1993; Ibarra & Kitsuse, 1993). Because of the need for broad-based data in legitimizing social problems, theoretically grounded analytical criteria for the use of narratives in problem construction are limited.

For those of us working in student affairs at colleges and universities in the United States, the use of the death story to represent the complex problem of heavy episodic drinking in college was both a blessing and a curse. Although the constant retelling of the death story raised the level of awareness and interest in the problem from administration, parents, and the general public, it also concretized a public-health frame for the issue that would characterize all efforts at problem reduction as "neoprohibitionist" (Gusfield, 1996; D. J. Hansen, 1995). Within this frame, college drinkers—particularly those in fraternities—became criminals or victims. Neither label would prove to be sufficient for those trying to help young adults take on the promises and perils of "adulthood" in the United States.

In this chapter, I explore the theoretical basis of narratives in social-problem construction and suggest that an effective tool for analyzing their use can be found in the notion of the "representative anecdote" (Burke, 1969). From this perspective, I examine the use of death stories, including the death of Scott Krueger, in the construction of the collegiate "binge-drinking" problem in the United States. I end the chapter with theoretical and practical implications of the death story and the use of Burke's representative anecdote as a methodology for future study.

## NARRATIVES IN SOCIAL-PROBLEM CONSTRUCTION

### Narratives as Moral Reasons

In his 1996 text, *Contested Meanings*, Gusfield wrote:

> As a rhetorical device, the concept of "social problem" is a claim that some condition, set of events, or group of persons constitutes a troublesome situation that needs to be changed or ameliorated. Those who define the problem do so from a standard which involves them in the role of legitimate spokespersons for the society or public interest. Having defined the condition as a "social problem" there is then a legitimate basis for bringing public resources to bear on it in the manner defined. (p. 17)

As Gusfield implies, the "naming" of the problem is a critical first step in the reduction of a condition to a single resonant term. Narratives serve as terminology in action, a symbolic system that, as Searle (1995) suggests, "*mean* something or express something or represent or symbolize something beyond themselves, *in a way that is publicly understandable*" (p. 60, italics in original). Although "putative conditions" must be widespread to justify the use of significant resources, a dramatic example is essential to both capture public attention and to serve as a living definition of the problem's terminology, especially when told through the news media. As Best (1995) suggested,

> Beginning with a dramatic example is a standard technique in newsmagazine cover stories, television news feature stories, and newspaper articles. Because we encounter them first, and because they are vivid, these examples play an important role in typifying social problems. Examples shape our sense of just what is the problem, of what needs to be done about it. (pp. 14–15)

Narratives have long been studied for their rhetorical value. Fisher (1984) contended "Language action is meaningful only in terms of narrative form" (p. 7). Lucaites and Condit (1985) suggested that narrative "represents a universal medium of human consciousness" (p. 90) that, McGee and Nelson (1985) argued "is supposed to persuade: it alleges *facts*, and it aims no higher than *plausibility*" (p. 149, italics in original). In social-problem construction, the tragic story both defines terms and legitimizes claims of ill in ways that quantitative data cannot match.

Such theory suggests, then, that the choice of story told to demonstrate the existence of a condition plays a critical role in the construction of social problems. The story must be dramatic enough to rivet the attention of the public, and compelling enough to open the pocketbooks of institutional-funding sources. Most importantly, however, the story itself must provide a linguistic "snapshot" of the problem; it must serve as the definition and illustration of the terminology used to describe the condition in public discourse. Gusfield (1996) added, "The concept of 'social problem,' as an aspect of our language, in turn implies a general framework" (p. 35).

In essence, narratives used to illustrate social problems serve as both a representation and a reduction of the problem that simplifies our understanding of the problem into a single human drama. Ibarra and Kitsuse (1993) described this rhetorical device as "motifs" that "operate as shorthand descriptions/evaluations of condition categories" (p. 31). Ibarra and Kitsuse make the point, however, that these devices do not document the existence or magnitude of the problem. Instead, they offer moral reasoning; motifs provide a "moral vocabulary" from which the public can speak about the problem from within a set of cultural values.

## The Representative Anecdote

Burke (1969) identified this rhetorical shorthand as the "representative anecdote":

> And we thereupon begin to ask ourselves: What would be "the ultimate act," or "the most complete act?" That is, what would be the "pure" act, an act so thoroughly an act that it could be considered the form or prototype of all acts? (p. 61, italics in orginal)

The "prototype act," as Burke suggests, speaks for all acts that live within the category created by the terminology. As such, it both represents the vocabulary by putting an "action" to the term, while also reducing the problem to a single action. Harter and Japp (2001) argued that a representative anecdote "establishes parameters, norms and hierarchies while developing and reinforcing language and other symbol systems that will operate within its boundaries" (p. 413). In social-problem construction, the representative anecdote becomes far more than a metanarrative or dominant story, it serves as the essence of the social problem's label and pervades the discourse of the problem in both spoken and unspoken terms. As the essence of the problem, the representative anecdote serves to motivate us toward resolution as a moral obligation.

Using the representative anecdote as an analytical tool enables the critic to view the discourse through a specific lens or template in order to "sum up the essence of a culture's values, concerns, and interests in regard to some real life issues or problems" (Brummett, 1984, p. 164). Identifying the representative anecdote "allows critics to go beyond surface narratives or scripts and tap into deeper, more implicit themes that shape the discourse" (Harter & Japp, 2001, p. 413). Ibarra and Kitsuse (1993) argued that such analysis yields a depth of insight beyond conventional constructionist studies of social problems discourse by "providing a framework for discerning patterns in phenomena that appear 'from the outside' to be incoherent and in a constant state of flux, even as participants assert their claims to be intelligible concerns about conditions" (p. 30).

A cursory glance throughout the popular media indicates that college "binge" drinking has captured public attention as well as a significant amount of public-health resources. But was that interest sparked by the use of a representative anecdote, and if so, what master narrative emerged as a reduction for the entire college-drinking problem? What would enable the death story to resonate among policy- makers, public-health officials, and the public? How important is a death story to solving the college-drinking problem?

## NARRATIVE USE IN THE CONSTRUCTION OF THE COLLEGE-DRINKING PROBLEM

### Methodology

I obtained discourse for analysis through a general search of all major media coverage of "college binge drinking" from 1997 until 2003. Media outlets included city and college newspapers, national television news reports, and television news programs.

I used content analysis to collect case narratives within media reports. I separated stories of a specific college student who died from alcohol from stories that identified college drinking as a problem using general statistics. Media reports that exclusively covered the death of a student were used only as secondary sources for fact verification. The media reports had to focus on the college binge-drinking problem and use the death as an example.

Once collected, I categorized the stories by student name and length of narrative. I distinguished discourse that simply mentioned the death of a student from discourse that used the story of the student at length to illustrate the harms of alcohol abuse. I then identified descriptions from those collected stories by associational clusters (Burke, 1973), a form of semiotic analysis that connects commonly used terms within the text in search of a common language that suggests "the predominance of certain cultural values" (Heinz & Lee, 1998, p. 89).[1]

Following the analysis, I conducted a second search for "death" stories throughout prevention literature created specifically for college audiences (students, staff, and administrators). Discourse analyzed included reports, journals, books, Web sites and pamphlets that were nationally distributed to college prevention/student affairs professionals. A similar methodology was used to determine if (a) similar narratives "crossed over" from media to these materials, and (b) if associational clusters emerged in a similar form from media reports.

## RESULTS

### Results of Content Analysis

In both the national media and the college alcohol-prevention field, the story of Scott Krueger, the freshman at MIT who died of alcohol poisoning, became the most commonly used narrative to illustrate the collegiate binge-drinking problem in America. Well over 700 articles between the years of 1997 and 2001 in periodicals ranging from *Newsweek, USA Today, New York Newsday*, the *Boston Globe*, and the *Kansas City Star*, to the *Lincoln Journal-Star*, the (Riverside, California) *Press-Enterprise*, or the (Dubuque, Iowa) *Telegraph Herald*, along with television news programs, *20/20, Dateline NBC*, and *48 Hours*, included the story of Scott Krueger's death in their coverage of the "binge-drinking" problem. Second only to the use of the Scott Krueger story was the story of Louisiana State University student, Benjamin Wynn, who died just a month earlier. Wynn's death also occurred within a fraternity setting, and the story shared similar aspects of fraternity hazing, alcohol abuse, and coercion. Often, articles referred to both the Krueger and Wynn stories.

Most media news depictions linked the Krueger story as part of their coverage of national studies done by Harvard University School of Public Health showing that 40% of college students engaged in *binge drink-*

*ing*, a term they would define as consuming five or more drinks in a row for males or four or more in a row for females. Harvard's lead researcher, Henry Wechsler, capitalized on the media's association of student death using his *binge* label. Though the data from the Harvard study never measured the number of deaths of college students due to binge drinking, or quantified the level of risk for death based on the binge-drinking measure, reporters commonly used death stories as illustrations of the collegiate binge-drinking problem. *Newsweek* (McCormick & Kalb, 1998, June 15), raised the problem in an article titled "Dying for a Drink." Another *Newsweek* article on September 25, 2000, combined the Wechsler study with Kreuger's death in an article entitled "Colleges—Drinking and Dying." An ABC Newsmagazine *20/20* story on binge drinking also featured the deaths of Krueger, Wynn, and several other college students, complete with a quote from Wechsler that would serve as the story's title: "Fraternities Are Drowning in a Sea of Alcohol." The story became repackaged and broadcast a total of four times between 1998 and 1999. Other news programs, including *Nightline, Good Morning America, 48 Hours,* and *Dateline NBC* ran similar stories that combined the Harvard study data with stories of alcohol-related college student deaths.

Although the national media's use of Scott Krueger as an illustration became less common after 2001, the college alcohol prevention field included the Krueger story in educational materials well into 2003 as the ultimate example of harm from excessive alcohol consumption. Universities and fraternal organizations regularly show the videotape produced by the International Fraternity of Phi Gamma Delta, which was created as a condition of their lawsuit settlement with the Kruegers, to new students, administrators, alumni, and Greek leaders, keeping Scott's story alive on campuses across the nation (Watt & Schuermann, 2002).

The association can also be found in a variety of research and scientific documents. The 1999 Educational Resources Information Center (ERIC) *Digest on Binge Drinking*, a summary of research on the subject, begins as well with the Krueger story (Kellog, 1999). Wechsler himself named his own (2002) book on the subject, *Dying to Drink: Confronting Binge Drinking on College Campuses*, including Krueger's story in the text as the ultimate example of harm.

The death anecdote also extended beyond the specific story of Scott Krueger, using more recent alcohol-related student deaths as the narrative illustration of the binge drinking problem. Later media stories highlighted the deaths of college students due to birthday celebrations (McGinn, 2000, November 27) and spring break excesses (Norris, 2002b). In each new illustration, the death story served as the representative anecdote, defining college drinking as a deadly act that robbed America of its future.

No other death story, however, received the media attention or recurrent telling as often or as completely as the Scott Krueger story. The drama of Scott Krueger's death serves as the ultimate illustration of the collegiate binge-drinking problem. More than a common illustration, aspects of the story constitute the representative anecdote for collegiate binge drinking.

Symbolically, the alignment of the Krueger story to the *binge-drinking* label intertwined the meanings of each to the other; "death" emerged as the assumed outcome of fraternal binge drinking, and all of fraternal binge drinking's harms were reduced to "death." The death of Krueger represents the potential death of all college students. In other words, the single death represents the whole problem rather than an isolated incident.

## Identification Within the Representative Anecdote

The title of ABC's *20/20* story broadcast on August 1, 1999—nearly 2 years after Krueger's death—sums up the representative anecdote best: "Why Did Scott Die? Binge Drinking—A Life Cut Short." A better question might be: Why did Scott Krueger's death story play so well in the discourse surrounding binge drinking?

Several answers emerge. Burke (1984) suggested "A well-rounded frame serves as an amplifying device" (p. 103). Scott Krueger fits within a set of expectations that many Americans have about college students. Scott's portrait in many media accounts shows him to be a vibrant, intelligent young man with a strong background and bright future. The media depicted him as typical of all first-year college students—bright, naive, and vulnerable. Burke (1973) defined this as "identification," where an audience finds familiarity with an element of the drama and, by doing so, draws personal meaning from the actor, act, agency or setting.[2]

In essence, Scott Krueger became our "reflection in the social mirror" (Burke, 1973, p. 227). In this MIT student, we frame all of our understandings of the hopes and dreams that surround a young man attending a premiere academic institution, making the loss more symbolically profound. Scott fits our understanding of college life, particularly within the fraternity, and amplifies our assumptions about the innocence (and folly) of youth, the privilege and pressure of achievement, and the dangers of growing up.

Yet the frame also amplifies our sense of social problems. Gusfield (1996) labeled the current period of alcohol prevention as existing

within the "public health" frame. In this frame, an important signification occurs where *morbidity* represents *responsibility*. In other
words, the story enables us to identify several characters in the
drama—the victim and the villian.

## Constructing the Victim and Villian

The first is the signification of the college student who died from alcohol abuse as the "victim." Media storytelling about Krueger's death
would show pictures of Scott with his family, and would depict the
young man's association to the fraternity as a housing necessity; the
ABC *20/20* report suggested that Scott joined Fiji because the Fiji
house offered an inexpensive place to live, not because he saw in the
men and their parties something attractive. Richard M. Schwartzstein,
M.D., the attending physician for Krueger at the time of his death, presents Krueger in a guest column for *The Wellesley Townsman* as hesitant and apprehensive, as if the evening 6 weeks into the semester
where alcohol is present is a sudden surprise: "There will be a fraternity party that evening and Scott has heard that the freshmen will be
forced to drink a large quantity of alcohol. He is apprehensive. He did
not drink in high school" (June 29, 1998, web archive).

Representing the death story as victimage adds an important element to the construction. If the fault for the tragic ending can be placed
outside of the victim's control, then external control must be provided
to protect the potential victim. As Burke (1970) suggested, the tragic
frame, in this case created by the representative anecdote, calls for a
sacrifice of atonement to complete the correction. MIT's solution—tougher policies, increased enforcement, limited choices for
freshmen—mirrored the "crackdown" framework that permeated colleges and universities attempting to save future victims. The President
of MIT, Charles M. Vest (1997), issued a statement on Tuesday, September 30 that also concretizes the "victim" frame:

> The death of Scott Krueger, a bright and talented young man, is a terrible
> tragedy ... For Scott's fellow students, and the faculty and staff who had
> come to know him, this is a dreadful loss as well, and the MIT commu-
> nity will do all that we can to see that this kind of tragedy never happens
> here again. (web archive)

As the aforementioned quotation suggests, the Krueger story added
another level of reduction in the anecdote. As an MIT student, Krueger
symbolized our romantic views about college students—particularly at
a premier institution—as "America's best and brightest" and "America's future." Such national treasures must be carefully protected,

which is why initial media coverage of the issue condemned college administrators for ignoring their responsibility as surrogate parents. Universities have long maintained a tension surrounding the expression *in loco parentis*, the relegation of parental responsibilities to college administrators that, despite the significant changes that occurred around "student rights" in the 1960s and 1970s, still clearly lives symbolically in the United States:

> The death of two students which occurred during drinking parties in 1949, and a third incident that year in which a student almost died while being initiated into a drinking club, stirred sharp condemnation of college administrators. Under the headline "Drinking Blame Put on College Rulers," the *New York Times* quoted the head of an intercollegiate fraternal organization as condemning irresolute college administrators for condoning much of the excessive drinking and moral laxity revealed on college campuses. (Strauss & Bacon, 1953, p. 38)

The story did not differ much in 2000, when *ABC News* of September 18 reported MIT's $6 million dollar settlement with the Kruegers as an admission that "inadequate alcohol and housing policies were partly to blame for the tragedy" (Durand, 2000). The message of the news item reified the association of college administrators as caretakers who, entrusted with America's vulnerable youth, should offer protection from lurking villains—even when the villains were, in this case, students as well. ABC News quoted Joel Epstein, a staff attorney for the Higher Education Center for Alcohol and Other Drug Prevention, as saying, "Increasingly, we are seeing a growing number of cases where courts, judges, lawyers and parents are saying this is absolutely outrageous we didn't know that there was this level of drinking—that it was this dangerous" (Durand, 2000).

The second symbolic bridge surrounds the construction of the "villain" in the representative anecdote, completing the *morbidity as responsibility* signification of the public-health frame. The Krueger story was sustained in the media largely because of its drama, as public health officials argued over who was most responsible for the tragedy. Criminal charges, lawsuits, and punitive actions shifted from the fraternity, to the university, to the environment, to students themselves. Harvard's research on binge drinking identifies multiple villains as ultimately "responsible" for the problem, from the alcohol industry to Greek organizations (Wechsler, Dowdall, Davenport, & DeJong, 1993, 1994; Wechsler, Dowdall, Maener, Gledhill-Hoyt, & Lee, 1998; Wechsler et al., 1999). The strategies recommended by Wechsler to reduce collegiate binge drinking—most of which follow a "control-of-consumption" framework (Hansen, 1995) that criminalizes both marketing and consumption of alcohol—fit well within this frame, and played well as responses to the Krueger story. Media tended to highlight singular solutions to the complex problem, despite existing alternative strategies that were given less public hearing and only found utilization following a more comprehensive task force report in 2001 on college drinking published by the National Institute for Alcoholism and Alcohol Abuse (NIAAA). An editorial in the *Milwaukee Journal Sentinel* begins: "Conventional wisdom teaches that college students drink and that there's not much their elders can do about it. Therefore, while deaths related to binge drinking, including two in Wisconsin this year, are tragic, these things happen. Conventional wisdom may be wrong" (p. 22).

*New York Newsday*, in a two part series on the issue, wrote, "The mounting death toll has rocked college campuses nationwide, prompting calls for alcohol bans and crackdowns on campus drinking and fraternity hazing rituals, initiation rites that sometimes include alcohol consumption" (Perlman, December 1, 1997, A23). A *USA Today* article (Marhlein, 1997, October) outlines the "new efforts" taken by college administrators as facilitating a ban on alcohol at university, fraternity, or dormitory functions. The *Boston Globe* (October 19, 1997) incorporates several of these terms when they wrote:

> Calls for an alcohol ban at Bridgewater State College, which began last May in response to an alcohol-fueled riot, have grown louder after a rape in a freshman dorm last month and recent alcohol-related deaths of students at the Massachusetts Institute of Technology and the University of Massachusetts at Amherst. State college and university officials across the state are under added pressure to crack down on underage and binge drinking after the state Board of Higher Education last week officially urged the institutions to adopt tough restrictions on alcohol use on campus. (p. 1)

In the Krueger story, however, and in much of the press coverage surrounding the Harvard research, the fraternity takes the blame as the ultimate villain of the binge-drinking problem. A string of studies indicate that members of male fraternal organizations drink excessively and engage in morally unacceptable behavior as a result of their consumption more than their non-Greek peers (Cashin, Presley, & Meilman, 1998; Friend, 1993; L. Goodwin, 1989; Wechsler et al., 1993, 1994, 1998), a fact consistently included in media reports on the topic of college drinking. Wechsler's "public" writing on the subject of binge drinking suggested that the fraternity system itself should be restructured, prohibiting college freshman from joining. "College and university fraternities," he and his colleagues wrote, "often bring few of the benefits they promise and cause more problems than they admit" (Wechsler, Kuh, & Davenport, 1996). Television programs such as

*20/20* and *48 Hours* focused segments exclusively on the fraternity as the center of the binge-drinking problem, limiting images and narratives of fraternal life to those that included intoxication, wild behavior, and irresponsibility. Moreover, the media spotlighted stories of young men who were "victimized" by peer pressure to drink heavily as a new member of the fraternity. The Krueger story, in painting a villain, ultimately tags the fraternal system as the culprit for Scott's death.

Not surprisingly, then, the fraternity has been the site of most control-based attempts to address the collegiate binge-drinking problem and is singled out above athletes or any other collegiate high-risk group for policies and other controls. The *USA Today* (Marhlein, 1997) of October 22, 1997 wrote:

> Alcohol abuse is the primary culprit, and campus-based education programs have been the norm. But with recent studies suggesting that binge drinking in college is often most likely to occur among fraternity and sorority members, some administrators are focusing new efforts on Greek Row. (p. 5D)

As a result of the construction, fraternal organizations across the country faced sanctions, disciplinary action, suspension, and lawsuits similar to Fiji whenever student drinking concludes with even the threat of harm. Many instituted "alcohol free" housing policies as a way to appease university administrators and parents (Russo, 1998). Yet, the association between death drinking and fraternity life is sealed. A letter to the editor by a fellow MIT student in the student newspaper *The Tech* (Cohen, 1997) of September 30, 1997, makes the point most eloquently when she writes, "Scott S. Krueger '01 and Fiji are now the names by which issues of under-age drinking and fraternity life at MIT will be discussed by students, administrators, and faculty members" (p. 4).

## DISCUSSION

### Socioecononic Class in the Representative Anecdote

Rhetors employing social problem constructions, however, rarely direct their efforts to students and faculty members, but to policymakers, who have significantly more political or financial power to enact changes or provide resources (Bridgman & Barry, 2002; Carstairs, 1998; Joseph & Kearns, 1999; Sharf, 2001). Evidence of the story's success in generating such resources confirms the fact that those in positions of authority identified with the story of Krueger's death. The American Medical Association and other national organizations labeled alcohol abuse as the number one health risk to college students (Delaney, 1998). University administrators are not shying away from the task at hand; the Network, a national organization of colleges and universities begun in 1987 by U.S. Department of Education to support alcohol, drug, and violence programs, now has over 1,400 members nationwide. Considering that college administrators, public-health foundations, and community leaders were the primary audience for the death story (along with the media-consuming public who adopted these cultural authorities), however, raises additional issues in the use of the Krueger story as representative anecdote.

It would be an easy guess that Krueger was not the only student getting drunk in America on the evening of Friday, September 26th, 1997. He was, however, the only one from a prominent institution of higher education recorded as having died that night because of it. The Scott Krueger/MIT story, though no less striking in its tragic waste of a young life, received far more references than the Benjamin Wynn/LSU story. MIT's very public response to the incident, involving significant policy changes across the institution, was far more overt than at Louisiana State, which received no national media coverage of its efforts to avoid future deaths.

Certainly, the identification of "college life" to Ivy League (rather than to a state institution) may have played best with prominent policymakers, those who most likely had similar backgrounds or privileges. Yet, it also may represent an important hierarchy within the United States that divides college students, like the rest of the population, into socioeconomic classes and places greater value on the lives of those in upper classes as opposed to those perceived to be in lower classes. In the bluntest of terms, the loss of a student at a private prominent institution may be a greater loss than that of a student at a public state institution. We, as a culture, expected great things from the MIT student, and assumed that great things were required to admit him into the institution.

Moreover, the use of the Kreuger story identifies binge drinking as a social problem unique to the college setting. No current funding exists for prevention programs to reduce binge drinking to young adults who are not currently enrolled in college. Would Scott's death from alcohol poisoning have become a national anecdote if he were not enrolled at a university—any university—and was simply out drinking with several other working friends who encouraged him to drink too much, too fast? Perhaps the resonance of the college-death story represents our collective value for higher education, where the university symbolizes our incubator for citizens of greater value who require special resources. Certainly, the sheer volume of media coverage of the college alcohol problem suggests that the lives of college students are privileged above other populations, and that the death of a college student represents a social loss that is greater than the loss of other members of society.

## Limits to the Death Story as Representative Anecdote

Several limitations to the use of the death story as the representative anecdote emerge and are worthy of note. Fisher (1987) suggested that stories that serve as "good reasons" for moral action must have fidelity, which occurs when the values of the story are "confirmed or validated in one's personal experience, in the lives or statements of others whom one admires and respects, and in a conception of the best audience that one can conceive" (p. 109). The representative anecdote for binge drinking, however, reduces all collegiate alcohol consumption as ending in death. This leads us to the first problem of the anecdote: Not everyone who drinks to Harvard's "binge" measure dies. Even the best estimates on college student deaths from alcohol use, published by the National Institute for Alcoholism and Alcohol Abuse (NIAAA) placed the number at 1,400 annually (Norris, 2002a). This number represents a dramatically small percentage of the students currently enrolled in U.S. colleges and universities, and is barely a significant percentage of some of the nation's largest campuses. Yet, a lack of strong statistical evidence of social harm may drive the use of the representative anecdote; when the sheer quantity of death lacks persuasiveness, the rhetoric may be more inclined to focus on the quality of the deaths.

Narrative fidelity also suggests that the storyteller has an ethos that assists in the development of the story's moral resonance. If the storyteller serves as a mouthpiece of the public health institution, then the culture may more likely reject the claims as carrying a nonresonant morality; it assumes another agenda. Controversy surrounding Wechsler's assertions have overwhelmed alcohol prevention in higher education. National fraternity leaders joke informally about Wechsler as having a personal grudge against Greek life. Students reject the binge-drinking label entirely (Workman, 2001a). Wechsler's book on college binge drinking, though treated as a "call to arms" by public health officials, received negative reviews and responses by several prominent practitioners in college alcohol prevention.

An ongoing battle over Wechsler's description of the problem continues to play itself out in prevention conferences and journals (Chapman, 2003). A town hall meeting held at the Department of Education's 17th Annual National Meeting on Alcohol and Other Drug Abuse and Violence Prevention in Higher Education focused exclusively on the terminology of the field, as researchers and practitioners argued about how the *binge drinking* label has helped or hindered problem abatement (Lucey, 2003). The American Medical Association's "A Matter of Degree" Program purposely uses the term *high-risk* rather than *binge* drinking in its title, as do a number of programs across the country.

Although funding was dedicated and a host of activities have been initiated in campus-communities across the nation to address the problem, Wechsler's own studies from 1993 to 2001 have concluded that little, if any, actual reduction has occurred in the binge drinking of college students (Wechsler et al., 2002). Taken together, these events suggest that, although the death story as representative anecdote clearly played a role in establishing the problem symbolically, the ethos of its storyteller and the lack of narrative fidelity explain why the anecdote has had little impact in sustaining the construction of the social problem or establishing a clear path for the adoption of solutions.

### The Death Story as Prevention Tool

Even though social problem theory never suggests the use of problem rhetoric for the purpose of actual behavior change, the death story has been employed countless times by social marketing campaigns and prevention materials targeted to students to reduce their alcohol consumption, such as the video presentation created by Phi Gamma Delta and a recent advertisement placed in college newspapers warning students of medical catastrophe should they engage in binge drinking on spring break (Associated Press, March 8, 2004). Narrative fidelity may also explain why, in the case of collegiate binge drinking, the use of the death story as a preventative tool is ill-advised.

The students at my university never tell the Scott Krueger story; no similar death story exists to "localize" the anecdote, yet I doubt that such a story would emerge in peer-to-peer storytelling even if it did. My own study of fraternity drinking stories found that students never shared tragic stories with each other, opting instead to tell only those stories about drunkenness that were ultimately inconsequential (Workman, 2001a). Stories of drinking events told by students incorporate themes of adventure, risk-taking, personal discovery, and drunkenness as entertainment—stories of survival, of mutual assistance and caretaking that avoids tragedy and enhances social standing. They contrast directly to the death story, and as such, serve as a barrier to the use of the death story as a motivation for personal change (Workman, 2001b).

On a broader scale, the stories communicated by a cultural authority, the media, or even peers never occur within a vacuum, but exist within the larger intertextual terrain, complete with a wide range of counternarratives and competing significations. Death stories are far from the representative anecdote for alcohol consumption provided by the alcohol industry and popular culture, which signifies alcohol consumption as a socially enhancing, gender-defining, and nonconsequential form of play (Workman, 2001b). No beer commercial ends with a funeral. Scenes of emergency rooms working full throttle to reverse alcohol poisoning have yet to make the many television shows, films, and music videos that incorporate college drinking into their stories. Like personal narratives about drinking shared by college students, "drinking" stories depicted in mediated popular culture rarely, if ever, incorporate the death story. Opposing stories, where the consequences of intoxication are far from tragic, abound within the culture, producing a counterrhetoric that limits the fidelity of the story.

In order for the representative anecdote to be used effectively as a prevention tool, it must be more than personally resonant to a specific audience. It must also be "intertextually resonant" within culture, existing in strands throughout the discourse. In the case of death as the representative anecdote for collegiate binge drinking, the signification drowns in its own sea of narratives that weaken the signification and ultimately, the ability of the construction to solve the social problem. Burke (1969) summed the issue best when he stated:

> If the originating anecdote is not representative, a vocabulary developed in strict conformity with it will not be representative. This embarrassment is usually avoided in practice by a break in the conformity at some crucial point; this means in effect that the vocabulary ceases to have the basis which is claimed for it. (p. 59)

For this reason, many of us working daily in collegiate alcohol-abuse prevention have focused away from death as the representative anecdote, concentrating on harms that are more salient to the stories that circulate throughout the culture such as embarrassment, regret, academic failure, or legal liability. Also growing in popularity is an entirely different approach characterized as *social norming*, which tells a positive story of student behavior by citing the prevalence of moderation among campus populations (Perkins, 2003). Under this very different frame, the death story serves as contrast rather than as representation. Scott Krueger's consumption, and rituals like the one at Fiji's "Animal House Night," differ sharply from the kind of drinking experienced by most students. Yet, using "normal" as the representative anecdote for college drinking has its intertextual resonation problems as well. Students with heavy episodic consumption patterns are equally likely to reject stories of moderation, especially when excessive consumption permeates popular culture.

## Theoretical Implications and Future Study

The successful use of the death story to elicit action and resources from public health institutions suggests that narratives play a key role in the construction of social problems, but much less in the prevention of those problems. More study is needed, however, to determine the scope of narrative use across complex health issues. Future research could determine if the death story is used as a representative anecdote in other social problems, particularly those that lack sufficient statistical evidence to establish harm.

Certainly, this analysis suggests that the identification of the victim as valuable to society, particularly in light of social hierarchy, is critical to the rhetorical success of the death story. This need for identification may possibly explain why other public health problems such as AIDS and tuberculosis have had less public support despite significantly higher mortality rates, or why the most significant story to impact the AIDS crisis involved Ryan White, a young hemophiliac boy who contracted the disease through a transfusion rather than a homosexual man or IV drug user. Like Krueger, White represents the perfect victim of a villainous disease rather than the villain who receives his due for his sins. In the same way, the story of an indigent who died from hypothermia may never carry the same rhetorical weight as a prominent actress who dies of ovarian cancer.

Another task is to determine the typology of narratives used in the construction of social problems. Are death stories the only genre than can be used to elicit action or resources, or are there other "putative conditions" (Ibarra & Kitsuse, 1993) that can serve as representative anecdotes of social problems? Although the social problem of excessive alcohol use has many potential harms ranging from the destruction of property to sexual assault (both of which occur at a much greater frequency than death), the death story remains the central anecdote for the problem. Tracing the stories used in other social problems may yield a broader set of narrative forms.

This analysis also suggests that Burke's (1969) theory of representative anecdote serves as an excellent analytical tool to examine the use of narratives within social-problem constructions. Accepting that stories serve as representations and reductions of reality provides a firm foundation for deeper analysis of the symbolic bridges forged within the anecdote. The methodology enables critics to explore issues of hierarchy in the formation of social problems, an element that is often missing in social-problem theory. Burke's notion of identification forces the analysis to explore the role of social hierarchy in the determination of which problems receive resources and which do not.

Perhaps the most important implication of this analysis is the distinction between the rhetoric needed for social-problem construction and social-problem alleviation. For practitioners, the rhetorical strategies needed to obtain resources and establish environmental policies might employ stories that are resonant only with policymakers, and will have little or no effect on changing the attitudes, beliefs or behaviors of college drinkers. Affected populations may not identify themselves with the representation of the victim or the death anecdote, particularly when the representative anecdote conflicts with stories across the cultural terrain. This finding suggests that rhetorical strategies employed to construct problems and raise resources must be separated from those designed to change behaviors. Given the intertextual nature of public discourse, however, message separation may be little more than a pipe dream. Practitioners benefiting from the resources gained by the death story must also distinguish themselves from the anecdote in order to find identification from those they seek to change.

For those of us working in college alcohol prevention on a daily basis, the story of MIT student, Scott Krueger, was a sad reminder that, when unchecked, alcohol abuse can and does raise itself to a life-or-death issue. As a representative anecdote, the death story assisted the Harvard School of Public Health and others in constructing college binge drinking as a significant social problem that deserved attention and resources in the United States. Yet, this very fact raises significant questions about the social hierarchy that privileges some death stories over others. In a culture where texts intertwine constantly, the death story does not live alone; it is surrounded by the many, many stories of intoxication that brought pleasure rather than pain and social life rather than physical death. As is true throughout the intertextual terrain, the existence of opposing stories creates a tension that ultimately limits the abilities of those attempting to solve the problem.

## NOTES

1. A complete description of associational clusters can be found in Burke (1973). Examples of the use of associational clusters as a semiotic method of analysis can be found in Heinz and Lee (1998), and Workman (2001a).
2. A complete discussion of identification can be found in Burke (1973).

# 7

## State-Induced Illness and Forbidden Stories: The Role of Storytelling in Healing Individual and Social Traumas in Romania[1]

ɶ

**Teodora Carabas**
**Lynn M. Harter**
*Ohio University*

> The struggle of man against power is the struggle of memory against forgetting.
>                                        —Kundera, 1981, p. 4

Collecting testimonies of past oppression, social struggle, and political disempowerment is a relatively new line of research in Eastern Europe (Harvey, 2000; *Analele Sighet* [the Sighet Files], 1995) and a significant area of study across academic disciplines (see, e.g., Cronon, 1992; Garro & Mattingly, 2000; Gugelberger, 1996). In the former communist countries of Eastern and Central Europe, most narratives of oppression emerged publicly after 1989, following the transition of Eastern and Central European regions from totalitarian to pluralistic societies. This chapter examines 53 published testimonies of oppression and 9 in-depth interviews with former political prisoners and deportees. The testimonies were given after 1990 by Romanian citizens of different ethnicities, individuals directly oppressed by the communist regime during the late 1940s, the 1950s, and early 1960s, and coerced—until December 1989—to conceal their suffering under penalty of additional incarceration or persecution.[2]

Throughout this chapter, we discuss, first, the ways in which illness becomes a tool for political oppression when inflicted by the state upon the undesirable bodies of political resistors. Second, we examine the degenerative role that the censoring of storytelling about state-inflicted illness plays in the lives of people who suffered horrendous physical and psychological traumas. We understand state-inflicted illness to be the physical, psychological, and social affliction that results from the violence of incarceration, torture, forced labor, deportation, clandestine living, economic deprivation, as well as from varied discriminatory practices that a state adopts against marginalized people (e.g., those who engage in acts of political opposition). The suffering that emerges from state-induced political violence includes a host of traumas—from pain, anguish, fear, loss, and grief, to the destruction of a lucid and meaningful reality (Kleinman, 1995). In the case of Romania, state-inflicted illness was induced physically and psychologically (i.e., the bodies and psyches of political resistors became incapacitated) as well as socially and symbolically (i.e., state-induced illness vilified the presence of those who bore its marks and transformed these citizens and their families into pariahs within their communities).

In cases when the state also censors the stories of induced illness, a community's sense of identity suffers damage; as a result, state-inflicted illness is manifested both at individual and community levels. State-induced illness serves to discipline the bodies of those it persecutes and erases their voices from the public space, thus ensuring the entire community's silence (Foucault, 1975, 1995). Consequently, state-induced illness functions as a docilizing mechanism that excludes already marginalized groups and individuals, secures the physical and symbolic thwarting of political resistance, and maintains the state's ability to punish its citizens. For these reasons, the consequences of state-induced illness are political.

The act of censoring narratives about state-caused illness—what we call "forbidden stories"—increases the psychological trauma of persecuted people and augments the stigma attached to their bodies. We use the concept of *stigma* as developed by Goffman (1963) to point out the ways in which state-induced illness restructures social relations by configuring outsiders and others and imposing these characterizations on diseased individuals. As a stigmatizing process, state-inflicted illness defines and labels specific groups as *undesirable, unproductive, dysfunctional,* and *potentially dangerous* (Goffman, 1963), and (re)produces the differential acceptability of various groups. The process of labeling (e.g., the *resistor* label) is a powerful rhetorical lever that can be simultaneously considered a genesis to and outcome of stigmatization. Classic conceptualizations proffer that stigmatization results in the devaluation of individuals and groups in society (e.g., Goffman, 1963; Katz, 1981). More than a mere indicator of certain attributes, stigma should be seen as "a language of relationships" (Goffman, 1963, p. 3) that emerges in the day-to-day activities of agents. Shame, embarrassment, and distrust evolve through the process of *othering* that stigmatization performs, and are embodied in people's life narratives.

What we identify as state-inflicted illness and forbidden stories are not unique to the Romanian context. Kleinman (1995) asserted, "Political violence carries the most ancient provenance. Wars, executions, and torture have been the authorized forms of asserting state power throughout the historical record" (p. 173). Every power structure neglects, deprives, and silences marginalized populations. Although individuals may not always be physically incarcerated or tortured, they are victims of state-induced neglect at best, and destructive politics at worst. Certainly, Western history indicates that the potential to harm the health of citizens exists in all political structures. For example, the Tuskegee Syphilis Experiment consisted of a 40-year study of untreated syphilis among African American men sponsored, in large part, by the United States Public Health System (Harter, Stephens, & Japp, 2000; Solomon, 1985). Notably, such stories have been suppressed in this case as well, at least in earlier sanitized versions of our history books, with disastrous consequences for the individuals affected (and/or their descendants) and the entire society (Jones, 1993). Various instances of state-induced illness and repressed stories—the internment of Japanese Americans during World War II (Yoo, 1996), the internment of Jews in concentration camps (Schwartzman, 2001; Sicher, 2001), or the racial inferiority experiments conducted on people of African descent[3]—illustrate the complex intersections between oppression, health, stigma, and the narrative (re)construction of subjectivities and collective memory.

Given the significant role that the censoring of narratives plays in complicating the consequences of state-inflicted illness (in its physical, psychological, social, and symbolic dimensions), it is only cogent to investigate the politics of illness in conjunction with the politics of storytelling. In this chapter, we discuss the epistemological and therapeutic importance of narratives, and illustrate the ways in which illness and storytelling (or the lack of storytelling) have political, social, and economic consequences. As stories once forbidden by state authorities, we investigate narratives that (a) represent individuals' attempts at coping with and making sense of traumatic experiences, (b) bear testimony to the repression of private citizens by a totalitarian political regime, and (c) aid in the construction of an alternative collective imagination.

## NARRATIVE AS AN EPISTEMOLOGICAL FRAMEWORK WITH THERAPEUTIC IMPLICATIONS

Narrative's importance lies in its being one of the main forms through which we perceive, experience, and judge our actions and the value of our lives and the world around us (Ochs & Capps, 1996; Somers, 1994; White, 1980). Historians, anthropologists, political scientists, sociologists, linguists, and communication scholars alike acknowledge and problematize the central role narrative plays in the way we construct knowledge, interpret experience, and define morality and human agency (Ahearn, 2001; Couto, 1993; Cronon, 1992; Garro & Mattingly, 2000; Johnstone, 2000; Krylova, 2001; Ochs & Capps, 1996). Because stories serve as the narrative frameworks within which we make our experiences meaningful, one of the primary functions of storytelling is to negotiate and mediate the plots we co-construct with others and within institutional discourses (Bochner, 2002).

Across our lifespans, human conduct constitutes a storied experience. Indeed, to have a self is to have a story (Bruner, 1986; Carbaugh, 1996). From an epistemological standpoint, stories do not simply describe the self; they are the self's medium of being. The constellation of narratives we construct, discover, and resist allows us to maintain a sense of coherence and continuity over the course of our lives. At times, we may find ourselves in stories we would rather not enact; at other times, we construct new story lines so that we can exert control over life's possibilities and limitations. In fact, Frank (1993) argued that a rhetoric of the self as a project for change characterizes Western public and private discourses of the past century. Within this rhetoric, certain events and experiences are understood as occasions for changing the self; illness is a prime example.

Storytelling functions as one of our most powerful forms for experiencing, expressing, and enacting sorrow and pain (Frank, 1995; Harvey, 2000). Storytelling is pivotal in the process of sensemaking, allowing individuals to cope with chaotic, equivocal, and confusing conditions of everyday life, including illness and suffering (Weick, 1995). Likewise, narrative scholars agree that the very voicing of an illness experience in story format is itself an act of agency and healing (Bruner, 1986; Sharf & Vanderford, 2003; Vanderford & Smith, 1996). Frank (1995) positioned illness as a call for stories and suffering individuals as "wounded" storytellers. Using a term coined by Ronald Dworkin, the *narrative wreck*, Frank explains that illness stories carry "some sense of being shipwrecked by the storm of disease" with repeated storytelling functioning as "repair work on the wreck" (p. 54). Thus, whether or not ill people want to narrate their stories and recount over and again how illness interrupted their lives and remapped their existence, the presence of the disease triggers the act of storytelling as a "dual reaffirmation" (p. 56) of one's relationship with others and with one's self.

The theraupeutic value of narrative popularized by White and Epston (1990) and Frank (1995, 2000b) is situated in poststructuralist discourses that force a reevaluation of traditional psychological approaches. Narrative as therapy is premised on Wittengenstein's (1953) arguments that language can blur, alter, or distort experience as we tell our stories; as such, it can condition how we think, feel, and act and can be used purposefully as a therapeutic tool. If storytelling can function to therapeutically and symbolically connect the self both to others and to the persona of the storyteller, then the absence of storytelling isolates the ill person, thus increasing his or her traumatic experience, as is the case with once censored testimonies of oppressed Romanians. We argue that, however painful the repeated narration of illness can become, the absence of this repetitive narrative act (or the impossibility to narrate one's illness story even once) deepens the sense of being "shipwrecked" and interrupts the act of dual reaffirmation.

We approach narratives as inherently sociopolitical performances, as sets of practices inscribed by power relations. Indeed, the often unrecognized potential of narrative as a form of interpersonal inquiry is revealed through its ability to render credible the voices of previously marginal and silenced individuals and groups (Clair, 2001; Langellier, 1989). As Foucault (1975, 1995) reminded us, some knowledges are subjugated—buried, hidden, disguised, masked, written out by revisionist histories—or denied space to perform adequately. The erasure of resistors' memory from the public space of Romania manipulated the symbolic force of the nation's collective imaginary and reinforced political propaganda. Phelan (2001) argued that a "national imaginary" embodies a community's dominant "cluster of images and rhetoric that, however inadequately and imperfectly, signal to a population who and what it is" (p. 7). The erasure of "undesirable" and "infectious" voices from Romania's public sphere no doubt influenced the kinds of images, symbols, and rhetoric that, in part, formed the nation's conception of self. The censoring of dissidents' storytelling made it easier for officialdom to render resistors as enemies, terrorists, or traitors because most dissenters' stories did not reach the public ear and could not have an impact on public imagination. Resistors' silence thus enhanced the stigma attached to political dissidence and helped the state propaganda to position resistance as a sign of illness and moral decay.

State-induced illness and the censoring of narratives contributed to the stifling and, often, defeat of political resistance in Romania. In recovering lived experiences of oppression, we can rediscover an entire

history of struggle and conflict, and challenge the effects of the central-
izing powers of institutional discourses. In 1989, when the stories of
Romanian resistors started to become part of public conversations,
the liberation embedded in the storytelling act brought to the resistors'
ill and stigmatized bodies a therapeutic victory and contributed to the
formation of a new personal and social identity. As Carbaugh (1990)
reminded us, people achieve a sense of "*shared identity*" and "*common means and meanings*" (p. xv, italics in the original) through the
communication of their experiences. After 1989, narratives about
state-inflicted illness started to function as "counterstories"
(Lindemann-Nelson, 2001) that shaped a new national imagination
and created *common ground* by rewriting a history of oppression and
silence. The agency embedded in the narrative act reformed or
reframed the meanings of events through these counternarratives. In
the form of testimonials, individuals in Romania reclaimed the capacity for telling their own life experiences and, through the act of telling,
transformed personal and social suffering. Those who had been objects of others' reports started to tell their own stories and rewrite official history in the first-person singular.

Our analysis begins with a discussion of the politics of illness and
then explores how the censoring of illness stories—what we call "the
politics of storytelling"—serves degenerative roles in the lives of political victims and their families (and ultimately in the lives of communities). Our chapter concentrates on the narrative testimonies presented
at a conference in June 1995 by former deportees and political prisoners (or their family members). The conference was held in Sighetu
Marmatiei, a city in Northern Romania. These testimonies were later
published by a Romanian nongovernmental organization, *Fundatia
Academic Civica*, under the title, *Analele Sighet: Instaurarea comu-
nis-mului—intre rezistenta si represiune. Comunicari prezentate la
Simpozionul de la Sighetu Marmatiei (9–11 iunie 1995). [The Sighet
files: The initial stages of communism—between resistance and repression. Testimonies presented at the Sighetu Marmatiei Convention (9–11 June 1995)].*[4]

Additionally, the first author conducted and transcribed nine in-
depth interviews. She interviewed five members of her family who
were either imprisoned or deported between the late 1940s and early
1960s. In the other four interviews, she spoke with family friends
who had similar experiences.[5] Both authors worked together to
co-construct a story about the political aspects of illness and storytelling and develop the key theoretical arguments presented throughout the chapter. When including narrative excerpts from public
testimonies, we include the source's name, the testimony's year of
publication and page number. In the case of interview data, we in-

clude the interviewee's initials followed by a notation of "personal communication."

## THE POLITICS OF ILLNESS

Weber (1996) argued that a state can, and should, be sociologically defined in terms of its means (rather than its ends), in terms of what it does to achieve certain purposes. Weber defines a *state* as a "human community that (successfully) claims the *monopoly of the legitimate use of physical force* within a given territory" (p. 43, italics in the original). The notion of *territory* (a unified geographical space) and the concept of *force*—or legitimate use of force—comprise the most critical characteristics of a state, according to Weber's definition. Implicit in the definition is the role that fear plays in commanding citizens' obedience. The state's "right" to use violence against its own citizens is generally grounded in the legitimacy and power that a particular community vests in its government. What happens, however, when the state ceases to represent the community's interests? What happens when the state makes vague and abstract references to "the people" (McGee, 1975) while using violence against those same people in order to maintain its power? In other words, what happens when the state draws its legitimacy from its own right to use violence and commands citizens' obedience by virtue of the fact that it can use force to achieve its ends? The testimonies of political oppression we investigate speak for the ways in which, in conditions of acute political conflict between state and citizens, the state makes use of its right to utilize violence and therefore cause illness in order to subdue citizens' bodies. The state's right to use violence extends from its ability to inflict physical, social, and symbolic pain on people who oppose its ideologies.

The state's "power to punish" (Foucault, 1975/1995, p. 74) its own citizens is manifest in the existence of a number of state institutions, among which the prison (or threat of imprisonment) is probably the most common. Throughout history, states have made use of their right to incarcerate people not only because individuals were a threat to a particular community but because they were a menace to the state itself (or to a set of practices and public norms endorsed by the state), a ... the political prison. When the power of the ... community that the state al- ... environment of terror, ... hoc military execu-

... we examine ... regard for human ... ng the late 1940s, the 1950s, and the early 1960s accompanied various discriminatory tactics (e.g., the seizing of detainees' goods, the censoring of all contact between inmates and their families, or the inmates' complete isolation from the outside world). Oftentimes, political prisoners' houses were burned, demolished, or simply confiscated together with the rest of their belongings, and the detainees' families were either deported or forcefully isolated from the rest of the community. The stigma attached to the bodies of political prisoners and those of their families hindered the ability of prisoners' spouses to find jobs or for their children to continue their education. Many testimonies emphasize these patterns of oppression and describe the pain and suffering that such practices engendered:

> The children of people who were deported were denied access to regular schools, forced to get jobs as unskilled workers while attending night schools, whereas college students [whose parents were deported] were expelled for their "unhealthy origins." (Râpeanu, 1995, p. 406)

Discrimination stigmatized and isolated all those who were marked as unhealthy "others" and created powerful cognitive maps for what counted as acceptable and nonacceptable social origin.

The Romanian state purposefully engaged in stigmatization through discrimination to punish, degrade, and weaken the human body by creating feelings of guilt, shame, and fear.

> [In 1949] our parents were deported first to Blaj, two weeks later to Huedin, then to Gherla, and finally to Turda where they remained until 1963. The separation from our parents mutilated our childhood and our entire lives. We lived until 1952 with my mother's parents.... During these years we lived in fear and uncertainty about our future; these feelings haunted us for decades and surfaced every time we were asked to fill out employment forms that made references to our social origin.... To be able to go to college, I agreed to be adopted by an uncle.... In 1955 I was accepted into the College of Medicine.... the whole time I was a student I lived under the terror and uncertainty that I might be expelled.... My sister, Otilia [who was not adopted by anybody else], graduated from high-school in 1957 and was denied access into the College of Philosophy because of her social origin. She went to a two-year vocational school, got a job, and after five more years she was finally able to register into the College of Economics, which she later graduated from. (Pop & Nicoara, 1995, pp. 413–415)

As this testimony illustrates, individuals with spoiled identities had to manage social information about their easily discreditable life situation. In Goffman's (1963) words, individuals struggled: "to display or not display; to tell or not to tell; to let on or not to let on; to lie or not to lie; and in each case, to whom, how, when, and where" (p. 42). Just as inhumane conditions of incarceration incapacitated the resistor's body, the additional practices of discrimination and economic deprivation adopted by the state created an "untouchable" condition intended to outcast the dissident's entire family. This "untouchable" condition instilled a social illness that rendered undesirable the presence of political resistors and their families in the public space; and, by extension, debilitated and stigmatized the resistance act itself.

Resistors experienced the most violent forms of state-inflicted illness, however, within the walls of political prisons and in concentration and forced labor camps. Inhumane conditions of detention and labor—with malnutrition and torture as part of the daily regimen—inflicted illness in very concrete, physical ways on Romanian political prisoners. Former political resistors describe the prison cells in which they were kept as insalubrious, their food as highly insufficient and inedible, and most of their guards as sadistic criminals. Here are several of their testimonies:

> In the Aiud prison the cells were for four persons; we used to have only a bucket for defecation and one for water in the room.... Here, at Aiud, a young man once came out at orderly time and told the guards that he was in great pains and could no longer stand it. They replied to him that his medicine was the barbed wire. He went straight for the wire and they shot him. (T. V., personal communication)

> Some of the prison cells I stayed in were quite big and the guards would put over 200 people in those rooms. Normally, only about 20 people could be accommodated in there but we were about 200. You can imagine what that was like!... The air was suffocating. In winter time, though we never had heating, the cell was always warm. During summers, however, it was hot as hell. We were wearing only our underwear, and we were always dripping with sweat. You can only imagine what that must have been like. (M. N., personal communication)

The two testimonies just cited illustrate the state's (or its representatives') utter disregard for human life and the extent to which physical and psychological injuries were induced in the bodies of political prisoners.

Hunger, harsh weather, and the permanent fear of additional persecution were among the most common and brutal tools for the infliction of illness, as the testimony to follow illustrates:

> The guards caught me once communicating in Morse and they wrote me down for isolation time. They did not take me right away, though. They let me wait for about three or four months until winter came. In this way they would, on the one hand, keep you under pressure all the time (be-

cause you were waiting to be taken away) and, on the other, they would have you spend your isolation time when the weather was harshest. Most of the time they would add up the days you had to spend in isolation so that you stayed there for as long as possible. When the guards took me to the isolation cell they asked me to take off all my clothes. The cell had no bed or anything else except a bucket for defecation. They would give you food only Tuesdays and Fridays. Nothing on the other days. On Tuesdays and Fridays only you'd get some sort of soup, or whatever else they had on that day, and bread. About 100 grams of bread.[6] (T. V., personal communication)

Starvation generated physical and psychological injuries that had both short and long-term consequences for the bodies of political prisoners. Though atrocious, the physical manifestations of illness through starvation pale by comparison to their psychological counterparts:

The quantity of food that a prisoner used to get was ... no, not insufficient ... it was unimaginably insufficient. Men who used to be of medium or large size before incarceration now looked like ghosts. Some of the younger people—people like me, who had never been large—would walk around like drunk chicken. In such detention conditions, given that we had no heating in the cells (we never had any heating), no food, no medical assistance, I wonder how we survived.... It is impossible to explain how a man could survive on 6-700 or maximum 800 calories per day for long periods of time. Many died. Hunger was no longer something you felt in your stomach but, rather, something you felt in all of your pores, in all of your tissues. Many times you didn't even feel hungry because your tissues were completely ruined. It was a kind of hunger that is very difficult to express in words. It was almost ... I could say it was almost like an obsession coming from within. It wasn't mere mouth-watering or appetite but an interior warning signal that said: "Give me something! Do something or else you and I will both cease to exist!" ... The physical aspect of your being influenced heavily your psychology. The hunger obsession lasted a long time, for some it lasted many years after they were released from prison. This obsession was like a ... no, not a fingerprint because this is too nice a word, a euphemism. It was more like a red iron that burnt your flesh to the bone. (O. R., personal communication)

Throughout their narratives, all former political prisoners in this project stressed the physical and psychological traumas induced through inhumane conditions of incarceration (of which starvation is only one example). These traumas grew still darker through injuries inflicted through the direct and frequent torturing of prisoners' bodies.

The testimony below reveals how the secret police repeatedly beat a former political prisoner as part of an attempt to force the detainee to divulge the name of a woman (a medical doctor and one of the prisoner's relatives) who was suspected of subversive activities:

> The secret police interrogated me three times, while I was still being kept at their headquarters. The first time they did not beat me; the second and third time however they tortured me brutally to make me tell them the names of people I had recruited. The second time they hung me from the wrists, which were tied at the back, and whipped my bare feet. Those criminals! I had never seen something like that. They would pull you by the hair (I wasn't yet shaven because I was still under investigation) and you'd scream and scream! I did not tell them anything, however, no name, no name.... The second time they beat me they also started to ask me about Dr. S., who was my wife's cousin. They were suspecting her but they did not have any evidence.... Oh, how much I was beaten for her! They beat me so fiercely ... they ripped my shirt and all of my clothes. I looked like a corpse. Three or four beefy men beat me then. I was not even 24 yet, merely two years older than my youngest grandson now. Oh, how much they beat me for Dr. S.! I kept telling them that I didn't know anything, that she had done nothing! They left me alone and then took me again, a third time. Oh, how they tortured me! They threatened to leave me without food. I told them that they can shoot me if they wanted but I still didn't know anything! When they carried me back to my cell, I thought that if they took me a forth time I would not be able to handle it any more, that I would confess it all. Luckily, they didn't take me a forth time and that's how Dr. S. got away with it, the poor woman! (T. V., personal communication)

Political prisoners' testimonies emphasize the ways in which the state purposefully and legally inflicted illness on the detainees' undesirable bodies. The violence of illness and its inoculation carved despair and fear among political resistors in ways that would alter individuals' identities and minimize their self-esteem. Pain and humiliation became docilizing mechanisms that guaranteed the suppression of political dissidents' voices within prison walls and, by extension, throughout the entire community.

Arendt (1972) contended that state violence is "instrumental" (p. 145) and that it appears whenever power is in danger. As such, state violence has political ends and can be justified, in Arendt's opinion, only if it stops the decline of political power. The illness inflicted by the Romanian state on dissidents, we argue, was political, not only because it reinforced the state's power but also because it promoted a system of domination that endorsed the state's legal right to be the sole perpetrator of violence by dislocating people's sense of identity, humiliating the body, and fragmenting the continuity of people's roles within their communities. As such, this system of domination relied on the infliction of pain to disrupt and shipwreck people's lives. Illness functioned as the primary mechanism through which state violence maintained the regime's political power and imposed a matrix of oppression that restructured institutions of public and private life.

State-inflicted illness also operated on symbolic levels. The moral discrediting of political resistors reinforced the disconnect between resistors and their communities. A former political resistor describes the dissenters' moral tainting by the state in the following way:

> Oftentimes resistors were forced through torture to throw mud at the people they loved most, such as their parents and siblings. They were forced to write and sign things like: "my mother was a prostitute." Can you imagine what that meant?... Or, "my father was a drunkard; he taught me everything I know." Or, "my brother raped my sister." These defamatory statements were used by the state to taint dissenters. So that the state can then say "look who these political dissidents are and what kind of families they come from." (G. J., personal communication)

This testimony illustrates how the state used the symbolic force embedded in discourses about morality to position political resistance as a sign of inner decay. Metaphors that connected dissidence to immorality assigned resistors a symbolic guilt that purportedly explained their initial opposition to the state. From an official perspective, therefore, dissidence became a form of symbolic illness that originated in the moral pollution of "abnormal" individuals coming from "abnormal" families. As such, the symbolic illness derived from alleged moral decay worked to justify state-imposed "cures": inhumane conditions of detention, inmates' complete isolation from the outside world, economic deprivation, and practices of discrimination against prisoners' families. By contrast, the state characterized citizens' obedience to the state as a sign of health (physical, mental, and moral) to be kept in strict isolation from the "abnormality" of resistance.

Illness—in physical, psychological, social, and symbolic ways— functioned to identify Romania's problems, from the bodies and ideas of political dissidents to the country's history and traditions (the latter when failing to match the stories told by officialdom). Thus, the open political conflict between state and citizens transformed the bodies of political resistors into sites of ideological struggle and turned illness into a signifier of state–citizen conflict. Across time and space, physical pain has been employed by states, and sometimes church institutions (see, e.g., the Inquisition), as mechanisms that silence undesirable opponents. The false stories of immorality and the subhuman conditions of detention just illustrated, however, aimed at doing more than silencing opposition. Pain and illness disconnect the ill person from her or his life and from others (Frank, 1995) and can also function as correctional devices for the bodies they discipline (Foucault 1975, 1995). Kleinman (1995) aptly argued, "the experience of suffering is interpersonal, involving lost relationships, the brutal breaking of intimate bonds, collective fear, and an assault on loyalty and respect among family and friends" (p. 180). When oppressors inflict pain and illness for ideological purposes, they discipline not just the body and mind of political resistors but the bodies and minds of all the members of the community. By inflicting pain on individual community members, the Romanian state sent a powerful message to the entire group, a message intended to muffle political opposition and force compliance. Thus, state-inflicted illness, while enfeebling the bodies of dissidents, also paralyzed the entire community's ability to resist the state apparatus.

## THE POLITICS OF STORYTELLING

The censoring of resistors' stories in the community's public space augments the violence of state-induced illness. For example, one characteristic of life in Romanian political prisons involved the inmates' complete isolation from families, friends, and the outside world. This isolation increased the traumatic effects of political detention, and reinforced the state's colonizing power over its citizens. On one hand, by imprisoning people in inhumane conditions and isolating them from the external world, the state used illness to achieve control over the disobedient bodies of individual citizens. On the other hand, by censoring communication between detainees and their families and friends, the state not only kept under control the flow of information between the two environments (prison and the outside world), but it also used silence to increase the despair of people inside prisons and the fear of those outside.

The testimonies we examined detail varied ways (from direct threats to the signing of legal documents) in which government authorities controlled the flow of storytelling about state-induced illness even after dissidents were released from prison. One Romanian who was tortured by the police testifies to the ways in which his voice was muted and his story forbidden by his persecutors upon his release:

> [After torture I was told by one of the seargents]: "Look here! Go home and tell whoever asks you (the marks of the beatings were of course visible) that you fell from the train on your way from Bucharest. Don't tell anybody what happened here." (Ratiu, 1995, p. 149)

The threat of death, torture, or additional detention censored storytelling about government abuses, further tarnished the names of political resistors, and allowed the persecutors to construct an inauthentic public discourse that spoke primarily of citizens' unanimous loyalty to the state. This "sanitary" account of events severed the connections that storytelling would otherwise have established between resistors and the community around them, and created feelings of guilt and shame that silenced or weakened people's voices even in spaces where they could talk about their experiences. The techniques of political violence, then, work to disrupt the routines of everyday life, devastating families and communities.

Costin, the daughter of a former political prisoner, remembers how her father felt embarrassed and ashamed to share his detention stories in Costin's presence:

> I remember that one day, in February 1953, my father told a family friend the story of two prisoners who had escaped from jail. The prisoners were eventually caught and the guards kept them outside, lying on the ground on a snowy, windy day, from morning until late afternoon. I entered the room just as my father was beginning his story; he did not stop, but he looked embarrassed of my presence. I realize today, with regret, that so many things remained unsaid, unshared, and that these white spots in the lives of people we love will always be there. (Costin, 1995, p. 94)

As illustrated by Costin's testimony, the censoring of stories and the stigma attached to state-induced illness were so pervasive that they penetrated even the most private of relationships (i.e., between parent and child) and interrupted the sense of communion even in the privacy of one's home, leaving "white spots" in people's lives and memories.

Of particular interest is how the state censored the flow of information even when government abuses resulted in the deaths of those under investigation or in detention. Two Romanians (themselves former political prisoners) recount how the state guarded the news about the prison deaths of close relatives and how such important information had to be communicated discretely and/or clandestinely investigated by family members:

> In 1962, while I was still in prison, my cousin died. He was also a political prisoner. The following day, sergeant C. came to take us from the dining hall to the factory where we were working at the time. He knew me well so he came to me and whispered: "V., your cousin died last night, but keep your mouth shut." (T. V., personal communication)

> My brother died in prison. I was also a political prisoner at the time. I had been in detention for 10 years at the time he died. The death certificate says that he died in 1961 but it seems that the papers are fake.... In 1958 I heard from another prisoner that my brother died and at that time my parents received a letter through which my brother was agree-

ing to send all his personal belongings (a watch, an I.D. and a few other things) back home. We believe that the police sent his things home because he was already dead. But the police never acknowledged that he died in 1958, we don't know why. Later on, in 1961, when my release was approaching, they sent my brother's death certificate to my parents.... The body was never sent home. There was a common grave next to the prison where he died, where prisoners' bodies were being buried.... I don't know why his death was kept a secret or why the police never sent the bodies of political prisoners home. The family did not have the right to request the body. All we got was the letter that informed us of my brother's death; but we never found out why and how he died ... those things were never revealed. Not for any of those who died in prison. (G. J., personal communication)

Some of the resistors who died during police interrogations or political imprisonment were buried in collective holes; others were secretly interred in community cemeteries with no public access to their graves. Another interviewee, N. C., recalls her family's efforts to find the grave of her husband's brother who died in the late 1940s during police interrogations. After many physical efforts and the conspiratorial help of various cemetery wardens, they discovered where the dead body had been buried, but it was not until 1991—after the fall of communism—that they could finally relocate the remains of the deceased to the family crypt in a Bucharest cemetery.

The presence of a dissident's body—whether dead or alive—tells a story of nonsubmission and of civic disobedience. As such, resistors' bodies continue to be politically marked (and therefore censored by the state) even after the dissenter's physical disappearance because the stories that bodies tell possess the power to shape people's collective imagination and foster further disobedience. The state's strict surveillance of information about resistance and about the prison environment illustrates the political significance of storytelling. By not allowing people to share their experiences with one another, by censoring the physical and symbolic access of resistors' bodies into the public space of their communities, the state tried to atomize resistance, to bury it within the self of the resistor (a self that had already been tainted by the discourse of "abnormality" and immorality constructed by the state around the idea of political resistance). Through their capacity to build connections among people and convey a sense of community between storyteller and audience, narratives have the potential to reverse the atomizing power of state-induced illness. As such, narratives about state-caused illness are political because they threaten the state's "right" to be a perpetrator of "legal" violence, because they permit the rearranging of the cluster of symbols that shape a community's understanding of who it is and what it stands for, and, ultimately, because they reenvision the future grounds on which citizens can and do encounter the state.

## TELLING IT LIKE IT WAS: STORYTELLING AS A THERAPEUTIC ACT

For people who were coerced to keep their traumatic experiences hidden from everybody else around them (including their own families in the case of some Romanians), the act of telling previously forbidden stories of illness is an immense victory and a long-awaited moment of social justice. As Netejoru (1995), a former political prisoner, testified, supreme justice happened for him when "the Soviet Union disappeared from the world map, torn apart in dozens of pieces, whereas my comrades and I are still standing" (p. 396). The fact that these people "still stand," able to tell their uncensored stories of illness and persecution after years of silent suffering, constitutes both a concrete and a symbolic victory. At the concrete level, this storytelling sheds light on a dark and terrible national past; at the symbolic level, these testimonies open doors to healing the fear and guilt previously inflicted upon storytellers while also connecting the "I" of the narrator to self and others.

Stories sustain cultures, yet they remain as fluid as the people, languages, or societal practices that they reproduce and/or resist. More than simple vehicles for diffusing information, narratives bring together storytellers and audiences, thus building bridges by means of which alternative ideological meaning formations are created, maintained, and articulated. The previously forbidden stories of Romanian political prisoners and deportees now serve as counternarratives (Lindemann-Nelson, 2001), breathing new life into Romanian culture, rebuilding trust among people, and helping to reorganize civic life. Through counternarratives, individual and community experiences fuse together; and through the act of storytelling, diversity and authenticity emerge as markers of public life. The counternarratives of former political prisoners and deportees, in their capacity as signifying systems, function to articulate alternative embodiments of lived experiences as well as alternative ways of redefining a community's identity and relation to the state.

Individual and collective identities are narratively constructed and damaged (see Carbaugh, 1996) and identities can be narratively repaired (Lindemann-Nelson, 2001; White & Epston, 1990). The voicing of personal and collective counternarratives can liberate and heal just as dominant stories often marginalize. By telling previously forbidden stories, individuals resist the stock plots and readily recognizable character types of master narratives. In so doing, people readjust the cluster of symbols that signify to themselves and others who their community is and what it represents. Thus, counternarratives become a way for people to heal their personal and collective past and embark on a new beginning.

Many of the resistors who testified at the Sighet conference referred to the importance of memory and storytelling in paying homage to those killed or victimized by the state and in "opening [the community's] way into the future" (Blandiana, 1995, pp. 517–518). Most of the people whose stories we heard emphasized that memory serves as a form of social justice and that, by sharing their narratives, resistors hope to "fulfill a moral obligation" (Schafhütl, 1995, p. 421) and to heal their community's past by "making the truth known to future generations" (Pop & Nicoara, 1995, p. 415). Hager (1995), a former deportee, noted that "only a clear memory of the past can give people more trust in themselves and others" (p. 428), while Constantinescu and Daescu (1995) added that testimonies of oppression mark a "form of oral history that must be written and transmitted to future generations so that the past may never be repeated" (p. 448). Testimonials, as embodiments of previously forbidden stories, represent a significant mode of remembering and recording experience and struggle, and they help to decenter hegemonic histories and subjectivities.

History, then, cannot escape the perspective that dominates its narrative expression (Bruner, 2002; White, 1980). Feminist analyses, for example, have recognized the centrality of rewriting and reenvisioning collective memory (e.g., Mohanty, 2003). Counternarratives are significant, not merely as a corrective to the gaps, erasures, and misunderstandings of hegemonic history, but also because the practice of rewriting leads to the formation of politicized consciousness and self-identity. Discourse becomes a terrain of struggle and contestation about reality itself. Narratives allow us to rethink, remember, and utilize our lived relations as a basis of knowledge. Ana Blandiana, a Romanian poetess and dissident, notes in one of the essays that concludes the testimonies grouped under the title *Analele Sighet* that collecting stories of pain and suffering is an act of social justice and moral healing. By assembling together and making public people's narratives of oppression, the Sighet files work to reconstruct and reorganize a "civil society that had been systematically destroyed" (Blandiana, 1995, p. 517). The Sighet testimonies express "the need for truth and respect for human beings," and a "symbol of the importance and necessity of civil society and of a just state" (Blandiana, 1995, p. 517).

The sharing of testimonies sets in motion a search for meaning and offers "dramatistic" forays into social life (Burke, 1969). For one of the authors of this essay, Teodora Carabas, these illness stories are personally meaningful because they built connections between her and the rest of her family. As a child born after 1964, the year when political prisoners were officially released from detention, she had been protected through silence from the past of her own family. After 1989, Teodora found out that her family had suffered tremendous persecutions during the communist period. The state imprisoned her grandfather, his father, and several of his cousins for long periods of time (as long as 14 years in her grandfather's case) and confiscated all the family's belongings after the passing of the sentence. One of her grandmother's sisters lived for 5 years in deportation together with her husband, who also spent 8 years in various Romanian political prisons. Their first child was born during these years of deportation.

Teodora's grandmother and other women in her family were forced to be the sole care and food providers for their families and children, under severe conditions of job inequity as well as social and political discrimination. Teodora's mother and her mother's siblings suffered further persecutions as offsprings of political resistors. They were forced to go to night classes (instead of regular daytime courses) in high-school, work from young adolescence on to support themselves, and carry the stigma of being different. Though very close to her grandparents, parents, uncles and aunts, Teodora was born too late to witness the atrocities experienced by her family. Stigmatized by the state and desiring to protect the younger members of the family from additional state persecution, for 25 years Teodora's relatives concealed their experiences of oppression. She became aware of her family's tragedies only after 1989, when the voices of the people around her were no longer silent.

Stories cannot replace years lost or change the suffering endured by narrators; however, these testimonials can and should enter the collective imagination of a nation whose citizens were often brutally tortured, incarcerated, and silenced. Frank (1995) argued "The witness offers testimony to a truth that is generally unrecognized or suppressed. People who tell stories of illness are witnesses, turning illness into moral responsibility" (p. 137). The participants in this project are witnesses, telling once-forbidden narratives. These enactments of oppression function as counternarratives that construct individual and communal identities, render credible previously muted voices, and re-historize emplotments and configurations of character relationships. These testimonials build a new social reality that resists the long tradition of exclusion so characteristic of the state-articulated history of Romania, and powerfully illustrate the significance of alternative public narratives in countering the damage to identity formation caused by singular dominant narratives.

Ultimately, we draw attention to undertheorized aspects of health and well-being: state-induced illness and forbidden stories. We encourage health communication scholars to explore the politics of illness and the politics of storytelling as manifest in struggles between states and citizens. Concomitantly, health communication scholars can deepen our understanding of the therapeutic value of storytelling as embodied in the complex intersections between oppression, health, stigma, and the narrative (re)construction of subjectivities and collective memory. By approaching narrative performances as situated within and informed by sociohistorical discourses, we can offer richer understandings of the ways in which illness and storytelling (or lack thereof) have political, social, and symbolic consequences.

# NOTES

1. The authors would like to thank Phyllis Japp and Christina Beck for their insightful suggestions and careful editing of previous versions of this essay.
2. As a result of international pressures, communist governments throughout Eastern and Central Europe agreed to free all their political prisoners in 1964. Officially, after that date, the Eastern European states (Romania included) declared that they had stopped the persecution and incarceration of political resistors, but unofficially the practice lasted until the fall of communist regimes in 1989. From 1964 to 1989, however, instead of accusing political resistors of crimes against the state, the communist governments generally framed those who opposed them for misdemeanors or even serious civic offenses and indicted them on false charges. As Sharlet (1983) argued, political prisoners in Romania and the rest of Eastern Europe were turned into "surrogate criminals," who were being sent to trial

    on fraudulent charges for such ordinary crimes as currency speculation (Soviet Union and Romania), receiving stolen property (Poland), petty and malicious hooliganism (Soviet Union), resisting arrest and battery of a policeman (Czechoslovakia and Poland), drug charges (Soviet Union), homosexuality (Romania), and rape (Soviet Union). The object of these trials is to felonize the political behavior of dissidents while publicly demeaning their character in the process. (pp. 13–14)

    Homosexuality was illegal in Romania and the rest of the Eastern European bloc and therefore placed on the same level as rape or hooliganism. For considerations of space and clarity of argument, our analysis focuses only on the pre-1964 period. The post-1964 period deserves attention in a separate chapter at another time.
3. Sara Baartman's case is one of the most famous examples of racial inferiority research conducted on people of African descent. Sara Baartman was a Khoi Khoi woman who was taken from Cape Town, South Africa, in 1810 and displayed across Britain as an exemplar of "primitive" sexuality and racial imperfection. Taken from Britain to France, Sara Baartman's body continued to be the object of experimentation that provided "scientific" support to White supremacist ideas. After her death, Sara Baartman's brain and sexual organs were exhibited in Paris at the *Musée de l'Homme* until 1985

when, after 175 years of degradation, her remains were finally taken back to South Africa.

4. The convention that took place in June 1995 in Sighet is the third conference that aimed to collect testimonies given by former resistors and victims of the state. The previous two conferences took place in 1993 and 1994, and were held also in Sighet. The city of Sighet was chosen as the symbol of repression and resistance in Romania because it has one of the first prisons (now a museum) that was used against political resistors by the communist state.

5. All personal communication cited in this essay was conducted in Romanian and translated into English by Teodora Carabas. Excerpts of the original tapes and the transcripts of the interviews are available upon request. Please e-mail Teodora Carabas at Teodora.Carabas.1@ohio.edu

6. 100 grams is the equivalent of 3.5 ounces.

# 8

## Cross-Border Mass-Mediated Health Narratives: Narrative Transparency, "Safe Sex," and Indian Viewers[1]

**Arvind Singhal**
**Ketan Chitnis**
**Ami Sengupta**
*Ohio University*

Consider the audience effects of the following mass-mediated narratives that consciously incorporated health themes in their emplotments:

> In 1986, when a character on Cristal, a Venezuelan tele-novela [television novel or soap opera] was diagnosed with breast cancer, the number of women viewers requesting mammograms rose steeply in Venezuela. Later when the show was broadcast in Spain, similar effects occurred (Andalao, 2003).
>
> In 1999, when Soul City, the popular South African television series, modeled a new collective behavior to portray how neighbors might intervene in a domestic violence—that is, by gathering around the abuser's residence and collectively banging pots and pans, pot banging to stop partner abuse was reported in several locations in South Africa (Usdin, Singhal, Shongwe, Goldstein, & Shabalala, 2004).
>
> In 2000, when Camilla, the protagonist on Lazos de Sangre [Blood Ties], a popular Brazilian telenovela, was diagnosed with leukemia, the Brazilian National Registry of Bone Marrow Donors reported that new donor registrations increased by 45

*times the average: from about 20 a month, to 900 a month (TV Globo, 2003).*

*On August 3, 2001, when Tony was diagnosed with HIV on an episode of the popular soap opera, The Bold and the Beautiful, the number of calls to CDC's AIDS hotline within the hour increased 16 times over the previous hour (Beck, 2004).*

These four narratives exemplify a rising trend in global media programming, commonly referred to as the entertainment-education communication strategy. *Entertainment-education* is the process of purposely designing and implementing a media message to both entertain and educate, in order to increase audience members' knowledge about an issue, create favorable attitudes, shift social norms, and change the overt behavior of individuals and communities (Singhal, Cody, Rogers, & Sabido, 2004; Singhal & Rogers, 1999, 2002). Entertainment-education narratives generally consist of two types: Long-running mass-media programs (such as *Soul City* in South Africa) that are explicitly designed to promote particular health and development themes, or programs (such as *Cristal, Lazos de Sangre,* and *The Bold and the Beautiful*) that include certain health themes in the context of a larger plot. The latter approach, commonly referred to as *social merchandizing,* involves the conscious placement of a social message, often a health message, in a popular mediated narrative (La Pastina, Patel, & Schiavo, 2004).

The social merchandizing approach is increasingly gaining ground among media producers in Hollywood and in other countries. For instance, in 2002, over a thousand episodes of *telenovelas* produced by Brazil's TV Globo consciously incorporated a range of social issues, ranging from safe sex, to blood and organ donation, to caring for the environment (TV Globo, 2003). In an episode of *Lazos de Sangre,* Capitu, a young Brazilian woman, purposely pulled out a condom during a passionate romantic encounter, gesturing to her partner that sex would only occur if it was protected. Episodes of *El Beso del Vampiro* [Kiss of the Vampire] were timed for broadcast during the same week as the International Blood Donation Day, encouraging Brazilian viewers to donate blood. In Hollywood, social merchandizing began over 40 years ago when scriptwriter Agnes Nixon incorporated a storyline on uterine cancer in the popular soap, *Guiding Light.* Other popular Hollywood narratives in which health issues have been incorporated include *Maude* (unintended pregnancy), *thirtysomething* (cancer), *LA Law* (mental illness), *Beverly Hills 90210* (violence against women), *The Young and the Restless* (diabetes), *7th Heaven* (teenage drug and alcohol abuse), *Friends* (safe sex), and many others (Beck, 2004; Sharf & Freimuth, 1993; Sharf, Freimuth, Greenspon, & Plotnick, 1996).

Since the mid-1990s, the social merchandizing approach has further gained currency in Hollywood through "Soap Summits" in New York and Los Angeles, where Hollywood producers, directors, and scriptwriters gather to exchange experiences in incorporating health emplotments in popular narratives through the Hollywood, Health & Society initiative of the Centers for Disease Control and the University of Southern California which facilitates the incorporation of health storylines in popular entertainment shows and through the Sentinel for Health Award for Daytime Drama, presented to an outstanding Hollywood narrative with a health storyline (Tony's HIV storyline in *The Bold and the Beautiful* received this prestigious award in 2002).

What happens when a Hollywood-produced popular narrative with a health emplotment is broadcast in an overseas context? How is Hollywood's mass-mediated world of health-related persuasion, information, and entertainment interpreted outside its borders? This chapter analyzes how audiences in India interpret "safe sex" emplotments in the Hollywood-produced sitcom, *Friends*. Drawing on a cultural approach to audience interpretation (McQuail, 1997), our research is guided by Olson's (1999) narrative transparency theory and Fisher's (1984, 1985a) narrative theory. *Narrative transparency theory* posits transparency as "the capability of certain texts to seem familiar regardless of their origin, to seem a part of one's own culture, even though they have been crafted elsewhere" (Olson, 1999, p. 18). Narrative transparency allows audience members of different cultures to project their own stories, values, myths and meanings into a foreign text, making them derive meanings as if the text was locally produced (Olson, 1999). Fisher's (1985a) concept of narrative rationality, which examines the truth and coherence of a story, also holds important implications for audience members who interpret a foreign text. The present research investigates the degree to which Indian audiences interpreted the "safe sex" emplotment in *Friends* as being a "transparent" narrative, and the degree to which Indian audiences viewed *Friends* as meeting the requirements of narrative rationality.

## HOLLYWOOD'S GLOBAL FOOTPRINT

The global reach of media corporations enables people of different cultures to consume media products produced in foreign lands. These global media corporations, only a handful in number, are primarily based in the United States, mostly in Hollywood (Demers, 1999; Wolf, 1999). Consider the following: Worldwide, audiences are 100 times more likely to see a Hollywood film than see a European film; further, Hollywood satisfies 70% of the international demand for television narratives and 80% of the demand for feature films (*Home Alone*,

1997; *Star Wars*, 1997). Not surprisingly, Hollywood has been criticized for media imperialism and creating a globally dispersed Western monoculture (Boyd, 1984; McChesney, 1997). Past studies seem to suggest that when consumed over a period of time, American media products may influence how an audience member in a foreign country may feel, dress, and act (McMillin, 2002; Olson, 1999; Rogers et al., 2003; Singhal & Rogers, 2001). For instance, reception studies in India found that the conception of the ideal female body type shifted from round to thin, largely through heavy consumption of American television programs (Malhotra & Rogers, 2000). Singhal and Rogers (2001) also noted a shift in the depiction of Indian women in indigenous television programming from the traditional roles of motherhood to that of a modern woman, especially after the advent of foreign satellite channels in India in the 1990s.

Researchers have also found evidence of the growing popularity of local and non-Western media products. For instance, Cantonese soap operas are highly popular in Hong Kong, and Indian soaps draw large audiences in India. Hybrid programs, such as Kung Fu movies, modeled after James Bond movies, also are highly popular in Hong Kong and overseas (Ang, 1996). Mexican and Brazilian *telenovelas* are now exported throughout Latin America and in many countries of Asia and Africa. Despite such evidence of popularity of non-Western media products, American media products remain popular in most global markets. Olson's (1999) narrative transparency theory argues that U.S. media texts have certain attributes that lend them a global and cross-cultural appeal.

## NARRATIVE TRANSPARENCY THEORY

Narrative transparency theory, first propounded by Olson (1999), builds on Hall's (1980) seminal argument that audiences can derive multiple meanings from a text. Television allows for the production of discursive knowledge and the intended meaning of a message may thus change for different audience individuals. However, Hall's analysis does not explicitly deal with cross-cultural consumption of media products; neither does it investigate the attributes of the text in the meaning-making process.

Critical media scholars have attempted to explain what makes American media products popular in other cultures (Newcomb, 1984; Olson, 1999). The main explanations have centered on media hegemony and imperialism; few dealt with how audience members engage with foreign texts. Newcomb (1984) investigated the language of television and argued that the medium allowed for different interpretations of its main ideology. In doing so, Newcomb challenged the predominant hegemonic view of global consumption, but still did not investigate how American media products were interpreted in other cultures. Olson (1999) suggested that if certain programs (e.g., *Dallas*) are popular among audiences from different cultures, the media text itself provides at least part of the explanation of its global popularity. Olson argued that the message has a "universal" meaning because of the language (or narratological devices) used to create it.

*Narrative transparency* questions the claim that indigenous cultures are disappearing because of Western media onslaughts, and that the monolithic American culture dominates the world. According to Olson, "Although the same media products are reaching most people, people do not possess the same ways of reading the meaning embedded in these media products" (1999, p. 6). For Olson, the global media texts are "transparent," that is the text allows audiences to project their own indigenous meaning into the global media product.

As noted previously, Olson's (1999) argument built on the concept of *multiple meaning* of media texts as espoused in reception studies since the 1980s. Hall (1980) argued that, although a producer may intend a "preferred reading" of the message, the audience might interpret the text differently based on their social situation. Fiske (1986) suggested the notion of *polysemy*, which means that there can be multiple meanings given to one text. Olson extends this argument to suggest that a media text has the ability to transcend cultures. Narrative transparency argues that a cross-cultural understanding of the text may take place because the audience individual interprets a foreign text from their own transparent lens of cultural beliefs and values. Transparency theory thus claims that in order to understand the popularity of global media, one has to understand both the media text and the audience members who consume them.

For example, the *Gbagyi* people in Nigeria interpreted *Dallas* very differently from American viewers. Based on their cultural beliefs and ideas, they drew connections between the traits of J. R. Ewing, the central character, and their traditional myths. So J. R. Ewing was viewed as the trickster worm in Nigerian mythology (Olson, 1999). Similarly, Laotian refugees in the United States especially identified with news items that dealt with Ethiopian refugee camps (Conquergood, 1986). The Laotians felt they were "like" the Ethiopian people in the refugee camps. The identifying elements of reality and vividness were drawn from their own personal, lived experiences. Physical distance and dissimilarity in physical appearance were less important to the Laotian refugees than the larger issues (such as displacement, hunger and poverty) shared by both the Laotian and Ethiopian refugees. Viewers were able to push the apparently "foreign" elements of the text to the background, focusing on personality traits (as in the case of J. R. Ewing) or social realities (as in the case of Ethiopian refugees) that were common.

## Elements of Narrative Transparency

The basic premise of transparency suggests no unified meaning in a mediated text. Instead, audiences read the same text differently, depending on the cultural context. The embedding of myths in the narrative makes the text transparent. Myths consist of stories that a culture makes about reality. Although different cultures have different myths, the underlying premise of myths is the same: They satisfy human needs (Olson, 1999). Myths are derived from *mythotypes*, which are inherent human needs. Mythotypes constitute narrative structures that evoke primary human emotions of "awe, wonder, purpose, joy and participation" (Olson, 1999, p. 93). Although myths transcend cultures and can change and evolve over time and space, the universal mythotypes remain constant.

According to Olson, eight narratological devices[2] internal to the text can convey transparency: virtuality, ellipticality, inclusion, verisimilitude, openendedness, negentropy, circularity, and archetypal dramatis personae.

*Virtuality* is the creation of a psychologically convincing and electronically stimulating environment (Olson, 1999). Audience members of long-running serials develop "hyperreal relationships" with the characters. For instance, many viewers of the popular CBS TV program, *M\*A\*S\*H*, reported acute "separation" anxiety when the program went off air. The *M\*A\*S\*H* fictional family had become more real to the viewers than their own families (Olson, 1999). The sadness felt by fans of Ally McBeal when her childhood love and colleague, Billy, died, provides another example of virtuality.

*Ellipticality* refers to the narrative technique of leaving the details out (Olson, 1999). Ellipticality makes use of the mythotype of audience participation, allowing the spectator to speculate on what may be going on, and thus "completing" the picture in their own minds. For example, in the *Friends* episode that we shared with our respondents in the present study, audience members may wonder what might have happened in the bedroom when Monica returned to tell her friend Richard that they will not be having sex that night. Viewers may wonder whether or not they really could restrain themselves, creating an ending that fits their beliefs and experiences.

*Inclusion* in texts is a quality that gives the viewer a sense that they are participating in the unfolding of the plot rather than simply observing it (Olson, 1999). For instance, in *Friends*, writers consciously base each episode on situations that young audiences commonly face: sharing an apartment, petty squabbles and fights about cleaning and cooking, the pressure to go out on a date, falling in love with the wrong person, and struggling to find a good job. Such narratives involve audiences through the portrayal of universal experiences.

*Verisimilitude* implies that texts convey to the viewer a sense of truth and realness. These plots appear natural and not something that is "fantastic" or "way out" (Olson, 1999). The notion of narrative verisimilitude is central to Fisher's (1984, 1985a) theory of narrative rationality. Fisher argues that human communication is essentially storytelling and all humans are storytellers. Fisher (1984) defined *narratives* as "symbolic actions—words and/or deeds—that have sequences and meaning for those who live, create or interpret them" (p. 2). Fisher (1985a) espoused the notion of *narrative rationality*, that is, stories meeting the twin tests of narrative probability and narrative fidelity. *Narrative probability* answers the question, "Is the story coherent?" allowing individuals to gauge whether or not the story makes sense, is believable, and could be real. *Narrative fidelity*, on the other hand, deals with the degree to which a story fits in with the audiences' lives, past experiences, and present beliefs. Narrative fidelity gauges whether or not viewers see the stories as fitting into their worldviews, and whether or not these incidents could happen to them or someone they know.

*Openendedness* refers to narrative texts that have no end; hence there is no resolution of the plot (Olson, 1999). American soap operas like *Dallas* and *The Bold and the Beautiful* are examples of such plots. Openendedness, according to Olson, promotes the mythic qualities of the media by encouraging audience participation. Because the text has no definite ending, the viewer must revisit the program, hoping for a sense of closure.

*Negentropy* refers to the manner in which a television narrative can instill a sense of order among its viewers. By seeing the same characters in a familiar setting on a regular basis, viewers gain a feeling of reality, through the mechanism of repetition (Olson, 1999). For Olson, "Television becomes a mechanism for conveying sense and meaning in a world that otherwise appears senseless and meaningless" (p. 98).

*Circularity* refers to the nature of narratives, which makes the story return to where it began. Circularity restores balance to the narrative and places the characters in a situation similar to where they initially began (Olson, 1999). Olson provides the example of the grand return of Odysseus in Homer's epic, *Odyssey*, as involving circularity. Other examples of circularity include the storyline of *M\*A\*S\*H*, when the characters return home from Korea, and the final episode of *Seinfeld*, where the protagonists repeat the very dialogues that launched the program (Olson, 1999).

*Archetypal dramatic personae* are "authentic" characters that exist in each culture, for example, the fair maiden, the handsome prince, and the caring mother. Archetypal characters contain an affective component that can transcend cultures (Olson, 1999). The four key archetypal characters in Western epics according to Olson, consist of the fool, the wizard (or cleric), the knight, and the king. These archetypal characters belong to myths and legends in almost all cultures and hold universal appeal.

Based on the aforementioned review of narrative transparency theory, we investigated how the combination of the eight mythotypes contributes to the transparency of Hollywood's narratives. In so doing, we privileged the examination of the first four mythotypes—virtuality, ellipticality, inclusion, and verisimilitude—as they seemed to generate the most revealing insights for our stated purpose.

Our analysis also focused on the other four mythotopes—openendedness, negentropy, circularity, and archetypical dramatis personae albeit mostly for contextualization. Our investigation, specifically, was guided by the following research questions: To what extent do Indian audiences find the narrative of the Hollywood-produced sitcom, *Friends*, to be transparent? How do Indian audiences subject the text of *Friends*, especially an emplotment about "safe sex" to diverse mythotypic readings?

## METHODOLOGY

The present research, guided by an interpretive audience approach, explores how local cultures organize mediated communication as an activity, decoded content based on audience characteristics, and form spectator identities through media use (see related work by Lindlof & Meyer, 1987).

### Data Collection Procedures

We conducted fieldwork during April 2003 with 39 heavy viewers of *Friends*. These heavy viewers had watched *Friends* for at least two years, considered themselves as fans of the program, tried hard not to miss an episode, and avidly watched the show's reruns. The research procedures included 17 in-depth interviews (with both male and female viewers) and four focus groups discussions (which included 12 men and 10 female participants in total). All interviewees spoke fluent English and all interviews and focus-group discussions were conducted in English. We first asked all respondents questions regarding their perceptions of *Friends*. We then showed an episode of *Friends* with a "safe sex" , and interviewed on the content of that episode. The interviews were semistructured, allowing the respondents to express their individual opinions.[3]

## Respondents' Profile

All 39 respondents (20 men and 19 women) were heavy viewers of *Friends*, who hailed from three Indian cities—New Delhi, Chandigarh, and Hyderabad. Their ages ranged from 18 to 45 years. Most respondents were university students; others included homemakers and professionals, including engineers, architects, and social workers.

## The Object of Study: The Sitcom *Friends*

The Hollywood-produced sitcom, *Friends*, is set in Manhattan. It revolves around a group of six friends and their close interpersonal relationships: Rachel Karen Green, Monica E. Geller (Bing), Phoebe Buffay, Chandler Muriel Bing, Ross Geller, and Joey Francis Tribbiani, Jr. *Friends* began broadcasting in 1994 on the NBC Network and immediately become very popular in the United States. The final season was 2003–2004; *Friends* was the highest rated comedy program for American viewers in the 18 to 49 age group for 5 straight years in a row.[4] In India, *Friends* began broadcasting on the Star World private satellite channel during prime-time hours (8:30 p.m.) in the mid-1990s. In 2003, Star World broadcast it at 7:30 p.m. and at midnight on weekdays. Reruns of *Friends* are broadcast in India on the Zee English Channel on weekday nights at 10 p.m.

The episode of *Friends* that was viewed by our Indian respondents purposely promoted the message of "safe sex." It featured Rachel, Ross, Monica, and her boyfriend Richard (played by Hollywood movie star, Tom Selleck). Condom use was the main theme running through the entire episode (condoms were mentioned six times).

The episode begins with Rachel, Ross, Monica, and her older boyfriend, Richard (a medical doctor), relaxing in Central Perk, a coffee shop in New York's Greenwich Village. Monica says that she and Richard should sleep at her apartment that night. Richard says that he does not have his pajamas. Monica replies that he may not need them, thus hinting that they may have sex.

Richard and Monica arrive at her apartment, which she shares with Rachel. Rachel and her boyfriend, Ross, are shown in a separate bedroom, discussing how many men and women each had dated prior to their present relationship. Rachel lists her former boyfriends. She claims that all of the earlier boyfriends just involved "animal sex." Her present relationship with Ross, she states, is a romantic relationship, not based just on sex. A parallel conversation is shown between Richard and Monica. Richard admits that he dated only two women in his life. One was Barbara, his wife for 30 years, and the second woman is Monica. Monica is skeptical about Richard's statement. Richard thinks that Monica dated a large number of men.

Before sexual passions run over, both Monica and Rachel are shown heading to the restroom in search of condoms so that they can both engage in protected sex with their partners. Meanwhile, Richard and Ross impatiently wait for their girlfriends to return. In their common quest for condoms, Rachel and Monica realize that they have only one condom in the apartment. After trying to solve their dilemma in different ways, Rachel and Monica finally choose (through the "rock, paper, and scissors" process) and Rachel gets the only condom. Monica tells Richard, "not tonight," because they cannot have unprotected sex.

## Data Analysis

The data analysis consisted of coding and categorizing of the interviews and group discussions. We employed an open coding procedure through which emergent concepts were identified and their properties and dimensions were discovered in data. While coding the responses, the emergent categories and subcategories were delineated and linked to the specific mythopes that guided the audience engagement with *Friends*.

## TRANSPARENCY OF *FRIENDS*

Analysis of the data revealed that Indian audiences interpret some elements of *Friends* as being transparent and some as opaque as discussed in the following sections.

### Virtuality

As noted previously, *virtuality* refers to the psychologically convincing "hyperreal relationships" that develop between the audience members and the characters of long-running television programs (Olson, 1999). Indian viewers of *Friends* displayed elements of virtuality with certain characters of *Friends*. For instance, Harpreet stated: "I'd like to meet a character like Phoebe. ... she is the kind of girl I'd like to be friends with. Phoebe is free, always ready to explore. ... she's ready to participate ... take responsibility. She has this strong, independent streak about her, which I really like in a woman" (Harpreet, personal communication, December 2001).

Further, the characters in *Friends* were able to create a psychological sense of reality among the Indian audiences. Several viewers liked

Phoebe, both for her innocence and foolishness, which were seen as normal human traits. Many respondents found her "excessively silly"; some said that without Phoebe's recurring *faux pas*, the program would "lose its entire flavor." Adil appreciated Phoebe's innocence, labeling it as a "rare quality in a world filled with shrewd people." Even when viewers were critical of the actions of certain characters, labeling them as *dumb*, *silly*, or *irritating*, they still viewed the characters as real people, displaying real emotions.

Several respondents labeled Joey as their most favorite character primarily because of his "simplicity" and for his "logical behavior." Some liked Chandler, for his "level-headedness" for having the "spirit to go on" despite several traumatic experiences in life. Rekha liked Chandler because of "the innocence on his face."

Many of our Indian respondents related to the friendship portrayed on *Friends*. The notion of "sharing things" with friends as well as "fighting with them" was similar to their experience, and hence perceived as real. However, for some respondents, the bonding and friendship shown in *Friends* was seen as unreal: "What they show in *Friends* is good, the way people live together and spend so much time together. But we do not have time to always be with our friends. We manage to spend only a couple of hours with them." Adil, a graduate student in New Delhi expressed how he felt the friendship portrayed on *Friends* was not as deep as he had personally experienced: "*Friends* has not taken up issues such as standing up for each other in times of crisis. They have never shown a real-life crisis like running short of money."

In summary, the Indian audiences display virtuality with most of the *Friends*' situations, relating the relevance of the situations to their own lives to see points of convergence and divergence.

## Ellipticality

As noted previously, *ellipticality* represents the narrative technique of leaving the details out, allowing the viewer to speculate on what might be happening (Olson, 1999). When our Indian respondents were asked how they felt about Monica's decision to call off sex for the night because of the nonavailability of a condom, we noted how it evoked several speculative readings.

Amrik strongly believed that Monica's actions would not be possible in India. In India, the male partner "would not have been pushed aside so easily"; instead, he would have "forced himself and persuaded the girl to have sex." Meenu, a young female viewer, believed that an Indian man would have been upset, fought with his girlfriend for calling off sex, and not been as understanding as Richard. Rakesh also felt that if a man and a woman were spending the night together, it was impossible to "shrug and pretend to say that [it] won't happen." Several re-spondents felt that under the circumstances, sex would definitely happen. Harpreet, a male respondent, agreed that it is hard to call off sex: "Once you make a plan, you have to perform it. You cannot make a plan and leave it half way. I will be willing to take [a] risk." Even though Harpreet believed that using a condom was necessary to avoid preg-nancy, it did not mean that he had to forego sex.

Bala, on the other hand, felt that such a situation—that is, running out of condoms—may arise in real life, and by watching how the char-acters in *Friends* dealt with the problem, he learned how to possibly act when confronted with a similar situation. Rakesh also felt that in the absence of a condom, he would abstain from sex. In essence, for some Indian reviewers, the *Friends* episode opened speculative read-ings; for some others, the readings were more closed, whereby they ac-cepted the manifest content portrayed in the plot.

The different readings of *Friends* suggest that its narrative is trans-parent, allowing the viewers to fill in the gaps. In so doing, Indian re-spondents negotiated preferred meaning of "safe sex" differently. Some accepted it; some rejected it outright. Several Indian respon-dents emphasized the impossibility of discussing sexual issues openly. As Mrs. Vaish noted: "This is not part of our culture. If at all a couple would discuss sex, they would have to be married." So, in some ways, the sexuality theme was opaque for our Indian respon-dents, especially as they could not relate it with their cultural values and sexual mores. However, the ellipticality in the narrative allowed them to engage in speculation, fill in the gaps, and make sense of the unfolding plot.

### Inclusion

As noted previously, *inclusion* is a narratological device that gives the viewer a sense that they are participating in the unfolding of the plot rather than simply observing it (Olson, 1999). Dinesh, a New Delhi-based male respondent, for instance, felt that the *Friends* plot was "pretty close" to his reality. He emphasized that young women in Indian metropolitan cities were open-minded, relatively free with boys, and could talk about all sorts of things, including sex, much like the women characters did in *Friends*. Dinesh felt that he could directly relate to the program's content as many of his young women city-based friends openly discussed things with him. Atul, another male respondent, highlighted how he felt included in the *Friends'* plot: "I want to act like Joey with my friends ... the way he talks, he walks ... his mannerisms really appeal to me." So Atul actively participated in the *Friends'* narra-tive by closely observing Joey while the program was on, and then also in the post-viewing context, he modeled Joey's behaviors in his inter-personal interactions.

Rakesh, another male respondent, elaborated on how he and his friends used to constantly spend time together—much like the friends in the sitcom, and noted how two of his friends eventually decided to get married—akin to the plot of *Friends*. Rakesh felt that the sitcom's narrative included and elaborated on his own lived experiences, noting "*Friends* is so similar to the friendships I have ... there is no stopping me [from watching it]." Another respondent echoed a similar sense of belonging and association with *Friends*. He observed, "I am able to directly associate with *Friends*. ... We took a house on rent ... three people living together."

## Verisimilitude

As noted previously, *verisimilitude* refers to the textual quality that conveys to the viewers that the plot is natural, real, and true to life (Olson, 1999). Verisimilitude hinges on Fisher's (1984, 1985a) twin concepts of *narrative probability*—Is the story coherent?; and narrative fidelity—To what degree does the story fits with the viewers' lives, past experiences, and present beliefs?

The Indian viewers assessed the narrative probability of *Friends* based on their personal lived experiences. Most respondents were highly uncomfortable about Monica being so open and suggestive about having sex with her partner in the same apartment as her brother, Ross. Bala noted, "Sex before marriage is not acceptable at any level in India. You never disclose to your brother if it happened. It is not proper." Adil noted: "This never happens in India because here brothers are very protective of their sisters." Zaira agreed: "It is not possible to be like this with my brothers. It is impossible." Harpreet was categorical: "We [in India] cannot tolerate such a relation. ... I won't allow her [my sister] this type of behavior." In essence, open discussion about sex among opposite sex siblings, and the possibility of them (knowingly) engaging in sex in adjoining rooms, is inconsistent with Indian cultural beliefs.

Our Indian respondents also felt that the situation depicting Monica and Rachael fighting over a condom was inconsistent with Indian reality. Stated Mrs. Vaish: "Monica and Rachael are fighting over one condom. These things don't happen in India." Rekha concurred: "You have your own condoms in 'your own' cupboard, but negotiating a condom is a closed topic here." Zaira from Hyderabad was even more emphatic: "Give me a break. Absolutely no. No way. This is absolutely weird. This will never happen in India. I don't think this even happens in America."

Also, Indian respondents did not believe that Indian women would take the lead in procuring a condom and deciding about whether or not sex would happen. This aspect of the plot was inconsistent with the perceptual "image of an Indian woman." As one respondent noted: "It is not good for a woman to carry a condom"; if she does, "her character is not too good." Another respondent clarified: "If her husband allows her to carry a condom ... then no problem; but it is different is he is un-married." Some respondents, however, agreed that Indian woman should "take the lead" in protecting themselves from pregnancy.

Viewers also questioned the narrative probability of *Friends* regard-ing the notion that Monica would go out with Richard, who is 30 years older than her. This age incompatibility would be very odd in India. As Mrs. Vaish stated: "To be very frank, the first thing that will come to people's minds is that the girl has married for money. No one in India accepts that a girl can marry an older male for just love." Further, In-dian respondents could not relate to the idea of a girl dating so many people, and having so many sexual partners.

Our respondents also assessed the narrative fidelity of *Friends* based on their own lived experiences. Many respondents could relate to the living arrangement of the six main characters in *Friends*, as they too had either shared a dorm room with friends while in college, or presently shared an apartment with friends. However, certain aspects of the narrative resonated more with the Indian context than certain other aspects. For instance, viewers found the explicit and open dis-cussion regarding sex, especially the conversation of the number of previous sexual partners as distasteful. One viewer stated: "The can-didness is quite American. I don't expect this to happen in India." An-other respondent stated that it is unacceptable in India to disclose to your partner that you "had sex with that guy last night," while in the United States, this perhaps would be acceptable. Priya, a 21-year-old unmarried female respondent, noted: "Though some girls do have sev-eral sexual partners, they do not talk about it, as premarital sex is still taboo in India, so they won't share this with even a best friend."

Rekha, a young woman mentioned that things were "very different in India." A mother in her forties clearly felt that she, understandably, could not identify with the lifestyle portrayed on *Friends*. Mrs. Vaish, a New Delhi-based homemaker concurred:

> ... the kind of lifestyle they lead, we wouldn't dream of letting our kids live in such proximity with the opposite sex, or at least we hope they won't. But things have changed, so I won't be surprised or horrified if such a thing was to happen in my family.

Responses from younger Indian viewers were more liberal, compared to the relatively more conservative beliefs held by the married and more senior (in age) respondents. Younger respondents acknowledged that such "free-wheeling" sexual relationships with the opposite sex were possible, even if not very probable. Most respondents felt that sexual openness was not yet acceptable in India.

## Other Mythotypical Elements

Consistent with our stated purpose, in the previous section, our analysis of *Friends* in India focused privileged the mythotypes of virtuality, ellipticality, inclusion, and verisimilitude. However, for contextualization, we further analyze how the mythotopes of openendedness, negentropy, circularity, and archetypical dramatis personae influence Indian audiences' reading of *Friends*.

As noted previously, *openendedness* refers to the textual quality of no resolution, which forces the viewer to return to the program with a hope for closure. The plot of *Friends*, consistent with the sitcom genre, evolves episodically without an actual ending to the storyline.[5] However, the ongoing narrative of *Friends* brought relief to the Indian audiences at the end of each episode—as the characters resolve their tricky situations. In this sense, *Friends* is an episodically "closed" text, but as a genre ongoing and openended.

As noted previously, *negentropy* refers to the textual quality of instilling a sense of meaning and order among its viewers. Seeing the same six characters in familiar settings on a regular basis was meaningful to the Indian viewers of *Friends*. Several of our respondents commented on the "thick" friendships among the series' six (both male and female) characters, something that they wished for in their personal lives. Watching these virtual friendships brought a sense of order, or negentropy, to the lives of these viewers.

As already noted, *circularity* refers to the narrative quality that makes viewers return to where the story began. Circularity also means placing the characters in a situation where they initially began. Our Indian viewers noted that they "looked forward" to the theme song of *Friends*, for it marked the beginning of yet another date with the six characters of the programs. They noted that the *Friends*' plot would invariably begin in the Greenwich Village Central Perk coffee shop. This narrative return to the familiar setting was like returning to the old familiar launch pad, only to take off again.

As noted, *archetypal dramatic personae* are "authentic" characters that are found in each culture and evoke affective responses across cultures. For example, many narratives include the archetype of a medieval knight, usually in the form of valiant die-hard romantic who steals the heart of young woman; or the archetype of a court jester, usually in the form of a comedian who entertains through humor. Several Indian respondents, as noted, considered Phoebe's role in *Friends* as being "silly, dumb, foolish, and funny." She exemplified the archetypal personae of a court jester.

## CONCLUSIONS

The present chapter investigated how Hollywood's mass-mediated world of health-related persuasion, information, and entertainment is interpreted outside its borders. We drew on Olson's (1999) narrative transparency theory and Fisher's (1984, 1985a) narrative theory to analyze how Indian audiences subjected the ideological and "safe sex" narrative of *Friends* to diverse mythotypic readings. In so doing, we responded to the call by cultural studies scholars to explore the intersections between texts, audience members, and their contexts.

The analysis just presented clearly shows the value of applying theoretical lenses to investigating the popularity of global narratives like *Friends*, which may purposely incorporate health messages as part of a social merchandizing approach. Clearly, most Indians watched *Friends* for a variety of reasons. Their motivations and involvement in *Friends* support, in various ways, Olson's (1999) mythotypes of *virtuality, ellipticality,* and *verisimilitude,* and Fisher's (1984, 1985a) concepts of *narrative probability* and *fidelity.* Not surprisingly, Indian viewers used their own lived experiences in interpreting *Friends,* and negotiated meanings based on personal values, lifestyles, and prevailing cultural norms.

It was interesting how *ellipticality,* which involves audience members filling in the gaps in the narrative, engendered highly affective responses from the Indian viewers. Our viewers wrestled with the role of women in initiating (and calling off sex), flaunting their multiple partners in premarital sexual encounters, and the like. In most instances, either the audience rejected the narrative because it was foreign to their experience, or they strongly felt the characters should have been married, in which case condom use and sexual openness become permissible. In essence, audience members provided their own culturally reasonable and acceptable speculations and resolutions to the unfolding "safe sex" emplotments. This finding suggests that although transparency narrative theory allows for audiences to bring in their own cultural values to interpret a foreign narrative, in reality, the viewers can go beyond to change the plot's context in order to fit their own prevailing realities.

One of the most revealing facets of this study was the sense of "cultural difference" that was clearly articulated and elaborated by Indian viewers of *Friends*. The difference was encapsulated in responses such as "It happens in the U.S. but not here in India," "That is American culture not Indian," and "They [the U.S.] have no culture." These references to the cultural difference espoused by Indian viewers can be construed as an indicator of the opacity of the narrative. However, opacity does not lead audiences to reject the entire narrative of *Friends*, nor did it offend their cultural sensibilities to the extent that they would switch off the program. In essence, opacity was identified for some specific issues but not for the whole program. While enjoying the program, when appropriate, the audience simply told themselves that this was a "window on another culture; it was not their own." And, on certain occasions, viewers viewed this difference in the context of how things were changing in India, and may be in the future.

Interestingly, viewers acknowledged that what is shown on *Friends* may not happen in India at the present time but may well take place in the coming years. This finding was evident especially among respondents who saw a looming "generation gap" between the prevailing Indian values with respect to mixed-sex friendships and sexuality and what was openly depicted on *Friends*. For instance, none of the Indian respondents said that they would feel comfortable watching *Friends* with their parents, grandparents, or other family elders. Several young viewers freely acknowledged that they were drawn to *Friends* because they knew the program would be considered taboo by their elders, and by watching it, they got the vicarious pleasure of going against the norms.

Linked to the reality of intergenerational difference in engaging with the sitcom was the theme of an "emergent culture," a new Indian culture, which according to majority of the Indian respondents models American culture. Although subtle, this theme was evident in almost all responses. The viewers felt that India was gradually moving toward a free-wheeling, sexually open culture, especially among the urban, elite youth who ape fashions of New York and Paris, drink coffee and cappuccinos, and hang out in bars and nightclubs. However, even those who embody this emergent Western culture live in a culture where sexual mores, in general, are highly conservative. For them, and for others, the sitcom may fill a desired vicarious need.

Does the watching of *Friends*, especially its sexually explicit emplotments, create possibilities for new health and lifestyle narratives by audience members? Our data suggests that watching of American television shows such as *Friends* spurs conversation (even if in hushed tones) among Indian viewers about topics that were hitherto taboo. Without necessarily accepting the "foreign" messages, Indian audience members—through repeated and consistent exposure to mediated programs like *Friends*—gain familiarity with, and a lingo for, talking about taboo topics. Over time, it is likely that repeated conversations on taboo topics make them less problematic, gradually shifting social mores.

What value did our investigation of the "safe sex" emplotment in *Friends* in India add to our understanding of Olson's (1999) narrative transparency theory? Interestingly, humor, as a narratological device, emerged as an overarching mythotype in our respondents' voices, even though it is not exclusively singled out in Olson's schemata. Humor, overwhelmingly, was brought up as being the primary affective motivation that goaded Indian audiences to regularly tune into *Friends*. Even though not all the jokes and funny lines were completely grasped by Indian viewers, it was clear that most respondents watched *Friends* because they found it humorous and relaxing. Despite the cultural-situatedness of jokes, humor about sex (and sexual innuendos, in particular) seemed to transcend cultural boundaries.

Further, what value did our Indian investigation of the "safe sex" emplotment in *Friends* add to our understanding of how entertainment-education programs are interpreted by audiences? Although most entertainment-education initiatives are framed within a psychological–cognitive framework to purposely influence audience members' knowledge, attitudes, and behaviors (Singhal & Rogers, 1999; Slater, 2002), our research design and results illustrate the efficacy of employing a dialogic and sociocultural approach to assessing entertainment-education effects. Our study points to the importance of recognizing how media texts, audience members, and contexts intersect to create multiple polysemic readings.[6] Our Indian respondents, far from being culturally duped by a foreign text, actively engaged with *Friends* to achieve varied ends—including the mocking (and, in some cases, the outright rejection) of American culture. Such results could only be revealed through a dialogic approach to assessing entertainment-education effects. By exploring how individuals negotiated unique meanings about health and sexuality with *Friends* in their differentiated contexts, our analysis ultimately illustrates how texts become sites of struggle over "preferred" meanings.

When entertainment-education programs seek to engender "preferred" meanings among audience members, it raises various ethical dilemmas (Singhal & Rogers, 1999). These dilemmas underscore the difficulties of planning entertainment education in the United States (Slater, 2002), and perhaps especially so when they are enacted across nation-states in the global public sphere. The *prosocial content* dilemma arises when the message is construed as prosocial by certain audience members and antisocial by others. Although some Indian audience members may consider the use of condoms in a first-time sexual encounter to be desirable, others may view depictions of sexual activity as promoting promiscuity. The *source-centered* dilemma deals with who decides what is prosocial. Should Hollywood producers really be deciding how people in India should be managing their sexual encounters? The *unintended effects* dilemma deals with the undesirable and unintended consequences that may result from adopting a certain "solution" depicted in a media text. What if an Indian woman is beaten by her male partner because she unilaterally calls off sex because a condom is unavailable? So, on one hand, a transparent narrative might empower an audience member to actively engage with the media text and make choices based on their situated context. On the other hand, does this freedom of interpretation afforded by a transparent narrative lead to greater risks for audience members in comparison to a close-ended opaque narrative, where the path of action is prescribed? Ultimately, the ethical dilemmas of entertainment-education texts are decided by audience members, who choose (or not choose) to embrace a "preferred" reading.

In ending, our analysis of *Friends* helped us gain theoretically rich insights on how Hollywood weaves its global web of transparent mass-mediated narratives. When such Hollywood-produced mass-mediated narratives include health emplotments, they raise important questions for scholars interested in the role of narratives in enacting wellness in the global public sphere.

## NOTES

1. We thank the following individuals and organizations who helped support the present research: The Centers for Disease Control and Prevention, Population Communications International, and the Center for Media Studies, New Delhi. We especially thank Irwin "Sonny" Fox, Everett M. Rogers, Avinash Thombre, Mrs. P. N. Vasanti, Adite Chatterjee, Sanjeev Kumar, Alok Shrivastav, V. V. Sundar, Michael I. Arrington, Devendra Sharma, and Saumya Pant for their inputs to the present project. A previous version of the present paper (Chitnis, Sengupta, & Singhal, 2004) was presented to the International Communication Association, New Orleans, May, 2004. We also thank Drs. Lynn M. Harter, Phyllis M. Japp, and Christie S. Beck, the editors of this volume, for their detailed and valuable comments on a previous version of this manuscript.

2. In addition to these eight devices that embody the internal "structural" aspects of the narratives, Olson (1999) called attention to two mythotypes that represent the media text's external attributes and contribute toward its transparency: *omnipresence* and *production values*. Omnipresence refers to the constant presence of electronic media in our lives—whether at home, in a doctor's waiting room, or in a shopping mall. Production values include the budgetary and other technical inputs which enhance the audience receptivity of a media message. Olson argues that Hollywood products are globally attractive because of their mega production budgets and elaborate special effects.

3. The data collection was commissioned to a professional New Delhi-based media research organization, Center for Media Studies, which also transcribed the interviews.

4. Since its launch, it has been nominated for a record-breaking 55 Emmy Awards, including the Outstanding Comedy Series, a recognition it won in 2003 (www.nbc.com/Friends/about/index.html). *Friends* is presently broadcast in over 100 countries, including Slovenia, Brazil, Croatia, Australia, and India, and is especially popular among younger populations. An estimated, 500 million people worldwide watch the show on a weekly basis.

5. *Friends* had its tenth and final season (2003–2004) of broadcast in the United States; although through syndicated reruns, it will maintain its presence on United States and overseas markets for years to come.

6. In this sense, our research may hold implications for the growing body of literature on *interpretive communities* that arise when people sit together and watch a media program together (Beck, 1995, Biocca, 1988; Gunter, 1988; Lindlof, 1988). An interpretive community exists when individuals who count themselves as members of a viewing community collaboratively co-define the viewing experience (when cheering, e.g., for a particular football team; or when watching a soap opera).

# III

## Narrating and Organizing
## Health Care Events and Resources

∾

### INTRODUCTION

**Lynn M. Harter**
*Ohio University*

*It was a sultry and slow summer evening in Athens. Emma Grace and I walked to the mailbox. On our trip back to the front porch, I fingered the envelope from my folks, Rich and Bev Harter. A smile crossed my face as I opened the letter and read the enclosed newspaper article. "Senator Chuck Hagel went to the front lines this week to listen to the life-and-death concerns of those who watch and wait and worry as Congress tackles Medicare reform," the article began, accompanied by a photograph of the senator engaged in conversation with several health care providers and patients (Walton, August 6, 2003, p. 1B). As a House-Senate conference committee deliberated about potential changes in Medicare legislation, Senator Hagel conducted focus groups with people who have cancer in hopes of better understanding the complexities of health care delivery in clinics, cancer centers, and hospitals. My father was one of the participants. "As Congress searches for a political solution to the Medicare impasse, Rich Harter of Plattsmouth told Hagel he hopes it will be alert to the danger of 'unintended consequences' that could damage the quality of health care" (Walton, August 6, 2003, p. 1B). My smile broadened as I beamed with pride and reflected on the inter-textual nature of our storied*

189

lives, among other things. My Dad is usually the first person I show my recently published works, many of which draw on Gidden's Structuration Theory to highlight "unintended consequences" of discursive practices and patterns.

I flashed back to August, 1997, when my father was diagnosed with multiple myeloma. The second year of my doctoral work had just begun. I had completed a course under the direction of Dr. Phyllis Japp on Rhetoric and Health, and was working as her teaching assistant in an Introduction to Health Communication undergraduate course. In punctuating key moments in my personal and professional journey in narrative and health, my father's battle (his metaphor of choice) with cancer remains central to the plot. Multiple myeloma is a rare form of blood cancer (constituting approximately one percent of cancer cases in the United States) in which cancerous plasma cells in the blood form tumors, termed myeloma, in bone marrow. My father's co-constructed and ever-evolving story of cancer includes multiple treatments, from five years of chemotherapy to an experimental stem cell transplant to daily doses of various potent steroids, thalidomide and narcotic pain medications; multiple side-effects and emergency interventions, including surgery to have part of his colon removed; diverse settings of care including cancer clinics, hospital settings, and home health care; and a cast of characters including health care providers, family, friends, participants of an online support group, former colleagues, and members of the local Catholic parish.

An ambient, opaque silence enveloped my father's initial diagnosis and increased our collective sense of chaos, dislocation, and loss. Initially, and then intermittently over the subsequent seven years of treatments, words failed to capture our fear. Yet, in other moments, storytelling emerged as a resource allowing us to reconnect, weave webs of significance and cohesion, and create meaning out of what otherwise might have remained an unbearable sequence of happenings. I've learned more about my father—his tour with the Army Special Operations command in Southeast Asia, his calling as a trial attorney, his painful first marriage—in the past seven years of coping with this "terminal" illness than in the preceding 27 years of my life. My father's multiple myeloma continues to serve as an occasion for family members to re-visit past experiences and re-envision future priorities. Storytelling functions as a symbolic ritual helping our family, most of the time, to engage in sense-making, (re)construct identities, and live healthy lives in the midst of cancer and its symptoms, side-effects, and suffering.

The interconnectedness of narrative activity surfaces as an undercurrent of this book. Institutional settings of all sorts, including health care contexts, supply the narrative auspices under which selves come to be articulated. At the same time, individual and institutional stories reflect and create, or at the very least, contribute to, broader socioeconomic political conditions as they are expressed through grand narratives (e.g., capitalism, technology as progress). My father's story of multiple myeloma continues to evolve as a constellation of stories including our family's (re)history, institutional narratives, societal myths and metaphors. For example, our family narrates our experiences, usually unconsciously, using the dominant biomedical language of military warfare: My father "fights" the cancerous cells "armed" with the most "powerful" technology that money can buy and with a team of oncologists "leading the charge." When narrative theorists draw attention to webs of interwoven social forces—market patterns, institutional practices, lived experiences of individuals—the locus of observation expands to include the hegemonic and material constraints that often lie beyond the awareness of individuals, including organizational features that enable, constrain, justify, mask, and mystify the interests of particular individuals or groups.

Communication scholars commonly assert that organizations are both the medium and outcome of discourses, always in a state of becoming, grounded in symbolic action, and anchored in social practices (Fairhurst & Putnam, 2004). The rules and resources drawn on by organizational members are at the same time the means of system reproduction. Almost 20 years ago, Dennis Mumby (1987) positioned narrative as a principal symbolic form through which organizational structure and ideology are (re)produced and resisted. Mumby wrote:

> Narratives do not simply inform organization members about the values, practices, and traditions to which their organization is committed. Rather, they help to constitute the organizational consciousness of social actors by articulating and embodying a particular reality, and subordinating or devaluing other modes of "organizational rationality." (p. 125)

Narratives are central to how we bring order and meaning to our lives, and as such remain the coin and currency of organizational and community life. Indeed, collective life would be impossible were it not for our human capacity to organize and embody lived experience in narrative form. It is out of narrative rituals that we carve lives for ourselves—and organizational forms.

All social structures, including health care organizations, can be conceived of as narrative threads or fragments of broad discursive forms (e.g., bureaucratic forms). Providers, patients, and politicians alike consume these representations, reproducing and/or resisting them in the daily performance of their roles. In the focus group led by Senator Hagel just mentioned, patients and family members urged the Senator to prevent the restructuring of Medicare that would limit patients' access to cancer clinics by cutting reimbursement to clinics by $500 million dollars. One participant, Jerry Krupinsky, shared, "Cancer in itself is devastating ... If I had to go to the hospital, instead of coming here [a cancer clinic], not knowing my nurse as I do now, it would be even more devastating" (Walton, 2003, p. 1B). In this case, the resources (and vulnerabilities) bestowed on patients and their families through the potential restructuring of Medicare operate at odds with their lived stories. Participants' stories collide and compete with institutional and societal narratives that strive for efficient and fiscally sound ways of organizing finite health care resources. Senator Hagel entered the co-construction of these seemingly incompatible and clashing realities. "I don't want you to worry that we will take away Medicare reimbursements for chemotherapy in clinics or as outpatients," he said. "We're not going to do it. We're going to straighten this out. We won't let this happen" (Walton, 2003, p. 1B).

Narrative practices, including who is entitled to tell a story and when it can be told, reflect and establish power relations in a wide range of domestic and community institutions. A case in point: Multiple myeloma did not receive widespread public recognition and attention until June, 2001, when Geraldine Ferraro testified on Capitol Hill to the Senate Appropriations and Labor, Health and Human Services Committees (Ferraro, 2001). Ferraro testified, from a self-described position of privilege and power, about her own diagnosis of multiple myeloma, including her treatment protocol and how the cancer has impacted her personal and professional relationships. I celebrated when Ferraro, a prominent figure in our culture's political scene, drew Americans' attention to the debilitating and painful condition of multiple myeloma, and I supported her call for research about its causes and consequences. Yet, I remain aware of how political power and access are not exclusively benign processes—powerful individuals help to set agendas, influencing which diseases are highlighted and which are ignored. Health problems of grave importance to significant numbers of Americans remain unnoticed because of a lack of publicity (e.g., childhood asthma, prenatal care) whereas relatively rare conditions receive attention and funding because of the clout of public spokespersons (e.g., multiple myeloma, Lou Gehrig's disease [ALS]). Moreover, I would be remiss not to recognize that the visibility of Senator Hagel "on the frontlines" (Walton, 2003, p. 1B) with cancer patients fosters a powerful narrative about his interface with constituents generally and health care issues specifically.

The chapters in this section also illustrate how institutional and cultural narratives articulate possibilities and preferences that social actors invoke as they live their lives. In chapter 9, Bill Rawlins vividly portrays how narrative is fundamental to the everyday accomplishment of medical knowledge and medical work. Through dialogue with his father, Dr. Jack Rawlins, Bill draws us into the career of one family's physician. Dr. Rawlins' narration illustrates the often unacknowledged position of health care providers as characters within and co-authors of patients' life stories, and encourages readers to reenvision the professional discourse of medicine as co-constructed, intertextual, narrative activity. For example, Dr. Rawlins poignantly shares a story of how he learned from another doctor to look for birds in children's ears—a strategy that successfully alleviated kids' anxiety towards otoscopes. Whenever Emma Grace and I visit her pediatrician, we now look for birds in her ears, mouth and tummy. We hope Dr. Rawlins' lifework as a narratively competent health care provider will be understood, appreciated and co-performed by readers.

Jayne Morgan-Witte (chap. 10) also explores narrative knowledge among caregivers. From an ethnographic standpoint, Jayne observes webs of storytelling in contemporary medical backstages—nurses' stations. Jayne's insightful analysis illustrates how the narrative construction of knowledge by medical professionals endorses and enacts certain value structures. The discourses of the biomedical model, including the norm of "detached concern" displayed by providers in this study, represent institutionalized narratives about how people, labor, and health care delivery should be arranged and enacted. Participants in Jayne's study embody and normalize such narratives in mundane interaction and in so doing (re)produce particular identities. The biomedical narrative functions as a textual guide that directs the formation not only of individual identities (e.g., the health care provider as distant and objective expert) but also organizational form (e.g., the prevalence of structures that privilege instrumental rationality).

Sunwolf, Larry Frey, and Lisa Keranen (chap. 11) emphasize the therapeutic value of storysharing for multiple stakeholders in health care encounters. By foregrounding the importance of listening to narratives, Sunwolf and her colleagues illustrate possibilities for engaging in dialogic narrative practice and position narrative activity as central to the organizing of health care resources. They describe numerous exemplars of how storytelling and story listening have been employed therapeutically in health contexts ranging from chronic conditions such as cancer and asthma to cases of severe trauma.

By carefully documenting existing limitations in palliative care, and by extension the preparation of health care providers, Sandra Ragan, Tiffany Mindt, and Elaine Wittenberg-Lyles (chap. 11) present a compelling case for narrative medicine and the possibilities (and potential limits) of narrative-based medical education. Sandra and her colleagues situate narrative-based education in the broader humanistic pedagogical movement in medical schools and provide readers with an extensive collection of resources on narrative pedagogy and its ability to develop students' cultural sensitivity, listening skills, and abilities to recognize and wrestle with ethical dilemmas. When positioned within the legacy of studies about the professional socialization of medical students, this chapter points to the importance of situating socializing discourses within social, political, and historical moments (e.g., consumer ideologies have led to increased accountability of providers for the satisfaction of patients and families).

Narativity creates and maintains organizational life by (re)producing and resisting social orders. Such is the case in the organizing of health care resources—within and beyond the boundaries of health care organizations. Patrice Buzzanell and Laura Ellingson (chap. 13) co-construct the story of one woman, Tara, who encounters pregnancy-related complications and an unsympathetic employer. Patrice, Laura, and Tara candidly illustrate how personal narratives are embodied within (and shaped by) organizational and societal narratives—some of which are ambiguous and competing—and reveal the theoretical and practical potential of feminist analysis. Their analysis is suggestive of the political nature of storytelling in and about organizational life, activity that cannot be viewed independently of the ideological meaning formations and relations of domination within which they are communicated (e.g., entrepreneurial discourses). Meanwhile, the authors also highlight the power of counternarratives to reclaim moral agency.

Magdalyn Miller, Patricia Geist-Martin, and Kristen Cannon Beatty (chap. 14) likewise reveal the power of counternarratives to repair damaged identities—of individuals and communities. Magdalyn and her colleagues share a case study of the Tariq Khamisa Foundation (TKF), an organization that works to disrupt dominant narratives of teenage violence and aggression and promote nonviolent behaviors through pedagogies of peace. The mobilizing narrative of TKF illustrates how the structural properties of narratives (e.g., emplotment, characters) become powerful repertories of protest. Ultimately, the storytelling that emerges through TKF's pedagogies of peace demonstrate why narratives have long been a favored route to teaching moral and ethical behavior.

These chapters represent starting points for describing and challenging narrative practices and patterns. They provide us with visions for how to (re)organize health care resources in ways that dignify rather than diminish the human spirit. Moreover, they resist the temptation to position organizations as mere containers of narrative life. In some chapters, the organization is a primary character in the unfolding story—a protagonist or hero constraining or enabling humanistic and effective health care (see e.g., Buzzanell & Ellingson, chap. 13, and Miller, Geist-Martin, & Cannon, chap. 14). In other chapters, health care organizations emerge as settings that shape and are shaped by webs of storytelling among diverse stakeholders including health care providers and patients (see e.g., Morgan-Witte, chap. 10, and Sunwolf, Frey, & Keranen, chap. 11). Collectively, these authors and chapters illustrate the ability of communication theory–research-praxis to yield insights into complex patterns and relationships—analyses that, in turn, become resources for organizational and social change.

# 9

## Our Family's Physician

∿

**William K. Rawlins**
*Ohio University*

I'm 14 years old and my band, The Dynasty, is playing at the Seaford Summer Canteen. It's a fiercely hot and humid midsummer night—a "close" one, as we call it in lower Delaware. The junior high cafeteria is packed with high school students—the boys with Beach Boy hair cuts, madras shirts, and white jeans; the girls with shoulder-length "Cher hair," halter tops, and tight white cut-offs. We're doing "My Generation" by The Who, and I'm drummin' like crazy. I play football, basketball, and baseball for our school, but I have never sweated like this. Emulating Keith Moon's gnashing, frenzied drum solo beat keeping for the last four minutes of the song is pretty well tapping me out. I can't hit my cymbals for the last chord of the song because both of my arms are clenched to my chest, and I can't pry them open. Scared and upset, I shriek to my band-mates, "I can't move my arms!"

Bill Waller, our bass player, bolts to the pay phone and calls the family doctor. He knows the number well because that doctor is my dad. "Well, hello, Duck," my dad says. "Aren't you with Bill?" Duck Waller tells Dad about what's happened and how terrified I am. "Tell Bill not to worry. You're in the cafeteria, aren't you?"

Duck says yes. "Well, go over by the service windows where they store the salt shakers. Pour half of one into a Coke, and tell Bill to drink it down. He'll be fine in a matter of moments." Truer words were never spoken. We finish the gig without a hitch, and I still carry salt tablets in my drums' trap case to this day.

\*   \*   \*

Of course, this wasn't the first time my dad answered a phone call or made a house call with healing wisdom for me and nearly everyone else in our small town during his 40 years of practicing medicine, and it certainly would not be the last. In fact, I'm 51 now and called him a few weeks ago for two reasons.

"Dad, I was talking to one of my colleagues the other day who is editing a book on narrative approaches to medicine. She has heard me speak before about your life as a doctor. On many occasions, I have characterized you as 'The Last of the Marcus Welbys' and as someone who would rather talk his patients into good health than simply prescribe drugs. She wondered if I might be interested in interviewing you and developing a chapter describing your experiences as a family physician. I am excited by her encouragement because at the very least we would have a record of you similar to the one Cousin Jimmy made of Grandmother that we all treasure so much. But I am also confident that you have some terrific stories to tell that are very much in the spirit of the book and useful for folks in health communication to think about. When we come east after Christmas, maybe we could find some time for me to interview you. What do you think?" "It sounds fine," my dad replies. "Let's see how it goes." "That will be great. I've got some spiffy new recording equipment that they bought me when I came here to OU, and I think you'll find it intriguing. But I've actually got a medical question to raise with you as well ..."

For as long as I can remember, I've had the privilege of asking my dad "medical questions." The unspoken rule in my experience, however, especially when we are talking on the phone, is to label them as such. This gives my mom the opportunity to excuse herself from the conversation although we will call her back when the "medical talk" is over. In my estimation, my dad is an extraordinarily talented diagnostician with a rigorous yet comforting "bedside manner," even when he is talking on the phone. Although he has always been reluctant to diagnose conditions without physically examining someone and carefully qualifies what he says, he is very good at narrowing the possibilities and offering reassurances or suggesting immediate attention from someone else based on the "indications" he has to work with. In truth, it is difficult for me to convey to you the confidence I have in my father's judgment in all matters medical; it borders on absolute. Paradoxically, any limits I have ever placed on his judgment have occurred because he has judged himself to be limited with regard to particular questions I have asked him. In such instances, he sends me elsewhere while he also "looks into it further."

For a couple days, I have been complaining to my wife Sandy about my skin "burning" along the outside right ridge of my back ribcage. Perhaps because I was raised as a physician's son, I have developed my own diagnosis. For the past 2 weeks, I have spent an hour a night sanding and varnishing some oak closet doors. I started noticing what I perceived as pain in my muscles on the right side of my back. Over the years, one of the first things Dad says about muscular pain is, "What have you been doing that might be using your muscles in a different way?" So I decide this is a clear case of specific muscular strain (since I'm a right-handed sander and painter), and Sandy is kind enough to rub a liberal amount of Ben Gay™ into the muscles in question. Since I'm also finished with the doors, I believe that I will be fine in the morning.

However, the next day when we go Christmas shopping, I not only feel a burning pain on the skin on my back but also on the skin of my chest. Although it persists all day, I don't mention it because I don't want to be a complainer and because I believe it will pass. I recall that the Ben Gay™ really seared the night before when Sandy squeezed it onto my back; maybe I've had an allergic reaction to it or perhaps to the bleach in my tee shirts? Something.

The next morning I complain to Sandy, who gently suggests that I go to the doctor if it bothers me that much. Instead, I call my dad. After narrating to him the above sequence of events, my dad says, "There are a few things this might be; but let me ask you a few questions. First, is all of the pain on one side?" I say yes while also trying to get some credit for my own diagnosis. He acknowledges my efforts but also brushes them off, "Is this burning you feel close to the surface of your skin?" "Yes." "And how long have you been experiencing this pain?" After I reply, he says, "Bill, this could be a couple of things, but it sounds to me that the most likely possibility is that you have shingles." After explaining that he doesn't want to alarm me but that shingles are a skin condition with potential complications that may occur decades after a person has had chicken pox, he says, "I am going to want to examine you when you arrive here."

\*   \*   \*

While my family and I prepare to travel east to visit my parents, I give considerable thought to my hypothesis that the upcoming interview with my father will yield valuable insights and edifying stories for persons interested in the roles of narrative in health communication. My dad loves telling and hearing stories, but there is more to it than that. From growing up with him, I have witnessed, felt and heard from others about his person-centered approach to medicine, his empathic and tender regard for children needing medical attention, and his deep understandings of the personal and family circumstances of his patients. I also know that during his active years of practice, he combined intense respect for an up-to-date scientific basis of medicine with a timeless, morally invested dedication to helping, to caring for those who "were having a pretty rough time of it lately" and had turned to him. I have often felt that he experiences the story of his own life and his identity as a physician as interwoven with the stories of his patients' lives. Further, he adroitly used what he could glean from his patients' stories to help them, and many of his admonitions for healthier lifestyles and his descriptions of diagnoses and treatments were actually rendered as stories. My considered opinion is that my father, John C. Rawlins, M.D., embodied a narrative stance and exemplified "narrative competence" (Montello, 1997) in his 40 years of practice as a family physician. I believe that hearing him narrate his life's work will dramatize key commitments and practices of such a stance that will be worthwhile for contemporary theorists, practitioners, and laypersons involved with health communication to hear.

For example, although my dad has always been tight-lipped about the particulars of his professional activities and rarely revealed the names of his patients in any discussions, I recall a story my dad once told me that vividly attests to his narrative sensibilities as a physician. It seems that Burt Phillips (pseudonym), one of the more renowned partiers in town from my dad's generation, was getting ready to go out with his wife, Gertie (pseudonym) late one Friday afternoon when he complained of "not feeling quite right." When pressed to explain by his wife, he added that he'd also been feeling a little light-headed at work that morning, but "figured he'd get past it." She said, "Why don't you call Jack Rawlins? He's probably still at his office." When he did call, my dad advised Burt to "slip on by my office so I can check you out." Once Burt arrived, my dad performed an EKG on him and had some blood work done stat. Meanwhile, he asked Burt to tell him about "what he'd been doing with himself lately, and how he'd been feeling," as usual, listening very carefully to the yarns, jokes, and business ventures, interspersed with self-mocking quips and brief reflections on how Burt felt that composed his reply and brought them both up to the puzzling present.

A little later, upon receiving the battery of test results, Dad said that he couldn't identify anything "definitive." Feeling satisfied that he'd "done his duty healthwise" and standing up to leave, Burt said, "Well, Doc, I guess this means Gertie and I will be moseying off to the Country Club just as we've planned for tonight." However, my dad still felt uneasy about Burt's situation; "Hold on a second, Chief," he said. He told me later that a few things were going through his mind in addition to the "objective indicators." First, he knew Burt had an "appetite for life—including cigars, drink, and too many extra helpings of rich foods—that was potentially killing him." He also knew that Burt wasn't a complainer. So recalling that Burt had just let slip in the story of his recent days that, "I feel like an elephant is resting his foot on my chest from time to time," my dad reached a decision. "I'm sorry, but I don't think you're going to the Country Club tonight," he told Burt. "And you have two choices. You can let me call Gertie to come and take you to the hospital, or I am going to call for the ambulance to do it."

I always get cold chills remembering the rest. Burt made it to the hospital in time to have a heart attack right in the emergency room in full attendance by hospital personnel. A telling combination of medical science, discerning attention to the physical implications of the elephant metaphor and other features in his patient's story, and his familiarity with Burt's personal habits, allowed my dad to respond in a manner that saved his life. My dad related to me, "When I visited him in the hospital later that night, I told him, 'When we get this all straightened out and you get out of here, I am going to want to have a little talk with you about the way you've been living.' "

And now that I think about it, he actually may have been telling me this story these many years ago when I was a young man to convince me to mend my own partying ways at that point in my life.

*    *    *

Our children, Sandy, and I have arrived in Seaford and are enjoying our visit. We've gone out to dinner, watched TV, and spent an afternoon with my brother, Ron, and his wife, Barbara, laughing and telling stories to our children about growing up in this family. We've wandered around my parents' house, my childhood home, noticing what's changed and what's stayed the same and swapping stories about any of the keepsakes or pictures that catch our eyes. Dad has examined me, confirmed his initial diagnosis face-to-face and printed 5 pages from the American Academy of Dermatology Public Resources Web site for me to read about my condition. As a final precaution, he has discussed my case at length with the young doctor who joined him late in his career and then took over his practice when Dad retired at age 70. Dr. Smith has prescribed a regimen of medication and I'm feeling a little better. It's now my third day in the home of my youth, and Dad and I are settled into a recorded conversation— an interview—about my dad's life as a doctor.

I ask him, "Do you remember when you first decided to become a doctor? Are there any particular events that led you to become a doctor?"

"I was born in Quitman, Georgia, April the first, 1921, and grew up in a rural area, and ... in this town my dad was an automobile mechanic, which was a little unusual because there weren't that many cars. But as a child I had several different conditions; I had what they said at the time was facial paralysis and had to have treatment [for] the spasm and whatnot that was in my cheek. My mother often said how many times she used to have to put pads in to keep me from chewing on this for the short time that I had it. Subsequently, I had the usual childhood diseases, but I had particularly severe ear infections and went to see the doctor innumerable times. I also had a number of boils, which were local infections; in retrospect, it was staphlococcic infections, and in those days there were absolutely no antibiotics. So it was treated very, uh [pause] severely."

"And I can remember going up into the second floor office of the doctor with these sores on my legs, and he apparently put some type of thing that burned very much and irritated my legs. And then he would put collodion, some type of coating that stuck to the skin, which required another visit, which had to be peeled off, and this was most uncomfortable; but I went to the doctor. Then to top it all off, at age 6 I suddenly had acute appendicitis, and I was carried to the hospital at the neighboring town, which was about 20 miles away, and at that time they had to operate on me for the appendix. The hospital was pretty well filled and I happened to be in the bed close to the hall, and this is fairly important because my mother was allowed to bring in a cot and stay beside me. But the area became infected and then I had to stay in the hospital for a bit longer than usual, and then I had to have a drain for this area, and my mother would say, 'They had to remove a pint of pus.' But this obviously kept me back as far as progress, and I missed some schooling, but fortunately I made up for that."

Hearing these stories makes me realize that part of the reason my dad wanted to become a doctor and later was so dedicated to empathic pediatrics could be his own rather trying experiences with doctors when he was a youth. But I also know he was impressed with the social role of physicians in his home town. I say, "It seems to me you've mentioned Dr. Fox and Dr. Lynch from time to time that I can recall, did they mentor you?"

"I think I've told you the story; when I was in high school, I just kept telling people that I was going to be a doctor. And Dr. Lynch had just opened a little office and I was playing football, and I was probably about a hundred and fifty pounds, a hundred and fifty-five pounds, and I was, I think that was when I was a sophomore in high school. But at any rate, they put me opposite somebody on the line and uh, I got pounded a couple times, and I finally started developing [what] actually was a hematoma on my left lower leg. My mother put a heating pad on it which might have been too hot, [and I] developed a blister, so I had a blister on top of the swollen leg, and I went to see Dr. Lynch. And Dr. Lynch used ethyl chloride and kept freezing it and kept waiting to use a knife to open up this hematoma. And he kept saying, 'Do you feel that?'

And I didn't feel nothin', but I kept saying, 'Yes I feel it, I feel it, I feel it.' And pretty soon my leg was frosted all over. But finally he jabbed the knife in, released the blood, and amazingly enough, I was a little woozy afterwards."

"But I had kept telling him I was going to be a doctor. So he pulls some loose-leaf sheets out of some obsolete medical things he had and gave me, and he said, 'You might want to study this over if you're going to be a doctor.' And then I got up and I was a little woozy and he said, 'Do you know, on the other hand, maybe I ought to take you with me on some of my house calls.' What he was doing was making sure I didn't pass out in the street. And he drove me around through a couple areas and finally took me home."

So many images and stories are recalled to me as I listen to my dad that I can't begin to share them all with you. Just hearing the two words, house calls, in this story of his visit with Dr. Lynch brings an avalanche of associations. My dad made house calls for as long as I can remember. The phone could ring any time day or night, and my dad would respond. He took me with him sometimes during the days, and watching from his car, I would catch glimpses of the anguished, grateful faces that would meet him at their house's threshold, many of whom would later be smiling, even laughing when he left. I sensed then and know now that these countless calls were shining moments. I'm grateful to have witnessed a sprinkling of them. My dad always used the phrases "caring for my patients" and "giving my patients the best care possible," in referring to his work and he meant what he said.

I have three brothers, and we all liked cars. Assuming in the greedy way that children sometimes do that my dad made a lot of money because he was a doctor, we often wondered and carped about why we didn't live more extravagantly. Once I asked my dad why he was driving a bland '58 Chevy Biscayne. Why didn't he drive something sharp and sporty like Mr. or Dr. so-and-so? He looked me in the eye and said, "Bill, you've been with me when I make house calls. Many of the homes I visit don't even have indoor plumbing. I don't think it's right to go see my patients in some flashy car. This one starts fine in the middle of the night, and that's what matters."

Dad was careful not to wake us during the nights when he was called out, sometimes more than twice. He left his clothes and tie on a high-backed chair in the bathroom, his overcoat and doctor's bag in the closet right by the door to the garage. When he answered the phone and believed it was necessary to see the patient, he was on his way. Actually, I don't recall hearing or witnessing this drill as a youth because he was so quiet in leaving. But in my later high school and college years, often when I was coming home at say 2:00 a.m. from a date or playing music, I encountered my dad at some point in his cycle of making house calls while most of the world was enjoying a good night's sleep. Once in a while we would have a bowl of vanilla ice cream with Rice Krispies and talk before going (back) to bed.

Returning to the interview, I refresh my knowledge of my dad's education. He received his Bachelor of Science in 1943 from Western Maryland College as a Biology major and a Chemistry minor. He went to medical school at the University of Maryland, finishing in 3 years due to the 9 months on, 1 month off schedule followed during World War II. After 15 months of interning in two different hospitals in Washington D.C., the local boy who always said that he was going to be a doctor was making good on his promise. I ask my dad, "What do you remember about your early years as a physician? How do you go from being some kid in town to a town doctor?"

My dad replies, "When I finished and got ready to practice medicine, I thought maybe I shouldn't go back to my own home town at first, so I decided I would go close by. And I was given some pretty good offers; (chuckling) they weren't very good offers, but I thought they were. I had letters from the mayor and the chief of, fire chief from Mardella, and from Hurlock, and Federalsburg. And I decided I would move to Federalsburg, Maryland."

"And in Federalsburg, Maryland, I started having a pretty good active practice although my office was two little tiny rooms and they were heated by an upright oil stove. And I had no nurse, saw all these patients completely with nobody around, no chaperone, no nurse, no nothing. And I started having maternity patients; and I had a screen in the room where my desk was, and it was really a very primitive set-up. And uh, actually, office hours were $2 a visit. And after I'd been there a year, well during this time I started getting ready for my Delaware boards. So I spent one summer basically boning up to take the state exam for Delaware."

"And then, and I went to Easton, I did my, there was no hospital in Seaford, and I did my deliveries over in Easton. And that's where Ronnie was delivered, by Doctor Baker—who always thought that Ronnie had been named after him."

We laugh together because my brother's name is Ronald Baker Rawlins, Baker being my mom's maiden name.

"But anyhow, suddenly I realized that I'd missed a diagnosis—of pyloric stenosis, and I thought, You know, if I'm going to do family practice, I'm well-versed in obstetrics, and I'm good in these other things, but I didn't have very much training in pediatrics. So I decided I would go back to study, and through the influence of a doctor in Easton, I applied and was accepted on the staff at Johns Hopkins. So I went to Johns Hopkins to get some experience in pediatrics so I would be well rounded. And while I was there, they tried to encourage me to go ahead and continue to do nothing but pediatrics. In fact, somebody came from Salisbury—Dr. Rivers Hanson came and offered me to come move down to Salisbury when I got out of Hopkins, come down there. And I said, 'No, I want to go back to my hometown.' "

"And when I let it be known that I was going to come back to Seaford, Dr. Fox contacted me, and said, 'Hey, how about joining me?' And I said, 'No, I don't want to do that.' Well, he had a very upstanding, good big practice, and he said, 'Well, you ought to do that 'cause we can join hands and have kind of like an emergency room right in my own office, right in my own place.' I said, 'No.' I turned him down about three or four times; and the reason I did, I didn't want people coming to see Dr. Fox and having to see Jack Rawlins. If they were going to come, they were going to come see Jack Rawlins—in his office—because he was Jack Rawlins. So I wanted my own autonomy and that's the way I did it. That's what I insisted on."

"Dad, you were saying something very interesting. You said there was a diagnosis over in Easton that you didn't think you got right. So you decided to get some more education. Could you talk more about that?"

"Yes, and this is very interesting; the course was pyloric stenosis, which is a very, 'stenosis'—tight opening of the intestines at the end of the stomach—and it caused the baby to regurgitate, not do they just spit up but they (he makes a sound effect, 'swhew') projectile vomit. And I missed this case, and I felt very badly about it so I went to Hopkins."

"What do you mean, 'you missed the case?' "

"I just didn't make the proper diagnosis. I had assumed it was something else and eventually, as it turns out, it's a very simple procedure if you find that in a baby. They make a very small incision, and they go in and they just nip the side of the scar tissue, and it pops open, and that's good."

"Um, so I go to Johns Hopkins, I'm there for a year, busy, see all kinds of pathology, learned a lot of medicine, and about 5 days before I left, I saw my next case of pyloric stenosis; there hadn't been another case at Hopkins the entire year. And this one? Came from Federalsburg." "That's intriguing." "Eh?" he asks with a smile. "And you recognized it."

"I didn't say I recognized it (laughs in a modest way); I saw it there; I learned from it. But I didn't really promote my improvement on that particular case by my year's absence at, (pause) at nothing a month. The salary there was nothing a month. Room and board and nothing a month."

There's a long pause as we both reflect silently on the stories that he's just been telling. I ask, "Do you want to take a break? Do you want any water or anything?"

"Yeah, I'll take a break."

Listening now while I'm writing, the tape runs on as we get up and stretch. I hear myself say as we walk into the kitchen, "I'm learning a lot, Dad."

*     *     *

Some minutes later we're back in the living room. Checking my machine to make sure it's on, I quietly ask again, "Why did you want to be a doctor?" We both laugh at the simultaneous redundancy and importance of the question.

"Well, based on my experience as a child, and the fact that I wanted it first as it was strictly an objective because it was the main role model that I had ever had. But then the more I got into it, I liked it more and more because I liked to be with people, I liked to communicate with people, and by being a family practitioner, I felt I was part of the family. And in many cases, I've still been considered that way. This is a rare privilege to be in people's lives and be involved *with* them and be considered part of the family. And consequently, that made me feel that I had to be available to them at all times, and this same philosophy is what was carried out when I got a partner to assist with this, and the main reason for this was to make sure that we could give 24-hour coverage."

"The ... sometimes this had its problems because it's kind of difficult to have an adult and have a child in the same family and both of them having completely opposite viewpoints, and both of them having different activities, and to try to be honest with *both* of them was a little difficult." "Do you mean in caring for them?" "Um hmm. I guess only when it really got complicated was suddenly having the mother and a daughter come into the office expecting a baby and neither one knew the other was having one. But that worked out very nicely."

"How do you deal with a situation like that? That seems like a conundrum involving a tight web of relationships. How do you deal with it?"

"One day at a time." He laughs quietly with a little sigh of knowing resignation. "Each event at a time. And being the physician for *each one*. And really let them know that you are their individual physician. You're not the physician for the family total, but individually."

"Dad, this is really interesting to me. I mean I know you are a family physician, and I know that you have always been proud of that, as we all have. But this is the first time I've heard you state that being a family physician to you also meant being part of these families. That's a very important image of your work; I've never heard you say that before."

"Well, actually they open up their mind to you. [pause] They, of course, they show you their minds, their hearts, their bodies, and you're part of it."

*     *     *

This relationship could not be plainer as we go out to dinner at a local diner. There is nothing fancy about the place although the food is delicious, and it's warmly decorated for Christmas. As we walk by the soda fountain to the dining room, I notice a ceramic crèche displayed on the formica counter beside the chrome-plated napkin dispenser and salt and pepper shakers. From virtually every booth and table people turn and smile warmly at Dr. Rawlins and my mother, June. He shakes hands, pats shoulders and greets several folks, briefly introducing my family to a few people as we are led to our table. It's all coming back to me. I can't remember a time we went anywhere in Seaford or the vicinity that he wasn't welcomed like this and didn't treat each person he met with genuine acknowledgment.

But it's even deeper than this, and I understand it better now. Dad's greetings have a history and familiarity beneath their necessary brevity on this occasion, as I can recall them having on others. He jokes openly with some folks and is gently knowing and solicitously tender with others. He even chides a couple of men as they hide their cigarettes for Jack Rawlins is notoriously against smoking, and everyone he cares for knows it. He truly seems to be regarded as family by these former patients even as he was (and always will be) their physician. And he knows a life's worth of things about each and every one of them that is only ever revealed or implied by the ways he treats them now and the ways he responded in the past when they needed him. He's delivered their babies, cared for their flus, their accidents and aching joints; he's eased the final days of their dying parents. I know these truths without him actually ever telling me; they reach my family through others; they are his legacy. Swelling with pride, I also reflect on the immense burdens that such knowing and confidence must entail.

* * *

"You've mentioned a specific sort of example of how your involvement with the family also involves a dedication to each member of the family as an individual ..." "Right." "Is there any way you could discuss that further? I mean, it sounds like you would advise and care for each person *as* each person, however the events unfolded in terms of them becoming aware of each other's condition. It's up to them?"

"Well, it's very difficult for a physician who has set views on what is the difference between right and wrong healthwise. It's very difficult to *not* preach, and this is what you *can't* do because you have to put out the facts and let them make their own decision. You try to give them the pros and cons. Course, I usually think that's what you should do anytime with anything that crops up. But you can't be the, uh; it's very unusual for me to have to do that with a person when you have someone you know what they're doing is wrong, and you know it's going to affect them adversely, and yet you want to continue to look after them. So you can't really completely say, 'I don't condone this at all.' You have to say, 'This exists and this might happen.' And then you let them ..."

Interrupting himself, he says, "Don't think that having been in practice as long as I have that I don't look back now and see people as you wander by and think, Hey, maybe if they had done this, they would have had a different life. Uh, maybe if they had done this, they would be a lot more successful. But, uh, it's not in the books apparently. You can only do, go so far."

Turning a little bookish myself, I make a mental note about my father's role as a trusted co-author of his patients' life stories. I'm going to want to come back to the affinities I see between the convictions my dad voices here and some of Mikhail Bakhtin's (1984a) sturdiest admonitions about the ethics and responsibilities of authorship.

My dad continues speaking, "Now, this is what I think makes the difference between a family physician who is interested in the unit rather than all the specialties that there are regardless of how skilled a person is when they are centering only on one thing. And, once again, by knowing the family as such, when certain kinds of symptoms come up and certain types of diseases, not diseases as such, but conditions come up, you can pretty well explain it because you know the environment. This is one of the advantages of house calls, too, going into somebody's house and seeing *how they live* just one time can make you a better physician for them for the next 10 or 15 years. You have to know what someone's habitat is."

"This was the, this was the thing that I felt like ... was a little different when I was in Johns Hopkins. I had a number of doctors there who had been born with silver spoons in their mouths, and they had gone to the best schools, and they had gone to the best training, and now they were going to be the best physicians. And they had no compunction about seeing somebody in the clinic and look at, and see a woman there with four children, one of them having had a bad tonsillitis, and the child to get there they had to get on a trolley, they had to sit in the waiting room for an hour and a half, the children running over everywhere, and finally the doctor walks in, and looks, and says, 'Do this, come back tomorrow.' "

"Now the only reason he wants her to come back tomorrow is that he wants to see how the medicine affects this person in 24 hours. He *knows* what it's supposed to be; he's been *taught* that it's gonna do so and so, but *he* wants to *see* how it works. So he says, 'Come back in 24 hours.' So here this woman has to take her children, go out, go through the thing, get on the trolley, go back to the house, and so forth and so on, and goodness knows how much they have to put up with to come back the next day. This to me was an example of someone who is only interested in the technical mechanical side of the medical practice, and not interested in the family as a whole. So, [pause] and it still exists."

"Now, to be a general practitioner and a family practitioner, you're trying to meet all of the needs of the patient. And it was always estimated that you could handle about 85% of those; that 15% you might have to get someone else to help. And as far as I was concerned, it is the mark of a good physician who is going to certainly recognize his own limitations and was very quick to find someone else who had better knowledge and better skills, and different techniques. You always welcomed people asking for consultations because, if you're incorrect, you're certainly—and you're interested in the patient's welfare just as much as the patient is—so if it's better for the patient to have someone else's opinion, so be it. It also didn't hurt at all to have a consultation, and for the patient to find out you were correct, and that the diagnosis had been made properly."

"One of my favorite stories along that line has to do with a child that was ill, in the hospital—I won't go into the diagnosis and whatnot—but she was getting the attention that she needed, and was very, and was doing fairly well but not spectacularly. Doing fine, but it so happens that the family had a relative who was a good friend of the head of the Department of Pediatrics at the University of Maryland, and so they wondered if they could get him to come over and see the patient. And I said, 'That'd be fine.' "

"And so the doctor took a whole afternoon to come from Baltimore to Seaford, saw the patient, agreed thoroughly with everything that had been done, reassured the relatives. And I thanked him profusely for coming because I learned something from him. And what I learned was that when he looked in a child's ear, lo and behold, he could see birds! And he would make the sound of a bird twittering when he looked in the ear. And I adopted that in my practice and then used it the rest of my career [laughs]. Puts the patient at ease, and so this was a consultation I considered very worthwhile."

"Eureka!" I say to myself. So that's where that came from! I can't convey to you how much this innocent strategy figured into my dad's rapport with children. I can see him taking the otoscope out of its small brown case and placing a sterile plastic sleeve over the cone that he will stick into the child's ear. It's still an intimidating device—cold, chrome and powerful looking, and it projects an intensely bright light out of its small opening. What's he going to do with *that* thing!? But now I remember something else ... "*My*, that's a bright light!" my dad would say to the child. "Do you think you could blow that light out for me?" Warily, the child would slowly shake her head and turn to clutch her mother's skirt. "Well, I'll bet you could!" Dad would blow at the otoscope and the light would go out. The child would pull her head out of her mom's skirt with the faintest hint of a smile. "My goodness, that light has come on again! Would you blow it out for me?"

After a few more successful gusts of wind from my dad, the child would try to extinguish the light. Then she would giggle proudly and say, "Do it again!"

At this point, my dad might make a little whistling sound, the only bird sound most of us can make, and the child's ears would perk up. "I think I hear a bird," Dad would announce, and before too long he was gazing at it in the child's ear, describing its colors and markings. When this bird watching was done, he was on his way to diagnosis and eventually the right prescription for addressing the child's symptoms and relieving her fever and pain. What's funny to me now is that my mom used the same technique when she cleaned our ears as children, finding all kinds of branches and nests that needed to be swiped with her trusty Q-Tips™. As silly as this sounds, I recalled this memory once again at my annual check-up last week, when Doctor Raju observed that I had a "pretty impressive build-up of wax in my right ear." He's going to dissolve it and clean it out when I return next week.

*   *   *

"When you think of your years as a physician, what made you proudest as a doctor?" "In my practice of medicine there have been a number of different little uh … We had a very interesting case, I had got a call, when I came to Seaford, Dr. Gray was the obstetrician—I think she delivered you …" I nod and smile. "And she ended up turning all of her babies over to me. That's why I became the pediatrician of Bridgeville and knew everybody in Bridgeville and so forth, but then gradually I started delivering her babies for her when she wasn't around. Suddenly she calls me up and tells me she has a child who has a pretty high fever, and so I admitted the child to the hospital and ordered the lab work and so forth and so on. But it so happens that we had tickets to go see the Harlem Globetrotters in Philadelphia. You've heard this story …" "No, I'm not sure." "So we took off to Philadelphia and saw the Harlem Globetrotters; it was a big deal in those days, I mean it was, and we saw them play, and then we got back home. And so about two or three o'clock [in the morning], I stopped off at the hospital to see this child. And lo and behold, the child's temperature was about 104 or 105, and yet the pulse rate was slow, and the white count was not too high. And what I had was a case of typhoid fever. Now typhoid fever, no one really wanted to believe that, but that's what it was. So where did we get typhoid fever? We back up a little bit, and then all of sudden I get a call, it turns out the child's mother has a high fever, so we admitted her to the hospital."

"At the time the treatment for typhoid fever was *chloromycetin.* Chloromycetin was one of the first antibiotics. But as usual one of the dangers of medicine, chloromycetin being one of the first antibiotics after penicillin, suddenly it was being used for everything, all of the, every infection people had they were given chloromycetin right and left, and all of a sudden they found it was affecting the blood work. So it was (he makes a 'swook,' sound effect and rapid pulling gesture) pulled off the market. But *this is the treatment* they were using for typhoid fever. So you call over to Baltimore, talk to a guy who is known all over the world for this treatment of chloromycetin, and tell him you have typhoid fever in Sussex County and he says, 'You must be kidding!' I said, 'No, we're not kidding.' So he supplied all of the chloromycetin for us. And we took care of the patient."

"Now where'd the typhoid fever come from? It turned out, that outside of Bridgeville, there was a woman, who had a cow, and she had a hired hand who milked the cow all the time; I don't know how many, whether she had more than one cow or not. But lo and behold, the hired hand got sick, and she milked her own cow—twice. And she was the carrier. It so happens that a lot of people can have typhoid fever and be carriers and never be sick. And if they don't take care of themselves properly and sanitarily, and handle food, they have typhoid."

"Did the hired hand have it?" "No he didn't; the owner had it. She had the typhoid fever, the germ, and milked the cow. Her germs went to the milk, to the teats, into the milk, and the people who drank the milk got the typhoid fever. And I called up the Public Health Department; the Public Health Department went out to see this woman, and, 'She didn't know who that new doctor was down in Seaford but he certainly had no sense in taking care of his patients.' [laughs] She was a little upset. So, they were the only two cases that we had."

"Are there any other moments you would point to?" "There have been a lot of small triumphs, Bill; there's no big deal that I that stands out. There are things that probably are more important to you or to someone that I'm talking to than it did seem to me. But I always thought it was a triumph just to win over a child who didn't want to come, didn't want to be examined. And to win the child over just to examine them. And you learned a lot about children that way because I got so that I would ignore them if I could, and then finally I would get them on my side. And after you got them and then get to examine them and whatnot, that's what made medicine to me worthwhile."

"The same way with the worst patient that comes into your office, to try to win them over, not try to yell them down but try to actually convince them that they might need help. And those are the triumphs, the things that occur from day to day. This is what's so unfortunate that people, looking at family physicians and think that maybe they are not quite up to standard because they are not using the most up to date technique, uh, they miss the point. In medicine, you're dealing with a different personality as a challenge every 15 or 20 minutes. You're seeing people that are—some people are very concerned about their big toe, whereas somebody else is real concerned because they're pregnant. Somebody else may be concerned because they are afraid their eyebrows are growing too thick. And you have to balance this because whatever is important to the person should be important to the *concerned* physician. [The longest pause of the interview transpires here.] I don't remember a day I didn't want to go to my practice; I really don't."

*    *    *

I've always known my dad as a good storyteller and as someone who appreciates a good story. I've also always revered my dad as a gifted physician, a devoted healer for the people of his community. Only recently have I truly recognized the indelible connections among these qualities. My brothers and I used to get impatient watching television with my dad. However complexly an episode was framed, regardless of whether it was a western, a detective or courtroom mystery, or one of the many spy shows popular during the Cold War—at some point my dad would predict the ending, saying, "I may be wrong but ..." "We'll have to see what happens, but if what he just said is true, then ..." And he was usually correct. Hunter's (1991) brilliantly argued book on the narrative basis of medical knowledge convinces me that my dad probably was diagnosing these fictional stories using sensibilities and skills he had honed in his practice of patient-centered medicine in the narrated contexts of their family's unfolding lives.

Hunter pointed out that while formidable scientific knowledge of the body is essential for practicing medicine, the challenge of effective diagnosis and treatment is to ascertain how the objective indications and deductive possibilities are playing out in each individual's subjective experience and bodily circumstances. She observed:

> The effective grasp of a patient's particular manifestation of a malady often depends not only on a careful written account of its physiological progression but on a recognition of its roots and its meaning in the life story of the patient. Narrative is essential to both of these tasks. (Hunter, 1991, p.106)

Hunter likens the effective diagnostician to Sherlock Holmes, someone with a storehouse of prior cases to draw on, rigorously deductive in ruling out possibilities, while skeptically receptive to the particularities of given cases and to contextual clues. Such details are the stuff of patients' stories.

My father's account provides several related lessons about a narrative stance toward practicing medicine. *Committing oneself to understanding patients' health concerns and observable symptoms in and through the contexts of their own lived stories is foremost.* Any person's health, disease, and treatment are thoroughly contextual and contingent experiences. Accordingly, familiarity with someone's unique personal history, habits, and values, where and how the patient lives, and the nature of his or her relationships with family and other persons is crucial for comprehending troubles and ills. I was impressed with Dad's reference to house calls in this regard: "... going into somebody's house and seeing *how they live* just one time can make you a better physician for them for the next 10 or 15 years," as well as his well-versed uptake of one man's allusion to an elephant's foot in narrating his worrisome recent days.

*Regarding patients in this storied way envisions them as significant characters involved in meaningfully unfolding situations, as opposed to mere objects of examination.* As Mattingly (1991) emphasized, embracing a narrative stance enjoins the health care practitioner to treat the whole person in his or her presence versus focusing principally on the disease. After depicting the centrality of particular individuals in all of his stories, my dad pointedly narrates the "small triumphs" of his years as a doctor in terms of helping specific people. With defining details he asserts, "In medicine, you're dealing with a different personality as a challenge every 15 or 20 minutes" and "whatever is important to the person should be important to the *concerned* physician."

*Valuing and portraying patients as characters in their own stories cultivates empathy and respect for their points of view.* There are multiple standpoints composing any health care narrative; to insist on the primacy of the physician's is to neglect the validity of other perspectives. I've often noticed my dad's attempts to see his patients as well as himself through their own and other persons' eyes. Recall how his concern for his patients' perceptions and feelings played out in the very car he drove to make house calls. Throughout our conversation, my dad's stories dramatize multiple points of view, that is, different sides to the "same" story. A telling example is his description of the Hopkins physician's versus the mother of four's possible standpoints on that doctor's instructions to bring her child (which would require bringing three siblings as well) back to the clinic the following day. Rita Charon (2001b) argued that such narrative competence is necessary for delivering empathic care because what is needed to tell a good story about a patient's situation derives from and informs empathy with that person.

Granting this penchant for empathy connected with narrative sensibilities, I am especially impressed with my father *recognizing as a physician his own potential roles as a co-author and a character in his patients' life stories.* He understands that he was potentially co-authoring the future plots of persons' lives when he presented them with options for treatment or alternative behaviors in addressing the conditions that were causing them physical and emotional distress—what Mattingly (1994) termed *therapeutic emplotment.* Although he accepted the responsibility for laying bare the contingencies and options before them and was clear in making his recommendations, he was adamant in our conversation that he believed his patients had to make their own choices. I am reminded once again of Bakhtin's (1984a) indictment of authors who abuse their responsibilities by attempting to dictate the experiences and actions of the characters they are creating and engaging through the dialogue of writing. Bakhtin insists that we respect the subjectivity and agency of all the characters we encounter and assist in narrating their lives. Charon (1993) echoes, "What, in fact, do doctors and patients do together but to create between themselves a many-staged narrative, sharing the roles of teller and listener, moving through a series of rhetorical strategies toward, ideally, accuracy and freedom?" (p. 87). I believe these co-authorial challenges presented to my father as a family physician were multiplied (even as they were informed) by his familiarity with the families he cared for and his commitment to preserving each member's trust in his judgment and discretion.

Numerous plots thickened and interwove in the unfolding of my dad's own life story as a physician. As a fellow member of the community, he interacted in multiple settings with these persons and families living in relationships with each other over time. Here he is years later, encountering people, many of whom he has guided, cured, helped, and treated with beneficial results. By his own convictions, however, he has had to allow others to make certain decisions that may not have proven to be in their best interests. Both he and these patients have had to share the responsibility and live with the consequences. Hunter (1991) held that *uncertainty*—the gap between knowledge and practice, laboratory principles and lived experience—simultaneously haunts and fascinates medical professionals. In her opinion, "their response to it is a hallmark of the physician's character" (p. 30).

I questioned my dad about how he dealt, for example, with the conundrum of simultaneous cases within the same family that were at odds with each other and required discrete and confidential handling. I admire his reply, "One day at a time. Each event at a time. And being the physician for *each one.*" With his concept of the *once-occurrent event,* Bakhtin (1993) reminded us of the ethical responsibility of answering every single moment of our lives for its unique possibilities and fallibilities, even as we might recognize its commonalities with other ones. *In voicing his responsibility to care for each person who called upon him in his or her physical, temporal, and existential particularity, my dad concisely articulated the ethical responsiveness living at the heart of his narratively composed practice of family medicine.*

My dad examined, viewed, and cared for his patients in terms of their own life narratives and not merely through the lens of available scientific knowledge. In doing so, he shouldered extensive responsibilities, many of which he believes are avoided today by physicians who engage in increasingly specialized foci and/or who base their practice primarily on technologically derived indicators of bodily functions. All physicians seek appropriate diagnoses and curative or palliative therapeutic regimens; for the narrowly focused, however, accomplishing these aims typically brings closure to the medical story at hand (Hunter, 1991). Not so for my dad and others who envision themselves as co-authors and curators of their patients' health narratives as continually performed within the enveloping contexts of their families and their communities.

                                    *     *     *

I think Dad liked it some years ago when I used a word I learned from Bellah, Madson, Sullivan, Swidler, and Tipton (1985) to refer to his life's work. The word is "calling." He was considering retiring and reflecting on how much his practice, his relationships with patients, and his opportunities to care for them meant to him. He told me he had explored the possibility of donating his time one day a week to serve as the physician for a local nursing home. Indignantly, he observed the possibility was "scotched" because he would have to pay the same premiums for malpractice insurance to contribute for free in this capacity once a week as he would practicing full-time as a professional. He also considered opening up a "translation service" for people emerging baffled and anxious from contemporary visits with specialists. "The thing about your approach to your work as a physician," I said at the time, "is that you've never lived it as merely a job, or even a career. You've lived medicine as a calling—a rich morally imbued identity—a lifetime of fulfilling promises to your community and in doing so, to yourself." That wording resonated with him so much that I wanted to say it to him again in this narrative.

My brothers and I were concerned with how my dad would handle retirement after decades of pursuing his calling with consummate dedication and energy. There are a few things we should have remembered. For one, he has never stopped learning and critically reflecting—activities I find tremendously inspiring as an educator and lifelong learner myself. He still subscribes to journals, monitors diverse Web sites concerning medical science and practice, converses with fellow physicians, and attends conferences, seminars and talks. For another, he rarely left for any significant stretch of time the community in which he grew up and practiced medicine. Upon retiring, he remains the doctor a large number of people look to—in spirit if not in fact. Finally, if there is anything that he loves more than medicine, and there is, it's my mother. Sixty years into their marriage, folks around town will see Jack and June Rawlins "cuttin' a rug" at local dances and benefits, or riding their bikes together down Nylon Boulevard—and then they know something's still right with the world Seaford-way.

Narrating my trip back home with my family to visit my parents, hearing my father's stories, and receiving his care have been deeply gratifying experiences for me. (And my shingles are long gone.) Writing this chapter has allowed me to share with you a number of touchstones among one man's lifelong devotion to the practice of family medicine and an array of ways that a narrative stance composes and potentially contributes to health care and well-being. Kathryn Hunter (1991) wrote:

> Attention to the patient's life story is not a nostalgic return to an idealized pretechnological time when social and personal details were entered into the medical record. On the contrary, this recognition of the patient's story is a new requirement of a mobile, urban, fragile society that lacks a binding communal religious belief and has come to expect much more of physicians, haloed by technology and the large sums of money they are paid. The medicine of neighbors that once augmented the physician's knowledge in a small or stable community now must be the object of special, reconstructive attention. (p. 172)

In closing this gift to my father, Dr. John C. Rawlins, my mother, June, and my brothers, Rocky, Ron, and Terry, Hunter's words confirm my belief that this narrative is not merely an exercise in sentimentality but a consideration and model of values and orientations that are still vital to concerned medical practitioners.

# 10

# Narrative Knowledge Development Among Caregivers: Stories From the Nurses' Station

∾

**Jayne Morgan-Witte**
*University of Northern Iowa*

The prevailing modern-day equivalent of the water cooler in medical settings arguably would be the nurses' station. Caregivers of all sorts gather around this central hub, certainly to engage in task-related interactions, but also to gossip, tell stories, mock patients and co-workers, crack jokes, play pranks, and discuss their personal lives. Together they spin, in this cultural web, a storytelling culture—where these various forms of tale telling string together to form a sense-making structure that at once is instructive regarding social norms and task procedures, reflective of work and personal relationships, and supportive of specific ideologies of caregiving.

Yet in our research of health care settings, we know little about these stories, what they sound like, why they are told, what they mean, or how they structure knowledge about caregiving. Researchers have discussed the importance of caregivers developing narrative knowledge to better understand their patients (Charon, 1993, 2001a), but have not considered fully how such knowledge is created and maintained in the medical backstage (Ellingson, 2003). Stories away from patients enable caregivers to discuss and express ideologies of caregiving. Caregivers, in turn, bring these ideologies into patient encounters as biases or lenses of perception (Geist & Dreyer, 1993).

As storytelling frames patient behaviors and conditions in certain ways, the nature and quality of care are affected accordingly (Mattingly, 1998). It is therefore vital to study the origins of narrative knowledge

217

development to explore potential outcomes for patient care. In addition, studying caregiver storytelling in real time shows glimpses of the *process* of narrative knowledge development often discussed but rarely captured through empirical study. These glimpses offer brief yet holistic backstage performances of what it "might be like" to be a member of the culture (Geertz, 1973; Mattingly, 1998), and underscore basic assumptions of "what it means" to play the role of nurse, doctor, or technician in these settings (Goffman, 1959). Caregivers learn, among other things, about group identity, ingroups and outgroups, and the proper way to show (or hide) emotion so as to be "professional" in their roles (Morgan & Krone, 2001). An investigation of backstage storytelling, then, reveals how narrative knowledge developed through caregiver interaction guides "appropriate" behavior, not just in terms of delivering care, but in multiple realms of caregivers' work experiences (Mattingly, 1998).

In this chapter, I view the nurses' station as a storytelling centerpiece in the work lives of caregivers in two different health care settings: a cardiac catheterization lab and an emergency department in a hospital. From these narrative centerpieces emanate sensemaking networks that are formed and informed by member interaction. Observations of these two sets of caregivers support the idea that medical settings are narrative creations in substance and form (Hunter, 1991). I explore the different functions of storytelling in these settings and how they have real consequences in terms of caregiving beliefs, actions, and outcomes. In addition, I illustrate how sensemaking structures create and maintain certain ideologies while obscuring or suppressing other ways of thinking, acting, and providing care.

## NARRATIVE KNOWLEDGE IN HEALTH CARE ORGANIZATIONS

Stories in organizations perform a variety of functions in the social construction of reality (Brown, 1985). Stories provide insight into various organizational events (Boje, 1991), manage meanings by giving members an outlet for individual and collective sensemaking (Brown, 1987; Currie & Brown, 2003), and facilitate members' identification by providing them with shared organizational information and similar lenses of perception (Hansen & Kahnweiler, 1993).

Emergent narrative networks reflect values of the organization's dominant culture and the multiple, stratified subcultures that develop in organizational life (Helmer, 1993). Members share stories, and in so doing embody their understanding of events within the organization (Boje, 2001). Thus, stories reflect the employees' understanding of essential norms and beliefs as rooted in the organization's traditions (Shaw, 2000). Stories provide culturally derived explanations about what organizations are, how they operate, and how people enact their roles within them (Kreps, 1990). In turn, storytelling is a primary means for individuals to share how they perceive their relationships with co-workers, patients or clients, and the organization (Tangherlini, 2000).

Underneath surface indications of power imbalances lies a grand narrative that speaks to the overarching ideology of doing business, or in the case of health care settings, giving care. Certain voices and interests are valued in the culture whereas others are muted or otherwise neglected (Mumby, 2000). As expressions of culture, stories are therefore not neutral as they support and maintain dominant ideologies of a work group or organization (Mumby, 1987). Extraorganizational sources of ideology also are influential in this context, as general preferences for a biomedical model in the health sciences are reinforced often in Western medical organizations (Goldstein, 1999). For example, caregiver distance or detachment, along with preferences for rationality and technical, scientific discourse, have predominated ways of caregiving in traditional health care organizations (Geist & Dreyer, 1993; Good, 1994; Hafferty, 1988; Lupton, 1994). This ideological position guides caregiver behavior toward exhibiting certainty, objectivity, and technical competence (P. Atkinson, 1995; Daly, 1989; Haas & Shaffir, 1982) in ways that are deemed professionally appropriate (Morgan & Krone, 2001). This perspective often suppresses a dialogic, emotional, narrative model of caregiving that places the patient as a whole person at the center of the medical encounter; where stories of illness are heard, understood, and validated (Cassell, 1991; Charon, 1993; Geist & Dreyer, 1993); where "detached concern" (Lief & Fox, 1963) gives way to "engaged concern" (Charon, 2001a) or empathy (Halpern, 2001).

Caregivers who do attend to others' stories are considered to have "narrative knowledge" of their patients (Charon, 2001a). A series of studies have addressed the importance of narrative knowledge in the caregiver–patient relationship (e.g., Charon, 1993, 2001a; Charon, Greene, & Adelman, 1994) but we know little of the narrative knowledge developed through stories told among caregiving staff in the backstage (Ellingson, 2003). Capturing storytelling segments in real time foregrounds how narratives frame perceptions of patient and co-worker encounters, influence medical action, and gain "rhetorical powers" in convincing others to adopt similar worldviews (Mattingly, 1998, p. 5). I offer a backstage glimpse of the perceptual framing process inherent in the construction of narrative knowledge by considering "lessons learned" about group identity, power, emotion, and, ultimately, caregiving ideologies. The questions considered were: How is narrative knowledge constructed in backstage caregiver storytelling? and How are ideological meaning formations (re)produced in backstage caregiver storytelling?

## LISTENING IN

Stories in this analysis were drawn from ethnographies performed in two different organizations in different locations, where the initial focus was on caregiver emotionality (Morgan, 2002; Morgan & Krone, 2001). I decided to approach these settings from a narrative perspective when it became clear early in my observations that the nurses' station served, literally and figuratively, as the hub of communication for caregivers. It is a backstage place where participants create, share, and maintain narrative knowledge.

### Participants and Settings

Caregivers in the catheterization lab (CL) included 14 cardiologists, one lab manager/nurse, four registered nurses (RNs), two licensed practical nurses (LPNs), and two technicians. The cardiologists were removed, spatially and symbolically, from the nurses' station activity. In fact, they did not walk behind the counter. I, too, remained on the fringe of the nurses' station, standing beside either one of the side walls, but never behind them. In contrast, I became fully immersed in the activities behind the nurses' station at the emergency room (ER). I tried to stand in unobtrusive spots (i.e., near the copier or fax machine), but the crowded and busy nature of the space often propelled me to the center of activity. I bobbed and weaved around the quick movements of the staff, and I suffered, on occasion, a glare or snide remark for being in the way during a busy time.

The ER doctors, too, were involved heavily in the nurses' station. Interestingly, however, many ER doctors stood on one side of the nurses' station while nurses congregated on the other. Two doctors in particular, though, interacted fully with the nursing staff on the "nurses' side" of the station on a regular basis. Also behind the counter stood a receptionist who answered incoming calls and contacted other parts of the hospital per doctors' orders. Paramedics, X-ray technicians, lab technicians, and hospital volunteers stayed outside the boundary of the nurses' station. Only paramedics (ambulance and flight crews) engaged in storytelling with the ER staff; the other groups appeared task-driven and did not interact socially with people behind the station. Paramedics shared their "juicy" field stories with the ER staff, and detailed the journey to the ER doors. All told, 8 emergency physicians and a group of 46 nurses and technicians worked in the emergency department. Any given shift featured two or three physicians and seven to ten nurses, with any number of technicians and paramedics happening by.

The settings also differed in their environments and opportunities for storytelling. The patient load dramatically differed between the two. In the CL, the staff worked with as little as four and a maximum of eight patients in one day. They experienced quite a bit of downtime at the nurses' station as the patients, once comfortable in the recovery rooms, required little attention most of the time. As the catheterization procedure was performed repeatedly throughout the day with few surprises, the staff followed a regular, unambiguous routine. Staff often congregated behind the nurses' station during downtimes between procedures. The atmosphere was relaxed and often upbeat, as staff mostly talked about their personal lives.

Contrast the CL with the absence of a patient schedule in the ER, where staff cared for 75 to 100 patients with various ailments and injuries every day. People from different races, classes, and age groups came to the ER with problems, large and small, real and feigned, life-threatening and mundane. The ER staff encountered many more fluctuations in their daily schedule than did the CL crew. Their shift could be quite hectic, yet staff members also enjoyed clear periods of downtime. When the ER was busy, it could appear chaotic (to an outsider), with multiple conversations and events occurring at the same time. Collisions of messages and actions resulted in staff clamoring for charts, reaching over each other for the phone, and talking louder than the next person in hopes of being heard. But when the ER was slow, it felt very slow to observers and workers alike. Stories told during downtimes, then, worked to relieve stress after hectic intervals, and to stimulate activity during sluggish stretches of a 12-hour shift.

## Story Collection and Analysis

For this study, my observation logs became the primary source of data. Specifically, I spent 2 months observing in the CL, and 6 months observing in the ER. Observations in the CL were conducted 4 days a week for 2 to 4 hours of time at various times of the day. I conducted observations in the ER 14 times at an average of 2 hours per visit, from 3:00 p.m. to 10:00 p.m., thus including observation of both day and evening shifts. In both settings, I also conducted interviews and feedback sessions (see Morgan, 2002; Morgan & Krone, 2001, for detailed descriptions). Although not always directly revealed in this study, remarks made by caregivers in these interactions placed my observations in context. I used the interviews (9 in the CL, 6 in the ER) and feedback sessions (1 in the CL, 2 in the ER) to check my perceptions with those of the participants.

As I grew interested in the backstage communication in these settings, I took detailed field notes when in and around the nurses' station. I captured, to the extent possible, all of the color and context of the
stories shared. My ethnographic portrayal includes phrases of conversation verbatim to ground the narratives in the caregivers' own words.
I noted the content of the stories as well as how they were delivered and
by whom. The audience of the story became an important element in
my notes as I wrote down the reactions of the listener(s), and how the
storyteller adapted to those reactions. I also noted how storytellers responded to me as a listener, included me as a participant, or even
made me the subject of a story.

I sorted out more "traditional" stories and story chains along with
other types of narrative communication, including joking, gossiping,
venting, and mocking behaviors. The sorting process continued by
grouping like stories together in terms of, for example, their tone (humorous or serious), content (work or nonwork), and subject (patient
or co-worker). Ultimately, I decided to analyze and write about the stories according to their subject, and let the content and tone of the stories take shape in my descriptions.

In writing up the analysis, I found it important to reveal my presence
as participant–observer, not only to give the reader a better sense of my
involvement, but also as a matter of ethics. To "hide" my role while portraying others' words and actions would create an incomplete picture
of what happened, and demonstrate an unfair use of my power as an
author to reconstruct events. Instead, I used my "liminal" positioning
between the worlds of researcher and researched to extend and enhance the analysis and interpretation of the data (Eastland, 1993). In
this way, all voices, including mine as author, are equally represented
in the project (Geist & Gates, 1996), and the tension between the
"other" and the researcher is recognized and addressed (Geertz, 1988;
Schwartzman, 1993). The triangulation of methods, including interviewing and member checking in the feedback sessions, allowed for
the infusion of multiple perspectives in the construction of the analysis
(Lindlof, 1995). The following sections reveal stories told in these settings, and how they work toward forging a narrative knowledge framework that guides ideological (re)production and caregiver behavior.

## STORIES TOLD

The following stories serve as examples of different types of narratives shared in and around the nurses' stations of these two settings. I
highlight knowledge constructed in and through patient stories and
carework(er) stories. Both themes reveal how the construction of
narrative knowledge frames patients, co-workers, and even the orga-

nization in certain ways, and form behavioral guidelines and cultural role expectations.

## Knowledge Constructed in and Through Patient Stories

By far, and perhaps not surprisingly, the caregivers talked about patients the most around the nurses' station. As a backstage area away from patients, staff members vented, told funny stories, and mocked patient behavior. While some of the staff members' behaviors may appear crude or "unprofessional" to the reader, they likely resemble backstage communication that takes place among other service-oriented personnel (e.g., Fine, 1988). It may be that we think of health care providers as being on a higher plane when it comes to professionalism because they are dealing so intimately with people and their health. But time spent away from the patient, although not free from behavioral rules, functions as a time for caregivers to let masks of professionalism slip to some degree. Besides venting, they use the backstage area to support each other and develop a strong group identity. Caregivers often see a side of human nature that most of us do not see; such exposure binds them so closely together and makes their stories seem somewhat unusual to outsiders—a point they freely admitted to me. They even seemed to relish the idea that lay persons simply could not understand all that they see and do on a daily basis. Caregivers spoke of the heightened importance of co-worker relationships, as family and friends could not truly empathize with their work situations.

Certain storytelling sessions underscored the caregiving group's special or unique identity. For example, the longest chain of storytelling that I witnessed in the ER started after a patient came in with a foreign object up his penis. The man thought he had a kidney stone (although not officially diagnosed) and attempted to dislodge it himself. He used tubing similar to a fish aquarium hose, thrust it up his penis, and apparently tried to irrigate it so the "stone" would come out. The tubing had entered the urethra and was apparently knotted or kinked. He was sent to an operating room to take care of the matter. This patient became the subject of jokes as the story was retold to new people entering the scene.

Staff members then created a string of stories related to similarly bizarre incidents. First, a nurse recalled how a patient had taken a knife to his testicle, apparently to remove a pimple. She said his wife was "hilarious" because she was doing a crossword puzzle casually while telling her husband to explain to the triage nurse, "Go ahead, tell her what you did. Go ahead, tell her why you did it. Go ahead, tell her what you used to do it!" Another nurse added a story about a man who apparently had tried to kill himself by slitting his wrists, failed, and then decided to cut the major artery in the leg near the groin area. A doctor chimed in and said he remembered that case and how the man "did a number" on his testicle. The doctor went on to tell a story told to him by another doctor in a different ER. He said that a patient apparently was operating a remote control car, when he fell on top of it and the antenna went up his penis. He said the man came in still holding the remote control box. The doctor admitted that he did not "buy" this particular story.

A nurse then chimed in, "Remember when the guy came in with the broomstick up his ass?" The doctor asked in response, "Wasn't it broken in half?" The nurse said, "Yeah, it was." Finally, a paramedic jumped in with a story of a man who was impaled by a rod that went in through a buttock and up his back. It managed to sever the bowel, but everything else was intact. The staff members working on the man estimated how big the pole was, guessing it to be about one-half inch thick. Then the crew heard a voice at the head of the table, the patient, say, "Five-eighths." The nurse said, "You oughta know!" Hearty laughter emerged from the group on the delivery of this line. By the end of this sequence, no fewer than six stories were spun out of the original storytelling incident.

Humorous stories in the CL also sprung up around patients' bizarre behaviors. One day upon entering the CL, the staff immediately told me the story of "the naked man" who had been in Room 3. He had decided on his own to take his gown off and just sit there upright in bed, naked. He sat facing the door, with the door wide open. A male nurse apparently tried to get his female co-workers to walk in on him so they would be surprised and shocked, much to the delight of the rest of the staff. A nurse took me over to the room and said, "Look where the bed was." It was certainly in plain view from the hallway. A nurse completed this story by saying, "There's crazy people out there, but it takes all kinds I guess." Room 3 was called the "wacko room" as they talked about how other "loony" patients had been there, like "the religious lady," who asked the nurse and me about our religious affiliations and whether we attended church regularly. She repeatedly thanked the Lord for no blockages in her heart. Because I was in the room when this happened, I became part of the story as it was recirculated at the nurses' station for several days in a row.

These story chains reveal how stories are maintained across time and space, even across organizations in the case of the story from a different emergency room. They follow a familiar pattern or plot. In this case, the narrative frame of the "bizarre patient" or the "bizarre case" is supported through repeated tellings of the same story in combination with similar stories that fit the conventions of the theme. These bizarre patients and cases become the perfect fodder for storytelling because they are so unusual and represent a major departure from the "normal" cases that the staff encounters most of the time. These stories bind the group together and stake out an identity that says that they are special because they see this type of human behavior most people do not see. Caregivers announce their group membership simply by contributing a story. In terms of creating patient knowledge, these stories set up expectations about how "normal" patients look and act by portraying the opposite characteristics and mannerisms. Meanwhile, bizarre patients are framed as such and will likely receive different care than other patients who present with normal behaviors and problems.

A particularly vivid story of patient framing happened one night in the ER. As a patient was being brought in by the ambulance, the paramedics called in to say the man was "ETOH" (intoxicated), claiming to have been struck by lightning. He reportedly had been standing under a tree with a beer in his hand. The lightning apparently struck the tree, but he was "knocked on his ass," as one nurse put it. A nurse in the ER teasingly drew a lightning bolt on the board next to a little stick figure with its hair standing on end. When the patient arrived, more jokes flourished. He was wheeled past the nurses' station as a police officer said, "He didn't get struck by lightning—there's no burns." A paramedic joked they needed to look at the "Doppler radar" for lightning strikes. The same nurse who drew the lightening bolt later signed up to take the patient. She walked back out to the nurses' station with a solemn face. Everyone grew quiet as they thought that something might be seriously wrong. She then said, "We need to check pinpoint Doppler radar." The entire crew laughed. Minutes later, without thinking, I even participated in the joke-telling by saying it smelled like fried chicken (which it did) and people agreed. Then I paused and said, "Unless it's that guy." A couple of nurses really laughed at that point. Like the others, I was swept up in the humorous storytelling of the moment.

A little later, however, the ER staff realized (perhaps because of my presence as an observer) how the joking could appear inappropriate. A paramedic commented, although half jokingly, about the lightning bolt on the board saying, "That's not very nice." A little later, the nurse who drew the figure said, "I suppose that wouldn't look good if a patient were to see the board." However, right before I left for the night, the staffers continued to place bets on the patient's blood alcohol level. Even the doctor posted a number. A nurse told me that this was a stress reliever for the staff.

Although the storytelling may benefit the caregivers by relieving stress and presenting a humorous break from their work, the story implicitly frames the patient as drunk (even before being seen) and therefore without a valid complaint or problem. The narrative knowledge constructed over time is that ER staff may not take as seriously those people who are self-impaired through drugs or alcohol. Given the number of people who do come through the ER doors in such a state, one can see how such sensemaking is formed. The humorous nature of the story (including my spontaneous comment) coincides with and ultimately supports the jovial culture of the night crew. The influence of the culture is so strong, however, that caregivers likely do not recognize the impact of such storytelling on patient care.

Other stories involved complaining about patients, particularly when they did not follow orders by nurses or doctors. In the CL, a nurse was upset one day when a patient would not allow her to apply pressure to the catheter insertion point to stop the bleeding. The nurse said to a co-worker, "Today this woman popped her clamp off and said 'You're hurting me.' I thought, 'I'll hurt 'ya.' Almost let her bleed to death on purpose." One other time in the CL, nurses complained about a heart transplant patient who failed to show up for an appointment. The nurse manager stated that if a patient "can't commit to the pretreatment then she doesn't deserve to be so high on the list." Later this same story was retold between two different nurses, then from an administrator to the rest of the staff. Complaining stories in the ER also revolved around "medical noncompliance." A regular patient in the ER (dubbed a "frequent flyer" by staff) complained of having seizures, yet he had failed to take his seizure medication. The doctor gently scolded the patient by saying that he had to take his medications. Back at the nurses' station, the doctor made a comment about the overweight appearance of the patient and his wife.

Caregivers directed complaints like these in both settings toward patients depicted as contributing to their conditions by excessively eating, smoking or drinking, disobeying medical orders, or in some other way jeopardizing their own health. Narrative sensemaking from these stories reveals a preference for "good" patients who take care of themselves and respect medical authority enough to follow orders. As a result, caregivers expressed less empathy to patients who "brought on" their own problems or ignored medical advice. In turn, narratives featured "good" nurses and doctors as those who commanded respect based on technical competence and superior medical knowledge.

## Knowledge Construction in and Through Carework(er) Stories

Other forms of sensemaking centered on the nature of caregiving. Staff members expressed their concern for the patients in the backstage and, at the same time, reassured and supported each other about caregiving practices. The ER group, for example, told sad stories about lives lost, particularly of patients that they knew, either firsthand or by association. One night, the ER staff talked about a "code" that happened a couple of nights earlier. The victim was an 18-year-old man from a nearby town who was killed in a motorcycle accident. A nurse said that all the EMTs from that town were crying when they took him from the ambulance to get on the helicopter. She said it was tough for people in the ER, too, as the victim was the son of an X-ray technician in their hospital. They also talked of two nurses from the emergency department they had lost to cancer and a brain aneurysm. They reminisced about the nurses, cried a little, and consoled each other before being called back to work.

Other types of reassuring stories centered on patient treatment. In the ER, a nurse asked the doctor about a pregnant woman who had been in a car accident. She asked what the doctor told the patient about the baby she was carrying. He replied that he told the patient that her tummy was like a water balloon with a quarter inside it—the baby was perfectly protected. A reassuring story also happened in the CL after a CHF (congestive heart failure) patient developed an irregular rhythm for about 17 beats. One nurse in particular was concerned that she missed something or that she could have responded sooner or "done more" to help the patient. The nurses huddled together around the nurses' station to walk through what happened step-by-step. They reassured themselves that they followed all the correct procedures, and that they handled the palpitations competently and correctly.

Reassuring stories help caregivers make sense of situations and calm their concerns about patients. They identify appropriate strategies in managing certain illnesses and ailments, while at the same time construct knowledge about how to display emotion appropriately with co-workers. Through narratives, they defined emotion norms within their unique cultural context, as other stories indicated when nurses cared too much or cared inappropriately. Such was the case in the CL, when a nurse mocked another nurse's concern about the patient's family, specifically how she could schedule it so the family could go to lunch and be back in time to walk with the patient over to the hospital. After speaking aloud her solution to the problem, the other nurse answered back with mock concern, "Do you think that will work?" The others standing around the nurses' station immediately remarked "Oooo" in unison, indicating that the nurse had been insulted for caring about the patient and the patient's family too much. When retold, these stories indicate how much and what types of emotional display are appropriate for a given scenario. The construction of narrative knowledge is biased toward the display of intense emotion only in serious cases with close or personal connections to staff members. Showing concern over tangential issues that go beyond the realm of the patient's immediate physical care is framed as inappropriate according to emotion norms.

When not dealing with patient demands, however, the cultures of both settings preferred rather playful backstage scenes. In both settings, staff joked, told stories, and talked about movies and family life. The evening staffers at the ER, by their own admission, could become particularly goofy. A doctor mentioned how their humor would degenerate as the long evening hours wore on. They told me about a time when they found a tick by the nurses' station so they put it in a Styrofoam cup and fed it blood. They also were fond of shooting rubber bands and mini basketballs to kill the time. As one doctor explained, "When it's busy, it's fine, everyone's all business. But when it's slow like this, any patient interruption just interrupts our happy time." His remark referenced a patient's family member who kept coming to the nurses' station to ask questions and to repeatedly tell the staff that the patient had to go to the bathroom. The doctor completed his comment by adding that, when the 7:00 a.m. shift comes in, they do not understand the night shift's humor. He said, "They come in with their coffee, all fresh, thinking the world is great, while the night crew is cynical and worn out." The day crew, although also preferring a lighthearted backstage, exhibited a more reserved style of humor that aligned with administrative expectations.

The staffers in the CL likewise were jovial in the backstage setting, although their humor centered more on the practical joke variety. They told and retold the story about the time that they made up a bed to resemble a patient lying in a bed by stuffing pillows under the sheets and using a mop for hair. One of the nurses hid under the bed to "voice" the fake patient. They told unsuspecting staffers to go peek at a patient who looked like Santa Claus. Surprising and shocking fellow co-workers served as a main source of humor for the CL crew.

The good-humored cultures in both settings influenced storytelling behavior to largely fit within the boundaries of lighthearted fun. The knowledge gained about "what it means" to be a caregiver in these settings involves being able to "take a joke" and to "play along" when it is "happy time." More task-oriented, serious nurses and doctors, however, tended not to engage in such conversations, especially ones that turned to gossip or joke telling. These caregivers were at times marginalized by the group, as they were construed as cultural bystanders through the content and form of the storytelling.

Stories about co-workers in these settings also underscored status differences. Doctor–nurse status stories prevailed in the CL, where the physicians were absent from the backstage. Some of the stories involved patient care and the ways in which doctors often made decisions without consulting nurses. One story in the CL surfaced around a doctor who let a patient go home before the allotted amount of bed-rest. The nurses expressed dismay at how he could simply tell a patient to go home without following proper procedures. Numerous other stories surfaced about how doctors would keep patients waiting longer than necessary. A nurse told a story of how a doctor kept a patient waiting for 4 hours before making it to the room to declare the patient free to go home. Doctors' lateness in showing up for procedures and visiting recovery rooms prompted constant complaining and venting among the CL staff because nurses managed the brunt of patient anger and anxiety during the wait.

In both settings, doctors clearly expected nurses to perform their work correctly, swiftly, and skillfully. As one ER nurse mentioned to me, the ER doctors expect nurses to "know their stuff" and handle patients competently. Thus, doctors pressured nurses to perform their jobs with accuracy and professionalism. Nurses sometimes turned to each other in the backstage, then, to admit their mistakes in a more understanding and supportive environment. In the ER, a nurse made the mistake of giving a patient the same medication twice. She told this story to another nurse and explained that she did not want to tell the doctor what she had done for fear of looking bad in his eyes. The other nurse insisted that she tell the doctor about the double dosing—that he simply had to know so he could take care of the patient. The nurse finally complied, but she initially feared the doctor's reaction more than the consequences for the patient, perhaps with good reason. Stories abounded in the CL about doctors yelling at nurses for their mistakes. A story circulated at the CL nurses' station about a cardiologist loudly scolding a nurse for placing the doctor's foot pedal (used to operate the X-ray machine) in the wrong place. Recurrently, the CL staff members referred to standards as "unfair"—doctors could violate the rules of professionalism, but they could not. Maintaining a "professional" front when a mistake has been made, however, can be detrimental to patient care.

As a response to physician expectations and violations of professionalism, CL staff members ridiculed and mocked doctors' actions and intelligence in the backstage. Venting forges a group identity by uniting staff members against higher authorities (i.e., doctors), and demonstrates, at least in that moment in time, the staff members' superiority in knowledge and competence. A technician told a story of a doctor who opened a bag containing X-ray film, thereby exposing and ruining it. She turned to me and said, "If you saw a black plastic bag that said DO NOT OPEN on it, would you open it?" She concluded that doctors "have all this education, but they're dumbshits." Another nurse told a story of how he was paged to come in all the way from the hospital to locate a film that was shelved right in front of the doctor's face. One mocking scenario, in particular, ridiculed a doctor's lack of expressiveness. As one nurse claimed, the doctor was an "oaf of a guy." She then started making horse noises and stomping her foot while another nurse added in a neighing sound. Someone questioned what the nurse was doing, and she replied, "He sounds like a horse. Haven't you ever heard him do that under his mask?" Making fun of doctors, although providing amusement for nurses and technicians, both resists and upholds the role boundaries between the two groups, ultimately acknowledging and reifying status differentials. The resistance, out of sight from the powers that be, only serves to maintain the status quo.

Status stories also were evident among peer groups. In the CL, nurses and technicians of different education levels once swapped stories about dissection and how their experiences varied based on the level of their training. They one-upped each other with stories of dissecting larger and more complex animals. Even though they were considered peers working as one staff, they clearly highlighted status differences between technicians, LPNs, and RNs. Stories reflected frustrations about not being permitted to perform certain work because of their education levels. For example, CL technicians and LPNs sometimes complained about not being able to start IVs to administer medicine, even though they had the skills to do so. In medical settings where professionals display educational degrees prominently on nametags and professional dress, status becomes an explicit issue for storytelling. Knowledge about the organizational culture ties to the importance of a hierarchy established on the grounds of professional titles and seniority. In addition, those caregivers who worked more closely with technology and/or with the actual patient treatment were respected more highly than those who served primarily in a nurturing, recovery, or laboratory role. The complaints of LPNs and technicians disallowed to perform certain tasks, along with the one-upping dissection stories, highlight how the culture favors those workers who can show more technical competence than their peers.

Related to status issues, staff members told stories that marked the insider or outsider position of different caregivers. In the CL, the male nurses and male doctors spent much time together outside of work, and even set up fishing trips and other excursions. The fact that they called themselves "The Boys' Club" further demarcated their separation from female staffers, and ultimately excluded women from their social networks. In the ER, a male doctor and male nurse also engaged in off-to-the-side joke and storytelling if they thought that their stories were taboo for mixed company. Conversely, the women in the CL talked at great length about their family lives and, in particular, their children's activities. Notably, single men and women were silent during or absent from these storytelling sessions. In the ER, the night crew shared their sets of in-group stories that excluded administrative and day-shift employees. In these ways, we see how stories formed boundaries, not only around job titles or roles but also around informal communication networks in the organization. Membership into groups based on gendered interests and activities highlights how employees construct what it means to be a man or a woman performing their roles in the organization. Knowledge of who is favored and who is left out reveals to the caregivers appropriate ways of being and acting according to their particular subcultures within the organization.

## LESSONS LEARNED

Stories serve many functions, but chief among them is the implicit distribution of a message, moral, or lesson regarding member thought and behavior (Brown, 1985, 1987). As already argued, stories indicate the "appropriate" ways to act and think in a given culture (Mumby, 1987). I analyzed the narrative construction of knowledge among caregivers in terms of lessons implicitly learned about patients and their roles as caregivers. These lessons, although separated out in this discussion, clearly overlap, appear together, and influence each other in real time as knowledge frameworks.

### Lessons on Identity

Members etch out group identity through storytelling, as stories form the basis for belonging and feeling like part of a group that shares the same experiences (Van Maanen, 1992). The wealth of stories regarding patient behavior speaks to the very unique perspective of these caregiving groups. The medical dramas that remain hidden from the general public unfold in plain view of these caregivers. Caregivers observe all different sides of human behavior that most people simply do not see. This fact binds them together and makes their group special. Through this identification by separation (Burke, 1950), the medical group distinguishes itself by what it is not: the lay public. During medical training, caregivers explicitly and implicitly prepare to engage the identity of a caregiver and simultaneously reject the identity of a "regular" person (Hafferty, 1988). Storytelling about patients' bizarre behaviors or characteristics on the job maintains and solidifies this distinction. However, as stories stake out boundaries regarding concern for and involvement with patients (Totka, 1996), the resulting identity separation likely makes empathic communication more difficult.

Caregivers also draw identity boundaries between caregivers based on education, experience, status, title, gender, and any number of in-

and outgroups seen in the organization. In this study, group identities formed around both formal work groups such as physicians, registered nurses, and licensed practical nurses, but also around informal groups such as the "Boys Club" in the CL or the night shift employees in the ER. Only in-group members may tell stories that speak to a given identity. In the ER, the two male caregivers stepped to the side to share inside stories. Women in the CL could certainly not participate in stories involving the "Boys Club." Storytellers made exclusions in content and participation based on the people present in the scene.

Within identity groups, however, a great deal of sensemaking and comforting took place. Caregivers learned of expected behaviors and responses through the telling of stories that reflected the "wrong" way of acting and perceiving. As Mattingly (1998) argued, "Since the stuff of narratives is the abnormal, the improper, and other departures from the norm, stories offer rich vehicles for passing along cultural knowledge" (p. 13). Sensemaking about roles also formed around the nurses who provided reassurance and advice to other members of their group. Identification with the organization is likely heightened because employees often envision themselves as part of the organization by way of their immediate work group (Morgan et al., 2004). As caregivers forge attachments to each other and their workplace through supportive storytelling, the more they align behaviors along organizational expectations.

## Lessons on Power

Several of the stories told in these settings uphold power imbalances between the various caregivers. Storytelling emphasizes status differences and ultimately serves to keep them in place (Helmer, 1993). Mocking stories may be interpreted as a resistance to, and yet a reinforcement of, power imbalances. In the CL, several stories revolved around the mocking of doctors. By making the doctors look incompetent, the nurses overtly resisted the expectation that they should always behave competently in front of the doctor audience. By making fun of the doctors' supposed lack of skill, they positioned themselves as being superior in knowledge. Mocking that takes place backstage, however, maintains status differences precisely because the resistance remains hidden.

The mocking of patient behavior also may be viewed as an expression of status difference, because storytelling itself constitutes an act of power (Charon, 1993). As the patients become the subjects of the story, they become the objects of control. Several stories revolved around the disapproval of patients who did not behave along the lines of a "normal" or "good" patient. Caregivers responded to those patients who seemed to bring on their own plights or conditions with sarcastic remarks, or worse yet, an unsympathetic attitude. Staff brought frustrations that could not be expressed to the patient back to the nurses' station for discussion. Storytelling reifies the power distance between patients and caregivers.

## Lessons on Emotion

Both settings featured emotion rules tilted toward professional detachment (Lupton, 1994). The short-term contact between caregivers and ER and CL patients sets up a context more focused on processing and patching than nurturing care. The nurse who was mocked for showing too much concern for a patient and the patient's family revealed how an emotion rule of detachment operated within this organization. Professionalism was instantiated through rational, competent, and distanced performances (Morgan & Krone, 2001). On stage, the stories caution, the caregiver exhibits competence and skill, carefully avoiding too much involvement with the patient. Even humorous stories about patients imply the caregiver should keep an emotional distance. Making fun of patient behavior denied emotional connections, while also staking out and upholding boundaries in identity and power.

In the backstage, performers let down their "professional" masks a bit to vent emotion they are unable to release in front of the patient. The nurses' station becomes an emotion-safe "zone" (Fineman, 1996), where caregivers can express true feelings about audiences not present backstage. The CL nurse who vented about the patient whom she wanted to let "bleed to death on purpose" certainly could not reveal such frustration to the patient. Because of the "rational" nature of these settings, feelings of anger, joy, frustration, fear, and sadness all must be released in the backstage or kept inside. Backstage storytelling cultivates a very important collective form of emotion management that allows the caregivers to act in organizationally appropriate ways during onstage performances. The mocking of doctors backstage helps nurses to put on professional faces when performing in front of the demanding physician audience (Morgan & Krone, 2001). Humor, in general, also serves a venting function, and simultaneously underscores the pressing emotional demands of the onstage areas.

On one hand, backstage sessions serve as important coping devices; yet, they also speak to the organization's level of control over worker feelings (Hochschild, 1983). ER nurses occasionally did use the time backstage to console each other and talk about patient deaths, particularly of those people they personally knew. They expressed to me a desire for more storytelling opportunities, such as informal meetings established by the ER, to share their feelings. The emergency department sometimes met formally after trauma cases resulting in death, but these meetings focused on the procedures followed in treatment and potentially "what went wrong" as opposed to the emotional aftermath of the event. ER nurses mentioned how they used the drive home to deal with their feelings. The CL nurses told me they shared stories outside of work as part of their coping process. Pushing emotional storytelling to the backstage or offstage maintains the emotional order of "professional" caregiving, and the emotional burden remains on the shoulders of individual caregivers.

## GRAND NARRATIVE

The aforementioned lessons interweave to form a sensemaking structure that works as a grand narrative about caregiving. Patient and co-worker stories, retold and reframed, become part of the larger "medical story" (Hunter, 1991). Learning to be a caregiver means making sense of group-identity boundaries, status and power differences, and emotion rules of the organization and its subcultures. The narrative construction of knowledge embodies "what it means" to be a caregiver in relation to patients and colleagues (Goffman, 1959). Narrative knowledge informs caregivers what roles they occupy and how to play them for different audiences. Strikingly, these stories function to frame caregiver perception and, in turn, affect patient care. Stories act as lenses of perception or problem-setting devices (Schon, 1979) that shape action toward those frames (Mattingly, 1998). Notably, in the case of the "lightning strike" patient (who was immediately perceived as drunk and, therefore, not credible), caregivers framed the patient as such before he even entered the emergency room. The perception was strengthened as the story passed from paramedic to police officer, from nurse to technician. The consequences for patient care of narrative framing, then, can be quite dramatic. A patient who is not taken seriously likely is going to receive different, or lower quality, treatment than someone who is seen as having a legitimate complaint.

In this way, caregivers "spin" narrative knowledge into a "web" that enables and constrains (Geertz, 1973). Narrative knowledge enables caregivers in the sense that it provides guidelines for them to follow in the course of doing their work. They "know" how to behave in a whole host of medical and relational situations. Their uncertainty in these situations becomes comfortably reduced, which, of course, can benefit both patients and co-workers. Caregivers can act quickly and competently, with certainty and confidence in their actions. However, what caregivers "know" limits their perceptions of people and things in particular ways. Such institutional knowledge also works as a finite script for behaviors when another course of action may, in fact, be better—

medically, emotionally, or even ethically. The act of storytelling itself can persuade others to adopt similar perceptions (Mattingly, 1998). Alternative ways of doing, feeling, and being are obscured by what is considered to be the best or right way according to the grand narrative spun in the backstage.

Through the exercise of "appropriate" microlevel actions, caregivers uphold certain ideologies of caregiving as superior while suppressing alternatives (see also Mumby, 2000). The dominant ideologies in these particular settings lean toward the "traditional" Western medical pillars of the biomedical model. Rationality is exalted as the basis for professional, detached treatment focused on curing over caring (Goldstein, 1999). Hierarchy is maintained according to title and education, where status matters in making identity distinctions between groups. Preferential treatment is provided to the good, compliant patients (Treweek, 1996) who have legitimate conditions brought on by circumstances beyond their control. Backstage storytelling serves a venting function and may, at times, resist these ideologies; yet, dominant caregiving ideologies are maintained precisely because they are concealed backstage. Other stories directly support these ideologies by informing members how to act along expected lines in various situations for certain audiences.

It would be interesting to hear stories told in "alternative" medical settings where caregivers emphasize dialogic, emotional, holistic patient care. These stories would stand as a response and critique to biomedical approaches to caregiving. Beyond this, such stories could transcend the narrow margins of stale biomedical discourse (Mattingly, 1998) by way of valuing experience above science (Greenhalgh & Hurwitz, 1999), embracing multiple narrative perspectives (Geist-Martin & Dreyer, 2001) and ultimately allowing the voice of the "lifeworld" to be brought forth and validated (Charon, 1993). Narrative knowledge developed through this alternative ideology, in fact, may lighten the burden of "professional" demands for individual caregivers and align better with their own personal beliefs about what it means to provide care.

The fundamental contribution of this study lies in the retelling of actual caregiver stories, where we can see how narrative knowledge is developed and maintained in the medical backstage. We especially can see how stories chain together and form conventional narrative frames such as "the bizarre patient," "the overly concerned nurse," and "the inept doctor" that reveal a preference for the opposite scenarios: normal or good patients provided care by detached, competent caregivers. These frames serve as the basis for continued storytelling along the same lines, as similar stories work to support and uphold those themes (and their underlying ideologies). The description of story chains in this study adds to theoretical knowledge by empirically illustrating how storytelling is not a linear event with clear beginnings and ends, but rather a fluid, ongoing exchange of multiauthored texts that intersect and (re)cycle through a group of people who share a common bond (Boje, 2001).

On a practical level, this study offers a glimpse of what it might be like to be a caregiver in these settings (Geertz, 1973; Mattingly, 1998). Providers tell stories from which we might understand better who they are, what they do, and what assumptions guide their work. Stories and story chains have real implications for the way caregivers come to perceive the nature of patient experiences, illness and health, medical authority and identities, work relationships, and the organization itself. Researchers and practitioners can study storytelling to uncover these hidden assumptions, among others, to help members understand the sources of their relational and medical knowledge. Alternative ideological positions and their associated actions even may be explored through such an exercise. Reflexively, the readers and listeners of medical stories likewise would enhance and perhaps question their own knowledge of what it means to give and receive care.

# 11

# R$_x$ Story Prescriptions: Healing Effects of Storytelling and Storylistening in the Practice of Medicine

**Sunwolf**
*Santa Clara University*

**Lawrence R. Frey**
**Lisa Keränen**
*University of Colorado at Boulder*

*In West Africa, when a person in the village becomes sick, the Healer will ask them, "When was the last time that you sang? When was the last time that you danced? When was the last time that you shared a story?"*

—Cox, 2000, p. 10

*Now God sometimes tires of making people happy and always mixes some misfortune with good luck, like rain with sun. The queen fell ill, and neither the learned doctors nor even the quacks could do anything for her.*

—Excerpt from *Donkeyskin*, an oral folktale

The potential beneficial effects for those who are ill of telling their story has been long recognized in many cultures and has received attention from philosophers, social scientists, and medical practitioners alike. Illness, treatment, or death challenge those who are affected to construct meanings that create a tolerable narrative for what appears to be inexplicable; in such a context, storytelling is viewed as a form of communication that can help people successfully cope with and reframe illnesses and, thereby, create the paradoxical possibility of being "successfully ill." Frank (1995), a sociologist at the University of Calgary, argued that illness may be thought of as a call for stories, in that becoming ill often triggers narratives that help affected individuals to redraw their self-maps, in light of changed circumstances.

Children, in particular, may feel the need for constructing stories that help them to deal with their illnesses. C. D. Clark (1998), for instance, examined childhood imaginative narratives in the face of chronic illnesses. Fear of death was a universal concern shared during Clark's interviews with asthmatic children; a lack of breath always carried a concurrent sense of life-threatening consequences. Clark reported that one child had sheets on his bed depicting Teenage Mutant Ninja Turtles, which provided a basis for the child's imagined "what-if" stories, in which, should a nighttime emergency with his breathing occur, one of the Turtles would fly off the sheets and go to get the doctor, which calmed him during attacks.

The recognition of the potential power of narrative for those who are ill has led to a number of autobiographical and biographical narratives written about illness, treatment, and death, or what Hawkins (1993) called *pathographies*. As two illustrations, Gilda Radner (1989), the famous comedian, wrote a text that chronicled the final days of her life, and the poet Audre Lorde (1980) documented her 14-year struggle with breast cancer. Other pathographies emanate from health care providers' accounts of their encounters with ill patients (Brody 2003; Hunter, 1991) that recognized that "daily practice is filled with stories" (Hunter, 1991, p. 5).

The potential power of narrative to heal is now so widely accepted that it is being used as an intervention strategy by those in the medical community. Greenhalgh and Hurwitz (1999), for instance, trained medical students to adopt the perspective that the process of getting ill, being ill, getting better (or getting worse), and coping (or failing to cope) with illness can be best conceptualized as enacted narratives within the wider narratives of people's lives.

Although the potential power of sharing illness narratives has been well documented for those who are ill, relatively little attention has been directed toward how listening to narratives affects either those who are ill or their caregivers and loved ones. Storytellers, however, have long recognized the power of narratives to move listeners from the pain of the moment to a "happier ever after" (Sunwolf, 1999), with powerful narratives provoking intense flashes of insight for listeners who are ill (insights that may be invisible to a health care provider). Trauma, illness and grief create frightening forests of pain, with unfamiliar roads; in such a context, listening to stories suggests myriad pathways out of dark forests (Sunwolf, 2003).

The magical words "Once upon a time ..." that often start a traditionally structured folktale can induce a soothing, familiar light trance. Indeed, "holding an audience spellbound," is often used to describe an audience's altered state of listening to a great tale told well, and psychologists have claimed that storytelling performances contain many of the conditions necessary for inducing trances. A Boulder, Colorado psychotherapist–storyteller described such trances as an inner-directed state of consciousness, such that although listeners' eyes may be on the storyteller, their consciousness is turned inward (S. Martin, 1993).

This hypnotic effect alone might be enough to recommend that listening to narratives can be therapeutic. There is evidence, however, that the listening to oral tales can meaningfully penetrate even organic brain disorders, producing significant moments in people's lives. The experience of a storytelling troupe of middle-school students, sponsored by the California Arts Council, who began giving weekly performances at a day care center for senior citizens powerfully illustrates this point (Loya, 1997). Loya recounted the effects of those story performances on one of the senior citizens:

> Frank told amazing stories. With each passing year, however, his personality deteriorated, ravaged by Alzheimer's disease. By the third year he barely talked and never told stories. One day a young teller, Yarra, told about dancing. When she finished, Frank spoke for the first time in months. He had been a champion dancer, had won lots of competitions. Would Yarra like to dance? She accepted. They moved gracefully about the room in a wonderful dance, then he brought her back to her chair. As he sat down, the light left his eyes for the last time. He never spoke again after that. (p. 10)

Even health care practitioners themselves are beginning to recognize the effects that listening to their clients' narratives can have on them. Remen (1996), a psychooncologist and pioneer in training physicians in relationship-centered care, first encountered story as a part of her practice when a male hospital teammate asked her to visit his patient, who was crying. As Remen reported:

> I was no more comfortable than he in such situations but I realized early that this was part of my ticket to acceptance and so I would go and listen while someone shared with me their concerns and their experience of actually living with the disease we had diagnosed. At first, I was surprised that people with the same disease had such very different stories. Later, I became deeply moved by these stories, by the people and the meaning they found in their problems, by the unsuspected strengths, the depths

of love and devotion, the rich and human tapestry initiated by the pathology I was studying and treating. Eventually, these stories would become far more compelling to me than the disease process. (p. xxiv)

The story of illness narratives, therefore, is incomplete without a focus on the potential healing effects of both storytelling and storylistening. Accordingly, in this chapter, we explore both storytelling and storylistening in the context of illness narratives. We begin by explaining and extending Sunwolf and Frey's (2001) functional framework for understanding narrative to identify the functions or purposes filled by both storytelling and storylistening, or story sharing, as we shall call the *interaction of telling and listening to stories.* We then examine some of the effects of sharing stories for both tellers, listeners, and the communities of which they are a part. Throughout our narrative, we weave in research and real-life examples of how storytelling and storylistening have been used in cases of severe trauma, complicated grief, and/or chronic illnesses such as cancer, arthritis, renal failure, dementia, eating disorders, asthma, and AIDS. Finally, we discuss some of the ethics involved in story sharing and suggest future implications for health care narrative practices that value storied medicine.

## A FUNCTIONAL MODEL OF STORY SHARING

Human beings ponder, perceive, imagine, and make choices using narrative structures (Sarbin, 1986). Our memories, future plans, even our loving and hating, are all guided by internalized narrative plots; survival in a complex world would be problematic in the absence of skills to make up and to interpret stories (Sarbin, 1998). Stories offer a way of knowing and remembering experiences, and provide a powerful structure for binding together seemingly isolated or confusing events in a meaningful way (Sunwolf & Frey, 2001).

The sharing of stories between tellers and listeners provides a symbolic framework offering myriad connections between story, self, other, and experience. Langer (1942) argued that people demonstrate a need for symbols that form the basis for their understanding of the world. Humans, in fact, have been described as storytelling animals by MacIntrye (1981); Fisher (1987) suggested that people might be best understood as *homo narrans*, organizing our experiences into stories with plots, central characters, and action sequences that carry implicit and explicit lessons. If, as Fisher (1985b, 1987) argued, people inherently pursue a narrative logic, and all humans are essentially storytellers, the sharing of stories offers a powerful tool for both those who are ill and those who care about and for them.

Although we specifically invite reflection in this chapter on the two events of storytelling and storylistening, a cautionary note is necessary. *Story sharing* is a dynamic process in which stories are transformed in the telling, and, then, further transformed in the receiving. In effect, all shared tales undergo important change. An untold tale may be "owned" yet, the act of telling a story is always one of co-narration (and, hence, co-ownership), as listeners actively select, refocus, and reframe events or characters in the received tale. When we listen to a teller, we hear our own story. Within all people is the power of the remembered story that has been lost to consciousness, but may be triggered into memory. The story the patient tells is probably never the same story the healer hears (or vice versa), yet this is, paradoxically, the medicinal power of story. People receive the magical gift of being connected, through story, with their own healing wisdom. The medicinal parsimony of the right story at the right time for the right person is now emerging in health care scholarship.

The functional model offered by Sunwolf and Frey (2001) of sharing stories in the practice of medicine offers a framework for examining the multiple goals that stories serve for both storytellers and story listeners (see Fig. 11.1). The model suggests that the sharing of stories may function for both caregivers and their clients in five significant ways: (a) to connect people (relating); (b) to understand the world (explaining); (c) to create/recreate reality (creating); (d) to remember/re-member (history making); and (e) to vision/re-vision the future (forecasting).

### Stories as Bridges: A Way of Connecting (Relational Narrating)

Shared stories function to help construct the self (helping to answer the question, "Who am I?") and the community within which people are embedded ("Who are we?"). Many illnesses have both biological and psychological components. Eating disorders, for example, have severe consequences for physical health, but are increasingly receiving narrative interventions from treating physicians (Andersen, 1993a, 1993b). Andersen is a psychiatrist at the University of Iowa Health Care Center who regularly publishes vignettes of original tales in folktale format he has found effective in helping patients trigger behavioral changes and their relationship with food. Eating disorders are widely agreed to be one of the most difficult challenges for health care providers. Reconstructed fairy tales have been effectively used by Hill (1992) as a treatment intervention for young girls with eating disorders to break the harmful cycle that occurs when life transitions demand changes that a weak sense of self cannot accommodate. As Hill (1992) explained:

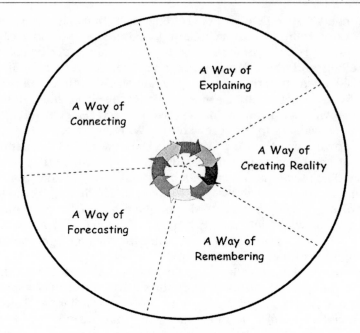

FIG. 11.1   A functional model of the effects of sharing stories in the practice of medicine.

Once upon a time there was a gentleman who married, for his second wife, the proudest and most haughty woman that was ever seen. He had by another wife, a young daughter, but of unparalleled goodness and sweetness of temper, which she took from her mother, who had been the best creature in the world. ... No sooner were the ceremonies of the wedding over than the stepmother began to show herself in her true colors. She could not bear the good qualities of this pretty girl. She employed her in the meanest work of the house. (p. 584)

Once told to the person, the fairy tale serves as a means to assimilate and accommodate desired aspects of the tale's characters at a prelogical level (Hill, 1992). One young girl, a binge eater, described visualizing what Cinderella ate at home and at the ball, and then what she might be feeling.

In addition to helping those who are ill to answer the "Who am I?" question, sharing stories functions to connect those who are ill with others and, thereby, answer the "Who are we?" question. Narratives are tools to access values and worldviews and are, thus, functional for gaining a holistic, culturally based understanding of the meaning of health interventions and illness in underresourced communities.

Cesario's (2001) work with tribal woman supported her narrative argument that because many tribes are matrilineal and women play an important role in both health care practices and decision making, the use of talking circles (comprised of 5 to 15 Native American women who gather to share information, support, and solve problems), in which storytelling is valued, is a key tool for health care providers. Scholars at the University of Washington's School of Nursing and the Yakama Indian Health Center found, through listening to stories, that illness tales for Yakama Indian women were part of a journey tale (Strickland, Chrisman, Yallup, Powell, & Squeoch, 1996). Cervical cancer was the leading cancer among Alaskan Native American women, who had a high incident of such cancer and the lowest cancer survival rates of any United States ethnic group (National Cancer Institute, 1993). Tribal leaders invited these scholars to work collaboratively with them after three of their respected elders died of cervical cancer in 1991. As a result of gaining access to the story circles of these women, the health care team discovered that the elders had the greatest influence on younger women starting the journey ("walking in grandmother's footsteps," p. 145); consequently, getting the Pap test was retold (by elders) as an important part of becoming a woman, much different than the Western approach to health teaching that focuses on videotapes, classes, and printed brochures.

Narrative interventions may simultaneously function to explore the "Who am I?" connection, as well as the "Who are we?" connection. A three-dimensional, multiuser computer environment was designed to help young people in the dialysis unit at Boston's Children's Hospital with renal disease (Bers, Gonzalez-Heydrich, Raches, & DeMaso, 2001). Users build virtual space populated with objects and characters that are programmed with storytelling behaviors, and, at the same time, they converse with others on dialysis in a virtual community. Comparing the use of this program by healthy children to the renal patients, Bers et al. observed that those on dialysis made more use of fantasy in creating their rooms and never used their own pictures or names, which the healthy children consistently did.

## Stories as Theories: A Way of Knowing (Explanatory Narrating)

The word "narrative" comes from the Indo-European root *gna*, meaning both "to know" and "to tell" (White, 1987). People have a need to understand their experiences, especially those experiences that are painful. Told stories function as *recipes* for structuring unfamiliar experience (Bruner, 1987) and, consequently, are not passively received by listeners. Health care issues inevitably involve the challenge of successfully coping with loss and grief, linked to "why" questions. Helping to make sense of life's disappointments, shared stories actively and idiosyncratically affect each listener, both at the time a tale is first heard and, subsequently, at unexpected reoccurring moments (Sunwolf, 2003). E. J. Taylor (1997), a professor of nursing and advocate of the use of storytelling in caring for the body as well as the spirit of those who are ill, argued that regardless of the type of story being told, the telling itself serves to organize, as well as shape, both experience and thought.

One psychotherapist imported interpretive folktales into her healing with women facing gendered issues of midlife and aging (Thomas, 1997). Thomas found the wisdom of folktales seemed to touch her female clients emotionally long after the tales were first told, as clients called or wrote to say, "Such and such was happening to me, and I remembered that story you told me about ..." (p. viii). Nossrat Peseschkian is a medical doctor who specializes in both psychiatry and neurology, notable for founding Positive Psychotherapy, using a transcultural approach. He is less known for his work in using Middle Eastern oral tales in psychotherapy (Peseschkian, 2000). One of his patients gained new self-understanding after listening to one version of an ancient Persian tale about a man's intolerable burdens:

> Once there was a traveler who was loaded with many burdens. Around his neck an old millstone dangled; a heavy sack of sand hung on his back; a water hose was draped around his body. In his hands he carried a boulder. Chains dragged heavy weights around his ankles. On his head, the man balanced a rotten pumpkin. Moaning and groaning, he moved forward but complained of the weariness that tormented him. A farmer met this traveler and asked, "Why do you load yourself down with this boulder?" The wanderer was surprised, "Awfully dumb, but I hadn't noticed it before." He threw the rock away and felt *much* lighter. Then he met a merchant who asked, "Tell me, why do you trouble yourself with the rotten pumpkin on your head and those heavy weights you drag behind you?" The wanderer was surprised again, "Awfully dumb, I'm glad you pointed it out." He took off the chains and smashed the pumpkin. Again, he felt lighter. *Yet he continued to suffer.* A housewife from a field watched him in amazement and said, "Tired wanderer, you are carrying sand in that sack, but what you see in the distance is more sand than you could ever want. Your big water hose is not needed, when there's a clear stream flowing alongside you." The wanderer dropped the hose and the heavy sand. Then he stood there and glanced down, seeing *for himself* the heavy millstone around his neck that caused him to walk bent over. He threw it into the river. Freed from his unnecessary burdens, the traveler wandered on, now delighting in the cool of the evening—and soon found both comfort and lodging. (Traditional Persian tale, adapted from Peseschkian, 2000)

This 42-year old mother of three had presented with severe depression. She listened to the tale from her doctor, then brought notes about her reaction to it to her next session, which were full of her personal connections with specific events and symbols, not just the "moral" of the tale (Peseschkian, 2000), delighted in newly emerging understandings about her condition. This care receiver was not only *collaborating* in her diagnosis through storylistening, but providing a powerful assessment tool for her therapist, sharing new perceptions about powerlessness and gender-role strain.

Storytelling has been used as a powerful tool between caregivers and their clients, as well as between those who are ill and their survivors. Using personal stories about cancer of elderly African American women (50 or older) in the southeastern part of the United States, six story types emerged that helped to change breast-health education (Williams-Brown, Baldwin, & Bakos, 2002). These researcher–health clinicians found that the stories associated with breast cancer and cancer screening for older African American women focused on loss, pain, suffering, fear and stress, death, and spiritual faith.

Uri Rueveni (1995), a professor of psychology at the University of Houston, described his work with chronic headache sufferers, who found their inner resiliencies drained by intense family commitments. The clients (a majority of whom are women) feel burdened and frustrated at an inability to control their headache pains, while at the same time guilty for not effectively carrying their roles as parent, spouse, friend, daughter, sister, or worker. One promising intervention is a combination of medical and psychotherapeutic intervention, which includes storytelling. Beauty and the Beast is a story that provides sufferers with novel connections to their modern lives (often described as being in a dark tunnel, rusty, with tarnished energy levels, and inability to regain their former human "form"). Fairy tales are rich resources for helping headache sufferers understand the real world enchantments they are tangled in, as "promises" made, kept or broken, and demanded haunt their worlds. Rueveni (1995) described the use of both individual and group work with stories to help clients connect with new options and maintain relatively headache-free lifestyles.

## Twisted Tales: A Way of Creating Reality (Creative Narrating)

The narratives people construct about being sick influence their healing. People face a painful dialectical choice in storying their health: If they deny the amount of actual disease/damage and its implications, they may not seek appropriate care but if they are overly involved in being ill, it becomes unnecessarily disabling. Lee and Dwyer (1995) described the bio-psycho-social complexity of a person's illness, discovering that health care professionals also influence and help to co-create their clients' stories of illness or wellness. They pointed out that the language of symptoms presented by the health care system creates the stories people absorb about their health. They explained that when some symptoms come on gradually, a person may step into a story in which the disease is sneaky; when the condition strikes in full force unexpectedly, the story is stormy with angry thunderbolts. Important to a symbolic functional standpoint, behavioral outcomes vary with the story; Lee and Dwyer (1995) reported that an individual's adaptive behavior ranges between denial of even the most grave and intrusive of symptoms to focusing on modest sensations, thus inviting a new story around the symptom context. They described an adolescent who wanted to be like his athletic brother and rejected the model of his passive, obese brother and, consequently, had become such a stoic hero in his own health story that no one else noticed the disease:

> Both David and his parents ignored his juvenile arthritis. Nothing was visibly wrong and as the condition gradually worsened, David compensated. It was not diagnosed until he was 14 years old, when spurs inside of his spinal canal made physical movement too difficult and painful to be ignored any longer. The physician was said to be amazed that David had kept silent and compensated so well. David's personal narrative now characterized him as a "Stoic." (p. 78)

Studying narrative effects with children suffering chronic illnesses, C. D. Clark (1998) reported the power of the story format to help change the painful present. In reframing his reality, a 5-year-old boy explained a narrative he had created that gave his favorite toy car magical qualities so that it could always take him to places outside the hospital. Maher (2002) reported finding that encouraging those with Alzheimer's disease in adult daycare facilities to "spin yarns" increased their verbal and nonverbal communication. A sense of hopelessness, with people closing down into themselves, is transformed with new possibilities of communication and connection to their families. Research suggests that the more people with Alzheimer's disease and related dementia can be kept communicating, the slower the process of decline. This is the premise for an organization called Time Slips (Maher, 2002), which employs storytelling as a vehicle for those with a diminished capacity to communicate their dreams and doubts about themselves and their new world, helping them to reclaim both their imaginations and their voices. Basting (1998) concluded, after working with groups of senior citizens and abandoning memorized scripts and focusing on spontaneous storytelling, that storytelling provided a transformational device for older people to change the way they and others think about aging, allowing even healthy seniors to assume new roles. Bastings's work exemplified the multiple functions storytelling fulfills; in addition to helping seniors, their families, and their care-givers recreate the possibilities of aging, she reported that memories are recovered in ways that families treasures.

### Flashbacks: A Way of Remembering (Historical Narrating)

The pain of holding onto stories with no audience to listen to them is acute for those who are ill. There was once a storyteller who was di-rected by a doctor to a man who had been in hospice care for more than 6 months, receiving no visitors, no mail, and not even a single phone call (Oceanna, 1998). By all medical standards, this person should have been dead. The storyteller told of sitting down and explaining who she was, yet this man said nothing, so they simply sat together quietly. She then began telling a tale. The man suddenly reached out his hand and touched her arm gently: "If you don't mind, I'd like to tell you *my* story, my life's story. I'm dying, you know, AIDS. There isn't anyone to tell it all to, and I can't die until I've told the whole thing. Will you lis-ten?" (p. 20).

They sat there for hours as his stories poured out. When the hospice nurse called the storyteller the next day to report that the man had died peacefully in his sleep that night, storytelling took on a new dimension for the teller, as she confronted the phenomenon she called "transi-tional storylistening." Oceanna's hospice work began to actively in-clude storylistening. She often had used stories to ease the transition between life and death, but she now realized that those who are dying often have a need to tell their own stories, to be heard and accepted by other human beings before they can let go of life. She began asking the people she visited if they wanted to tell her their stories. As she ex-plained, "One elderly English gentleman called me his personal bard. In his mind's eye, he said, he saw me singing songs and passing down stories about his life like the troubadours of old. He claimed it made him feel immortal" (Oceanna, 1998, p. 20).

### Foreflashes: A Way of Visioning the Future (Forecasting)

Storytelling facilitates new ways of imagining even unwanted futures, which is valuable for people with poor health prognoses. Freeman (1991), a family nurse practitioner who works with chronically ill chil-dren and adolescents, reported his observations of one 12-year-old Korean–American boy with cancer, who incorporated the stories he read into story sharing and story performance. One story the boy en-joyed reading again and again involved an adolescent superhero, Wingman, who could fly anywhere. When treatments were no longer working, and quality of life was the boy's primary goal, he went to an oncology camp, where, on the last day of camp, the children make masks and act out stories. As Freeman (1991) explained:

> Another important part of the retreat was the fairy tale play, presented annually by the children for the adults, when all the children made masks out of casting materials in which to act out their parts. At the second retreat, Roy utilized his storytelling skills by serving as co-narrator. And, that year, 6 months before his death, Roy's mask was the largest of all, a great blue heron with an imposing beak. When I first saw it, I didn't recall the story of Wingman, the superhero who left bridges below and who could fly anywhere by means of imagination. (p. 210)

## NARRATIVE HEALING: THE EFFECTS OF STORY SHARING

> *I will tell you something about stories*
> *they are all we have, you see,*
> *all we have to fight off*
> *illness and death.*
> —Silko, 1977, p. 2

How can stories help in the healing process? There is evidence to suggest that both storytelling and storylistening trigger healing (together with the dynamic of co-narration), and that these effects hold for both teller and audience, broadening our view of story as medicine and, thereby, the story of medicine.

### Healing by Creating New States of Consciousness

Indigenous people around the world still tell ancestral stories to evoke healing spirits and inspire change (Meade, 1995). Kirkwood (1992) suggested that stories function to open the mind to creative possibilities when the tales exceed people's beliefs, values, and experiences. Klingler (1997) argued that stories are effective during lengthy illnesses or healing journeys by providing distance from the stress and anxiety inherent in hospital settings and medical procedures. Some researchers explain the healing power of story by arguing that listening to stories allows the mind to enter a deeper, more imaginative state of consciousness. A former nurse-turned-storyteller explained that for both the storyteller and the health care provider, stories can help to establish a safe, slower paced, receptive human environment in which those who are ill can feel more relaxed and empowered to express questions, concerns, and needs (Klingler, 1997).

## Healing by Offering Examples of Success

Three studies were undertaken to explore the coping benefits and limitations of stories people listen to about others undergoing similar stressful events (S. E. Taylor, Aspinwall, Giuliano, Dakof, & Reardon, 1993). Interestingly, people living with cancer reported that positive stories about other people with cancer were more helpful than negative stories, yet negative stories were the most commonly told! Relatively few people were interested in seeking stories about other people living with cancer, although participants repeatedly reported that they had been told one or more stories about other people with cancer, usually by friends or relatives who themselves did not have cancer (two thirds of these stories were about others who had died or coped poorly with cancer). The source of a story may influence how it is perceived, even when the story parallels a person's own situation; S. E. Taylor et al. (1993), postulated that the most effective stories may come from similar others or experts. When the valence and source of stories told to college students facing midterm exams were manipulated, stories with positive endings and those relayed by expert sources were regarded more positively than negative stories and those told by nonexperts (S. E. Taylor et al., 1993). In a third study, three groups of students listened either to stories of another student's poor college adjustment, average level of adjustment, or excellent success; there were two additional story conditions (an informative story condition, containing information relevant to improving college adjustment, and an uninformative story condition). These findings showed that the perceived helpfulness of a story depended on the story's valence (negative stories made students feel lucky by comparison, whereas positive stories were perceived as offering a better role model and sense of hope). This suggests that illness tales from survivors of similar illnesses may have the most profound healing and comforting effects for people with newly diagnosed illnesses.

## Healing by Reducing Unhealthy Anxieties

The effects of storylistening have also been measured in medical settings. Although health care practitioners routinely rely on the self-reports of their clients to measure the healing effects of telling and listening to stories, one unique effort to quantify such effects is the use of a Death Anxiety Scale to gauge the degree to which an individual experiences anxiety at the prospect of dying. This scale has been applied in storytelling applications to help create emotional and spiritual healing at life's end (Stone, 1996). The Missoula Quality at Life's End Demonstration Project currently is finalizing results from a study in which two groups of 30 residents living in a congregate living facility participated in research over a period of 6 to 8 weeks. The Death Anxiety Scale was administered before, at the conclusion of the story treatment, and then 6 to 8 weeks later. A matched control group was led by a facilitator in general discussions about events of the day at the same time each week, whereas the experimental group participants worked with story exercises designed to facilitate reminiscence sharing (Stone, 1996). Another research project has examined the biochemical effects of story sharing, testing story listeners for the presence of an immune substance known as immunoglobulin A and the hormone, cortisol, both of which have been connected with the trance state associated with story listening (Martin, 1993).

## Co-Healing: Medicine for the Teller and the Listener

Cotter (1998) described the power that stories have to heal both the listener and the teller for chronic illness. Cotter, a farmer from Minnesota and professional storyteller, led a workshop on storytelling for 22 terminally ill people at Cape May, New Jersey (M. Cotter, personal communication, February 17, 2001). The location selected was powerful; a wildlife laboratory, where the enormous glass windows of the large room overlooked a marsh that fed into the Atlantic Ocean. Most of the people attending were suffering from AIDS or cancer; all had been waiting expectantly for this unique, unknown experience. Because of participants' fragile condition and the novelty of the approach, therapists, doctors, and nurses were present as well. Cotter's job was to tell his own most vulnerable stories, to create a safe place, and to help these people see the powerful stories embedded in their years of painful experiences. A circle of anxious participants and caregivers formed in the room, led by this farmer who had never lived more than 60 feet from the spot where he had been born more than 60 years before. Cotter pondered about which stories he should tell, finally settling on two stories about his life on the farm, both of which revealed in diverse ways his own uncertainties and vulnerabilities. Recognizing the challenge of leading listeners into the role of tellers, he focused on something that was simultaneously distant from their current fears and yet connected to the genesis of who they were: He asked each person to share the story of his or her name, something each person knew and could tell without planning. As Cotter (1998) explained: "When their stories began to come—hesitant at first, fragile and vulnerable, then with more power and humor and force—they came like a tidal wave. Sad, tender, at times humorous, they were the stories of people looking at life's end" (p. 4).

In enacting storytelling *with* one another, and making the transition from listeners to Cotter's tales to tellers of their own stories, participants seemed to gain a sense of mission, as they moved from names to individual life–dream identity stories. As Cotter (1998) elaborated:

> Of the 22 participants, 21 told their stories. An 11 year old boy with brain cancer just wanted his classmates to treat him normally. There was a young father of three whose six-year-old daughter had only known him as ill. That was the only kind of father she knew, though he longed to be a normal one to her.... There was a woman who lived in a setting surrounded by birds and trees and natural sounds. She told of having to go from the well world of nature with its sounds and colors, into the sterile shut-in sounds of the hospital where she had only herself and her fear and her pain. (p. 4)

The stories that day healed in unexpected ways. When the workshop was over, Cotter described a woman who had remained silent but found the farmer and poured out her story privately. It was such a powerful story that the farmer did some inner healing of his own, as he was reminded of a time when he had overcome a fear and helped his desperately ill young daughter (M. Cotter, personal communication, February 17, 2001).

## Healing the Practioner

Although the effects of storylistening have been studied, less attention has been paid to the impact that these tales have on health care practitioners. This is unfortunate, for health care professionals' days are filled with stories that must be successfully navigated. Again and again, those who are ill regularly tell stories to their health care providers, in response to such prompts as, "When did you first notice this?" and "How did this happen?" The ability to take in someone's illness story, to track and contextualize the meaning of its words, is, thus, a critical part of the health care professionals' job (Reynolds, 2003). Professional health care providers, in turn, re-tell their clients' tales to one that reveal the biomedical approach to medicine most often adopted in Western health care settings (e.g., "A 63-year-old, well-nourished Hispanic male presents with ..."). At the same time, every member of a health care team may soon be telling part of a different story, now structured as diagnoses, consultations, or treatment strategies. Even the bioethicist is now trained to write up cases in the traditional narrative "case history" form, which structures events and constrains interpretations of events (Chambers 1999).

**Healing the Community**

Finally, stories not only help to heal individual tellers and listeners but they also can help groups and communities to cope with illness. Illness not only threatens individuals but also the collectives within which those individuals are embedded. The Yakama Edlers, for instance, recognize that "cervical cancer robs a people of its childbearing women, its mothers, its elders ... its hope for survival and the passing on of the culture" (cited in Strickland et al., 1996, p. 141).

Within a collective context, Bormann (1986) argued, a story is a "creative and imaginative shared interpretation of events that fulfills a group psychological need" (p. 221). Adelman and Frey (1997), in their longitudinal study of communication and community building in a residential setting for people with AIDS, talked about the role of narrative and other symbolic practices (such as ritual) in helping residents to cope with their circumstances. Residents, for instance, were fond of retelling the story of Sean, a rather eccentric resident, who, because he was mentally disoriented in the latter stage of his illness, was found one day running around "butt naked" in the foyer of the house. As Adelman and Frey (1997) explained, such "illness tales" represent "collective interpretations that ease the stigma of deviant behavior and unusual symptoms due to AIDS by conversion to the absurd" (p. 41). Moreover "success stories and illness tales told over and over again become part of the Bonaventure House legacy. For both newcomers and veterans, these stories help create and sustain a unified rhetorical vision of BH as a community where people live, not die, with AIDS" (p. 41).

## STORIED MEDICINE FOR A MORE SUCCESSFUL JOURNEY FORWARD

The healing journey offered by story sharing carries with it significant ethical challenges. Both teller and listener must balance three related issues: (a) giving attention during story sharings, (b) offering feedback during and after story sharings, and (c) considering appropriate constraints on the retelling of someone else's story. Caregivers, in particular, must simultaneously do other care and self-care as they are consistently challenged by the dialectical tension they experience between wanting to establish healthy connection with and healthy disengagement from those they serve (Sunwolf, in press): "The very worst times are the ones when I have felt so much and hurt so long for a family that finally I can't feel anything at all" (Anonymous helper, cited in Larson, 1993, p. 58).

Caring helpers experience an exhausting struggle with professional burnout, with high empathy and helper stress being positively correlated (e.g., Stotland, Mathews, Sherman, Hansson, & Richardson's 1978 finding that high-empathy nurses were the first to leave the rooms of dying patients).

Both storytelling and storylistening involve choice. The teller must summon the courage to narrate, to find his or her voice, and to recognize receptive audiences. The listener must choose to remain open to someone else's story, offer attentive feedback, engage in appropriate perception checking after the telling, and honor the teller's perspective and privacy in any retelling of the tale. The choices involved in such acts are profoundly moral. In both medical literature and writings on moral philosophy, the dynamics of the relationship between teller and listener are increasingly expressed as a matter of ethical obligation. Kleinman (1988) described the ideal relationship between a healer and client as one that involved a deep existential commitment to being with the other that was predicated on empathic listening. *Empathy* involves both cognitive role taking and an other-oriented emotional responsiveness that allows helpers to imagine what it would be like to be in another person's predicament (Larson, 1993). Kleinman (1988) quoted William James as saying that "a doctor does more by the moral effect of his presence on the patient and family than anything else" (p. 227). Part of this presence involves listening, an act that can alter both teller and listener by establishing a mutual recognition of difference and connection that forges a common bond. The commitment to being with the other can be extended from caregivers as healer to caregivers as storylisteners, who willingly bear witness to stories of illness and suffering.

Storylistening also involves recognition of the identities of the other and the way in which those identities are shaped by illness. Storylistening often involves placing ourselves outside of the comfort zone of our own experience and into the experiences of another; as C. Taylor (1991) wrote: "the acknowledgment that our identity requires recognition by others" (p. 45). Listening and affirming is one way of demonstrating recognition of others. As Forester (1980) explained: "When we do not listen, we deny our membership in a shared world with others. We shirk the responsibility of responding genuinely when spoken to— as if we could extend into a way of living the perpetual refusal to respond when being greeted" (p. 221).

For Forester, listening "is an act of participation, nurturing a 'we.'" It is also a political act: "Just because we learn language and the world together, if we do not listen, we cannot have much of a world together" (Forester, 1980, p. 230). The ill, the well, the worried well—we all inhabit the same world, but without remaining open to the stories of the other, we cannot begin to find common ground. Eadie (1990) reminded us that "we need to make special effort to hear the voices of those who are not like us, to listen for their truth, and to celebrate both how we are similar and how we are different" (p. 3).

There are risks involved in both storytelling and storylistening, particularly when either is done with mixed intentions. Larson (1993), a psychologist who researches the challenges of giving hospice care, first spoke to healers about "the helper's pit." Larson's metaphor describes someone needing help as standing at the bottom of a deep pit, while a helper stands on the edge of that pit, reaching down. Larson explained the task of a "helper on the pit's edge" as one of attempting to provide caring service—without falling into the pit with the distressed client. If the helper slides into the pit, useful empathy for the client transforms into personal distress for the helper. To be sure, storytelling and storylistening are not a panacea for what ails individuals and society, but they are processes that help us to recognize the suffering of others as a first step toward healing.

Stone (1996) developed a guide to help health care practitioners elicit story memories from their clients, and actively conducts workshops across the country on topics such as (a) the healing power of humor in storytelling, (b) enhancing communication skills through the power of storytelling, (c) improving physician communication through positive listening attitudes, (d) transforming a hospital's culture through the power of storytelling, and (e) building a community of caring and support in health care institutions. His storytelling workshops are intensive and experiential, designed not only for nurses and doctors but also for therapists, social workers, volunteers, patient advocates, interns, and clergy—groups that constitute additional accessible avenues for eliciting stories from anxious people who are ill. Bristow (1997) developed a "storyboard" to aid in the process of putting together some orderly sequence to a patient's told story.

In the same way that a story may function as a bridge, connecting those who are ill to new possibilities in their lives, professional storytellers are now serving as bridges to hospitals, hospices, and health care providers. Workshops and collaborative teamwork offer therapists new possibilities for their own practices. The National Storytelling Network (www.storynet.org) has organized The Healing Arts Special Interest Group, offering references, resources, and networking for health care givers wishing to read and train in narrative healing or to connect with tellers who use narrative in health care settings.

Some national health care organizations now regularly offer training programs designed to help people heal through storytelling, including the National Hospice Organization and the Spiritual Caregivers Association. The growing use of oral storytelling by health care practitioners is predicated on the belief that storytelling is a natural outcome of speech, and that all people, therefore, are storytellers, whether they know it or not. Klingler (1997) offered a radical prediction, foreseeing changes in the U.S. health care system:

> Hospital settings and other health care environments should make room for institutional models of healing that incorporate storytelling and other art forms ... even traditionalists are opening themselves to the possibility that the quickest route to healing the body is through the psyche and the soul. Like shamans in tribal societies, storytellers may soon be walking the halls of hallowed medical institutions dispensing their remedies one tale at a time. (pp. 21–22)

Understanding the role of narratives in the context of wellness, in general, and in medical health care, in particular, thus, requires a parallel focus on both the telling of and listening to stories for those who are ill, their caregivers, and their loved ones. Although storytelling has received significant attention in the health care literature, the story of storytelling is incomplete without the recognition of the importance of listening and responding to and being affected by the stories that one hears. Although health care practitioners are receiving training in the use of narrative as an intervention strategy, such practitioners still too often are trained to listen for certain types of biomedical information, rather than to elicit narratives about the subjective meanings of illnesses. Although there are some important structural barriers to intense storylistening in the modern health care setting (e.g., time constraints and division of labor), continued efforts to train health care workers to listen and respond to elicited stories would potentially help the healing and health care endeavor. Of course, medical practitioners, such as physicians and nurses, do not bear the entire responsibility for providing opportunities for storytelling and listening. Volunteers, family members, friends, and others involved in the lives of those who are ill can contribute to the effort in a myriad of ways. Kleinman (1988) explained "If there is a single dimension of illness that can teach us something valuable for our own lives, then it must be how to confront and respond to the fact that we will all die, each of us" (p. 157). Storytelling and storylistening are twin processes that can help us all to confront this fact—together, one story at a time.

## ADDENDUM: THE AUTHORS' STORY CONNECTIONS

*It was a dark and stormy night on the oncology ward of a large children's hospital when I first stepped into story, as medicine. There was a room no doctors could enter, a room of sanctuary, where children knew they would be temporarily free of painful intrusive treatments.*

*The life battles these children confronted necessitated long periods of hospital-style incarceration—even the most engaging toys or creative crafts become too familiar. Late one night, on duty as the play therapist, I found myself surrounded by six bored adolescents. Caught in a moment of epiphany, I (who was not a storyteller) asked my patient–companions if they'd like to turn out the lights and tell ghost stories. I gave them a story my father had given to me, then a couple more that just seemed to show up. The shivers and chills, shared in the community of group, were far different versions of fear than the ones these children and teens faced daily. They laughed, screeched, giggled. A trial attorney by day, my logical brain went into action and I set up camp in the local library until I had unearthed every book I could find about storytelling. I knew more would be needed.*

*—Sunwolf*

*I was laying in bed one cold, snowy winter night in Chicago when I received a call from Mannie, a resident at Bonaventure House, the residential facility for people with AIDS that my colleague Mara Adelman and I had been studying for a number of years. Mannie was one of our key informants and a friend. He asked if I could come over and talk with him right then. I didn't want to leave the comfort of my home, but I could hear the desperation in Mannie's voice, so I drove over to the house. When I entered Mannie's room, it was clear that he was very sick. He told me that he wasn't feeling very well but "wanted to contribute to our research project one more time." We didn't really talk about research-related things; we just shared some stories about our lives, our hopes, and our dreams. When I left, I knew that would be the last time I would see Mannie. That experience taught me firsthand the power of sharing stories for both those who are ill and those who care for and about them. It also taught me, as Farmer (1992) said, "Research is very often an inappropriate response to suffering. In such instances, we may find that personal integrity and professional interest are best served by putting aside tape recorders and notebooks" (p. 315) and connecting as simply one homo narran to another.*

*—Lawrence R. Frey*

*My entrée into the realm of illness stories began in 2001 when, as part of a clinical practicum in bioethics, I stepped into an intensive-care unit on a hot and humid June day at a Pittsburgh hospital to round with the intensivists. Immediately, I was immersed in a technological realm. Alone at the nurses' station waiting for someone to notice my arrival, I listened to the blips and bleeps, and gurgles and swooshes of the machines that were keeping many of the patients alive. Eventually, a nurse brought human voice into the mix, decrying that a patient had had an accident in his bed. Soon, the nurse's voice was joined by a chorus of others who all added nuance to the "story" of the patient's life. Yet, the patient himself remained silent and inaccessible to me. I heard the medical resident's account, then that of the attending physician, and even the pharmacist. When I later sat with the patient's family as they made a decision about life-sustaining treatment, I was struck by stark differences between their stories and the others offered throughout the day. Although the patient was now unable to tell his story, his family's narrative pierced through the technological realm to infuse the patient's life with meaning.*

—Lisa Keränen

# 12

## Narrative Medicine and Education in Palliative Care

∾

**Sandra L. Ragan**
**Tiffany Mindt**
*University of Oklahoma*

**Elaine Wittenberg-Lyles**
*University of Nevada, Las Vegas*

*My initial experience of illness was as a series of disconnected shocks, and my first instinct was to try to bring it under control by turning it into a narrative. Always in emergencies we invent narratives. We describe what is happening, as if to confine the catastrophe. When people heard that I was ill, they inundated me with stories of their own illnesses, as well as the cases of friends. Storytelling seems to be a natural reaction to illness. People bleed stories, and I've become a blood bank of them. The patient has to start by treating his illness not as a disaster, an occasion for depression or panic, but as a narrative, a story. Stories are antibodies against illness and pain.*

—Broyard, 1992, pp. 19–20

These lovely words penned by Anatole Broyard, renowned literary critic for *The New York Times* for 19 years, did not prove an effective antibody against his death from metastatic prostate cancer; yet despite the pain he suffered in his dying, he continued writing his story until just weeks before his life ended. Stories have long been heralded as healing, and the publication of this volume bespeaks that. This chapter discusses how narrative literature can and should be a part of medical school curricula in order to inculcate patients' experiences of their illnesses and dying into medical practitioners. In particular, we emphasize the value of stories in teaching doctors about palliative care.

The face of medicine has seen drastic changes in the past 20 years. Among the technological and scientific advances, the basic model of medicine and patient–doctor relationships has evolved from a biomedical focus to a broader, more inclusive biopsychosocial focus. With this expanded focus emerge new roles and responsibilities for the health care team, such as seeking to understand and helping the patient balance the differing components of health—biological, psychological, social, and even spiritual and existential. Such understanding becomes particularly pressing when a patient is receiving palliative care, whether at end of life or during another phase of a potentially life-threatening illness.

Paramount to palliative care, according to the World Health Organization, is control of pain and noxious symptoms, as well as attending to the psychological, social, and spiritual problems associated with terminal illness and the dying process in the hopes of achieving the best quality of life for patients and their families (Billings & Block, 1997). End-of-life care became a popular topic in the 1960s following the publication of Elizabeth Kubler-Ross's *On Death and Dying* (1969), which proposed a five-stage model of dying. Her extensive research stemmed from the stories of dying patients and sparked much needed attention to the needs of the dying (Holleman, 1991). Overall, Kubler-Ross provided a framework for learning how to cope with dying and gave medical staff some insight on how to help those dying (Corr, 1993).

Since the introduction of palliative care into medical education in the 1960s, it has garnered much attention in medical journals and much discussion about the best possible approaches to its implementation into medical school curricula and into the practice of medicine. This discussion may have more of a presence in the journals than in the classroom, however. Many physicians and scholars criticize medical school education in palliative care as inadequate and/or virtually nonexistent (Billings & Block, 1997; Block, 2002; Doorenbos, Briller, & Chapleski, 2003; Gatrad, Brown, Notta, & Sheikh, 2003; Sullivan, Lakoma, & Block, 2003). In fact, in a national survey of medical students and residents, only 18% of students and residents received any formal education in end-of-life care (Sullivan et al., 2003). On average, only 1.59% of the pages in medical textbooks address end-of-life care issues (Block, 2002). Because of this educational void, many students and residents reported feeling ill prepared to address their patients' thoughts and fears about dying, and a majority reported feeling ill prepared to address cultural issues and spiritual issues pertinent to this care and to managing their own emotions or those of the family during the death process (Sullivan et al., 2003). In addition, despite the pressing need for death education, medical education curricula have neglected to provide communication skills training in building relationships and in decision making, two critical aspects of the physician's role in providing end-of-life care (Von Gunten, Ferris, & Emanuel, 2000).

The omission of palliative care in the classroom looms in the clinic as well, as the quality of end-of-life care provided by physicians has been described in the current literature as poor, insufficient, and/or in need of change (Billings & Block, 1997; A. Cohen, 1997; Curtis et al., 2001; Gatrad et al., 2003; Sullivan et al., 2003). Some argue that this inadequacy in end-of-life care results from the lingering, traditional view of death as a failure of medicine and the physician (Danis et al., 1999; Fins & Nilson, 2000; Sullivan et al., 2003).

With the advent of the biopsychosocial model of medicine also came new means of learning and acquiring a more humanistic focus in medicine. Although this transition is far from complete, the relatively new inclusion of the study of narrative literature into medical education bears witness to it. Beginning with the first appointment of a medical faculty in literature in 1972 at the Pennsylvania State University College of Medicine, nearly one third of American medical schools taught literature to their students a little over two decades later in 1995 (Charon et al., 1995; Hunter, Charon, & Coulehan, 1995). In fact, literature and medicine now receives recognition as its own field, with its own academic journals, professional associations, and graduate programs (Charon et al., 1995). However, as stated, this transition to the biopsychosocial model still lacks completion, and medical schools still remain reluctant to require the study of literature. The majority of such courses are elective (Welch, 2000) and offered during students' preclinical years (Hunter et al., 1995), when students do not interact with patients. Regardless, the study of literature is present in a large number of medical schools, offering a broader, more humanistic education.

The narrative medicine movement is currently in vogue, in part because of a felt need to counter technology with old-fashioned practices that include doctors really listening to their patients. As former dean of the University of Oklahoma College of Medicine, Dr. Jerry Vannatta explains, "[T]echnology has become a religion within the medical community. It is easy to lose sight of the fact that still, in the 21st century, it is believed that 80 to 85 percent of the diagnosis is in the patient's story" (D. Smith, 2003, para. 2). Sharf and Vanderford (2003) echoed this perspective in their discussion of illness narratives and reiterated that both the voice of medicine and the voice of the lifeworld, the patient's voice (Mishler, 1984), must be interwoven into a "consistent, mutually agreed upon story" (Sharf & Vanderford, 2003, p. 15). As Hunter et al. (1995) explained: "The study of literature was introduced into medical curricula not to provide 'culture' or to remedy the omissions of premedical undergraduate study but to enrich a narrow curriculum that was focused, almost exclusively, on the value-neutral transfer of scientific fact" (p. 788).

Medical schools incorporate fiction and nonfiction narratives into their pedagogy in two ways: first, through studying and analyzing the narratives (written and oral) of others, and second, through encouraging medical students to write their own narratives. Narratives offer invaluable benefits for those in the medical field, including a humanistic focus, narrative skills (defined and described in the next section), exposure to other experiences and realities, self-reflection, and emotional release. Each of these attributes is pertinent to—and vital to— the practice of effective palliative care. In fact, the study of literature can respond to many of the previously mentioned criticisms of palliative care.

## READING NARRATIVES

The very nature of narrative makes it a prime instrument for learning. Greenhalgh and Hurwitz (1999) pointed out that narratives are "memorable, grounded in experience, and encourage reflection" (para. 4). Because narratives highlight how individuals feel and experience their reality, rather than just what they do or what is done to them, they provide a more visual representation of the emotions and cognitions involved (Loftus, 1998), increasing both comprehension and retention. The study of literature can hone literary skills, such as tolerance for ambiguity and interpretation, empathy, and reflection; it also can illustrate cultural differences and can develop medical ethics.

### Narrative Skills

The study of narratives develops important skills within its readers, skills critical to the practice of medicine. These skills, termed *narrative skills*, include interpretation, empathy, and reflection. To understand the relevancy of these skills, one must first recognize the nature of medicine. Diagnosis is not purely an objective process, not a factual location of symptoms that lead to the truth; it is instead grounded in interpretation and evaluation. This notion conflicts with our traditional views of science and medicine and the role of the physician, as reflected in Charon's (2001b) statement: "Logicoscientific knowledge attempts to illuminate the universally true by transcending the particular" (para. 7). Narrative knowledge is particularly pertinent to this new biopsychosocial model of medical knowledge, attempting instead to "illuminate the universally true by revealing the particular" (para. 7).

Skelton, Macleod, and Thomas (2000) pointed out that, in literature, reality involves values, not facts, ambivalence, not reductionism, hence creating a world where everything is not amenable to experiment. This "reality," as it is constructed in literature, is much "like the life of a doctor" (p. 202). Ahlzen (2002) also acknowledges this nonscientific feature of medicine and the value of literature in noting, "Narratives give full justice to the crucial elements of clinical practice: ambiguity, complexity, paradox, and tragic choice—and capture the 'human life worlds, especially as they may evolve in and around illness and suffering'" (p. 148). Because of the presence of these characteristics in the body of the narrative, they hone within the reader (or listener) such skills as pattern finding, meaning making, interpretation, and evaluation, "attitudes and rhetorical frames that are essential to managing difficult or ambiguous information, skills, or situations" (C. Anderson, 1998, p. 282), and apt clinical evaluation (Charon et al., 1995).

Additionally, and importantly, literature can hone empathic skills. As Charon (as cited in D. Smith, 2003, para. 10) attests, "No medical school can train students in empathy. But we have a duty to equip them with the ability to see, to articulate, to grasp and comprehend the position of the patient." Physicians have long been taught detachment for survival, objectivity, and success. Emotions—whether within the physician or patient—remained a component of medical practice to be eschewed. This disconnect can be witnessed in the reduction of the patient in case studies and medical charts to "events in the exterior, objective world neglect[ing] or objectify[ing] subjective experience, including symptoms" (Donnelly, 1988, p. 823). Such emotional distancing can still be seen in modern medicine according to Greenhalgh and Hurwitz (1999), "Modern medicine lacks a metric for existential qualities, such as the inner hurt, despair, hope, grief, and moral pain that frequently accompany, and often indeed constitute the illnesses from which people suffer" (p. 48). The moving film, *The Doctor* (in which a brusque, uncaring cardiologist becomes a patient himself and experiences a dose of his own medicine before he understands that caring for the patient is critical to the practice of good medicine) graphically illustrates emotional distancing.

The advent of the biopsychosocial model of medicine calls for more empathy and understanding, as Greenhalgh and Hurwitz (1999) acknowledge:

The relentless substitution during the course of medical training of skills deemed "scientific"—those that are eminently measurable but unavoidably reductionist—for those that are fundamentally linguistic, empathic, and interpretive should be seen as anything but a successful feature of the modern curriculum. (p. 49)

Coulehan (1995) agreed that "[D]etached concern is a risk or failure of medical education, rather than an appropriate goal ... lead[ing] to ... a general discounting of the affective life" (p. 225). To exercise empathy and understand the patient, one must consider as important and legitimate the patient's experience beyond the physical symptoms. To aid in this discussion, Kleinman, Eisenberg, and Good (1978) distinguished between disease, the biological–physiological conditions that can be objectively and quantitatively assessed, and illness, the patient's experience of that disease.

Narratives offer physicians an invaluable opportunity to witness the human side of medicine, and to understand illness and medicine from the perspective of a patient. Unlike the case study, narratives are not bound to the restrictive notion of objectivity; they extend beyond the physical symptoms, allowing the reader to subjectively feel the experience as a whole, evoking emotions and discomfort (Wear & Nixon, 2002). As Trautman (1982) pointed out, narratives allow insight not only into the physical condition, but also into the mind of the patient. Particularly in palliative care, narratives serve as better illustrators of the complex care of the dying. A number of medical schools employ literature and drama to teach death education: "Rich with insight, meaning, and painfully accurate description, these stories have the power to shape not only the students' attitudes toward their dying patients, but also to shape their values, their character, and their attitude toward their work and their lives" (Holleman, 1991, p. 17).

Narratives can convey the "particularity and metaphorical richness" of the experiences of patients and the challenges and rewards for their physicians (Charon et al., 1995, para. 1). An understanding or empathy for illness and what it is to be a patient can help physicians accompany their patients through their illness "with empathy, respect, and effective care" (Charon et al., 1995, para 1). Additionally, as Charon et al. (1995) assert, learning the value of illness narratives can encourage medical students to listen to their own patients' illness narratives.

Finally, narratives sharpen another skill, reflection. The process of reflection can help medical students realize the clinical and nonclinical implications of their work, better understand their own complicated relationships with their work and patients, as well as comprehend what their work has done to them, offers to them, and what they can offer to medicine (Charon et al., 1995). Narratives "provide the means to understand the personal connections between the patient and physician, the meaning of medical practice for the individual physician, the physician's collective profession of their ideals, and medicine's discourse with the society it serves" (Charon, 2001b, para. 5). Additionally, some narratives offer the ability to reflect on—and accept—the *inevitability* of fatal decisions, as well as the *fallibility* of physicians and medicine (Ahlzen, 2002; C. Anderson, 1998). These concepts can create great stress and pressure for medical students, and failure to recognize this inevitability and fallibility can result in feelings of guilt and depression when patients die.

The emergence of this concept of *narrative skills*, such as interpretation, empathy, and reflection, also has led to the concept of *narrative competence*, or one's ability to effectively exercise these skills. Perhaps the most vocal advocate of narrative-based medicine, Charon (2002) described the integral role narrative competence plays with physicians, arguing "The effective practice of medicine requires narrative competence, that is the ability to acknowledge, absorb, and act on the stories and plights of others" (para. 2). She furthers, "Narrative competence enables a physician to practice medicine with empathy, reflection, professionalism, and trustworthiness" (para. 1).

### Cultural Views of Medicine, Illness, Healing, and Death

Particularly in the field of medicine, participants must be able to understand the stories of others, because culture, especially such components as ethnicity, race, gender, and religion, largely shapes views of medicine, illness, and death. Culture influences beliefs about the value of life in a debilitated state, the concept of a *good death*, whether or not individuals seek health information, how they seek this information, what information they seek, and whether the family or individual makes the decisions concerning health care (Danis et al., 1999).

Considering its integral relationship with health and medicine, culture greatly influences a patient's perceptions of, need for, and decisions concerning end-of-life care. For example, contradictory to the traditional Western notion of the patient's autonomy, Korean Americans and Mexican Americans often believe that the patient's family should make the decisions concerning end-of-life care (Doorenbos et al., 2003). Offering another example, Caresse and Rhode (1995) pointed out that, according to traditional Navajo beliefs, words have the power to create reality; hence, it is dangerous to speak of death, especially in relation to a particular patient. Similarly, death constitutes a taboo topic in traditional Chinese culture; speaking about death can be seen as casting a curse or quickening the dying process (Yam, Rossiter, & Cheung, 2001). However, more than just ethnicity affects one's construction of the meaning of death and needs relating to palliative care. A content analysis of 504 samples of free-form writing about death found that constructions of death also differed significantly depending on the subject's gender, health status, and personal philosophy (Holcomb, Neimeyer, & Moore, 1993).

Failure to understand and incorporate intercultural differences risks misunderstanding and cultural insensitivity on the part of the physician. In fact, Billings and Block (1997) asserted that much of the "dissatisfaction, stress, and dilemmas" associated with end-of-life care for the patients, their families, and the attending physicians results from the deficient appreciation of cultural diversity and intolerance of differing "attitudes, preferences, and personal styles among patients and families" (p. 736). Gatrad et al. (2003) criticized current palliative care for its Western assumptions: "Minorities must be understood before the establishment of an effective palliative care treatment program ... knowledge of different cultures is the key to understanding how they should die" (Gatrad et al., 2003, para. 1). Additionally, they argue for diversity in religious perspectives and understanding: "Training in issues to do with faith—a subject so important to so many people during their last days—need to be incorporated into professional training" (para. 6). Many other physicians and researchers have also recognized the importance of, and called for, the appropriate inclusion of culture—in the holistic sense of ethnicity, race, gender, and religion—into palliative care (Billings & Block, 1997; Caresse & Rhode, 1999; Curtis et al., 2001; Danis et al., 1999; Doorenbros et al., 2003; Fins & Nilson, 2000).

Narratives can enhance palliative care training by offering the study of and the understanding of culture's relation to medicine. Whether biographical or fictional, narratives written or told by members of a particular cultural, ethnic, or religious background can "situate illness within a specific cultural and spiritual understanding of the body" (Charon et al., 1995, para. 10), allowing the reader to enter into the lifeworld and illness experience of others. Narratives have the unique ability not only to envelop the reader in the situation and reality of others, but to allow the reader to experience this reality as if it were his or her own. Hurwitz (2000) contends, "Through stories, we are able to imaginatively enter into other worlds, shift viewpoints, change perspectives, and focus upon the experiences of others" (p. 2086). Narrative offers an invaluable experience for the physician or medical student that extends beyond what traditional learning materials, such as case studies, medical charts, and textbooks, offer. Wear and Nixon (2002) explained that, although the case study—and the same argument applies to charts and medical texts as well—maintains the current medical hierarchy, as well as the dominant culture, literature forces the reader to break away from the traditional caregiver role. Narratives enter into the subjective experience, vicariously immersing readers in experiences of culture, gender, race, ethnicity, social class, disability, or illness that they have not lived (Wear & Nixon, 2002). Reading narratives, then, can assist the physician or medical student in better understanding the intersection of patients and their illnesses—the patient's illness experience. For the patient, the experience of a severe or chronic illness is often difficult, stressful, confusing, fearful, and painful; these emotions may be exacerbated when patients receive a terminal diagnosis. Understanding the beliefs, attitudes, lifeworlds, and illness experiences of patients has never been more important than at this time.

## Ethics

Working with terminal illness and death poses new and unique ethical concerns, different from those in day-to-day medical practice. Medical-school training in ethics needs to address these concerns, and narratives offer a valuable tool. As Brody (2003) asserted, "ethical decisions (in medicine and in the rest of life) arise from and depend upon the narrative context" (p. 7). According to A. H. Jones (1999), narratives flush out ethical dilemmas by portraying them in a human context, "complicated by powerful emotions, and complex interpersonal dynamics" (p. 253). This further stimulates "ethical responsiveness and refin[es] moral perception, through showing—emotionally and cognitively—the presence of incommensurable values in our lives and the conflicts between these values" (Ahlzen, 2002, p. 148). A. H. Jones (1999) offered three ways in which narratives are important in developing medical ethics. First, they can provide case examples for teaching principle-based professional ethics. Second, narratives can provide moral guides for living a "good life." Finally, in providing their readers with experiential truth and passion, narratives "compel re-examination of accepted medical practices and ethical precepts" (A. H. Jones, 1999, p. 253).

As A. H. Jones (1999) described, narratives can help a doctor in consoling the ill by refining moral perception, as in a "kind of attentiveness that makes it possible for a person to discover the moral dimension of a particular situation," and hence be "finely aware and richly responsible" (Ahlzen, 2002, p. 150). Such moral perception inherently relates to the physician's ability to understand the culture and values of the patient. Charon et al. (1995) further elaborated on culture and moral ethics, as well as the role of narratives in nurturing moral ethics. Ethical quandaries within narratives occur within the character's moral perceptions, values, culture, and biography; therefore, developing skills in narrative ethics encourages sensitivity to morals and values as they occur in the clinical encounter and encourages physicians to incorporate inquiry about such values and beliefs into the normal encounter. This sensitivity facilitates better anticipation, understanding, and fulfillment of the needs and concerns of the patients. Doctors need such qualities, especially when they interact with chronically ill and/or dying patients and their families.

Additionally, through exposing the lifeworlds, beliefs, and cultures of others, narratives provide physicians the opportunity to recognize the values of Western civilization in the medicine that they practice. These Western values have set the accepted definitions for the good life and standard medical treatment, resulting in the curative- (vs. comfort-) oriented care that often insists on futile, allegedly curative treatment regimens, even as the patient is dying. C. Anderson (1998) asserted that narratives grant the opportunity to "ask and address questions that normative medical training often marginalizes or silences outright: Who should die? What is a good death? What constitutes success and failure in medicine?" (p. 289). Such questions can result in a recognition of the limitations of the traditional, Western context of medicine with the hope that such questions might get situated within new cultural contexts.

## WRITING NARRATIVES

Although not as elaborated in the literature, encouraging medical students and physicians to write their own narratives also offers valuable insight and knowledge for their authors, through self-reflection and emotional release. As Holleman (1991) asserted, writing narratives helps young medical residents "overcome psychological barriers and learn to express themselves" (p. 17). Abma (2001) concluded that such an approach "is grounded in the assumption that people learn and change through reflection on personal experiences and that change is a dynamic ongoing process within a complex context" (p. 273). Therefore, by recalling narratives, palliative care providers may analyze their own role in palliative care services (Wittenberg & Ragan, in press).

### Self-Reflection

Billings and Block (1997) argued that, although important and vital to effective medical practice, medical professionals experience little opportunity for personal reflection within medical school and subsequent medical practice. Much like reading narratives, writing one's own narratives offers the opportunity for reflection on the self and one's work, role, goals, ideals, and purpose. Reflection through writing leads to a better understanding of one's self. As Pennebaker (2000) explained, "The act of structuring stories appeared to be a natural human process that helped individuals understand their experience and themselves" (p. 3). Charon (2001a) pointed out that many medical schools and residency programs now ask trainees to reflect on their experiences with patients in narratives, particularly those experiences with dying patients. In fact, she herself has witnessed the effects of self-reflection. Charon (2001a) noted "The more I wrote about my patients and myself, the more confident I became that the act of narrative writing granted me access to knowledge—about the patient and myself—that would otherwise have remained out of reach" (January, para. 11).

## Understanding and Managing Emotion

Throughout medical school and medical practice thereafter, students and physicians face countless new pressures, situations, roles, responsibilities, and a resulting array of emotions. Smith and Kleinman (1989) found, in a study of first- through third-year medical students, that students experience a multitude of uncomfortable feelings, from embarrassment and disgust to arousal, as they interact in ways with their patients that, in the world outside of the hospital, would be considered inappropriate. No doubt, contemporary medical students continue to struggle with such feelings. Degner and Gow (1988) and Reifler (1996) further explained that, given the Western philosophy about death and the continuance of treatment and hospitalization until death, nursing and medical students include largely young adults who have been sheltered from illness, death, and the dying process. Yet, professors expect these students to adapt immediately to their clinical environment and to appropriately and sensitively respond to the needs of their patients throughout the entire illness and dying process. An analysis of the narratives of nurses who work with dying patients documents the emotional vulnerability of the students and the moral and emotional effects they experience, such as guilt, stress, sleeplessness, and burnout (Loftus, 1998). In another study, 44% of medical students described caring for dying patients as depressing (Sullivan et al., 2003). These feelings, roles, and responsibilities affect even the students' sense of identity. Charon (2002) asserted that, because of these new emotions, roles, and responsibilities, "When becoming physicians, medical students undergo dramatic personal transformations, often in a relatively short period of time, that render them unrecognizable to themselves" (para. 7).

Writing narratives can help students and physicians identify and interpret their emotional responses to patients; this process can facilitate their interactions with their patients (Charon, 2001). Additionally, emotional expression has been found to improve emotional and physical health. In a series of experiments, Pennebaker (2000) found that, as people wrote about their emotions, their physical and mental health improved markedly. This finding would appear to apply to medical students and their experiences as well. In fact, in 1995, a study found improvement in the health of medical students following narrative self-reflection (Petrie, 1995).

## CONCLUSIONS

As the face of medicine becomes more humanistic and more inclusive (in terms of a consideration of the psychological, social, and cultural aspects of medicine), palliative or comfort care in the United States has become more accepted. Concurrently, however, the practice of palliative care garners much criticism because it needs a much broader, multicultural emphasis (Billings & Block, 1997; Caresse & Rhode, 1995; Cohen, 1997; Curtis et al., 2001; Doorenbros et al., 2003). A major problem stems from the dearth of courses in death and dying and palliative care in many medical school curricula. The majority of graduating medical students describe themselves as inadequately prepared to administer palliative care, and most have never experienced any formal education in the field (Block, 2002; Gatrad et al., 2003; Sullivan et al., 2003).

Palliative-care education must become a priority. Narratives, because they enhance the development of the skills of interpretation, empathy, and reflection, as well as cultural understanding and ethical decision making, offer an invaluable tool in this training. Encouraging medical students to study, analyze, and reflect on the narratives of others, as well as to engage in writing narratives of their own, can assist physicians in practicing palliative care that considers the holistic needs of their patients. Additionally, many other health care providers can benefit from narrative instruction. Although often neglected in the literature, the study of narratives also can be useful for all involved in medical practice, not only physicians. Wilson (2000) asserted that storytelling plays a pivotal role in training hospice volunteers. Additionally, narrative medicine can hone similar skills for nurses as well as physicians. Durgahee (1997) found that clinical experiences shared through storytelling aided nurses in ethical decision making. Through reflection, nurses may become better able to analyze the "interactions and needs of the parties involved, leading to new understandings" (Durgahee, 1997, p. 136). Durgahee (1997) posits that narrative reasoning is part of the process of ethical decision making.

Several researchers suggest fictive literature that would be useful in palliative care instruction. For example, Charon et al. (1995) listed Franz Kafka's *The Metamorphosis* and Leo Tolstoy's *The Death of*

*Ivan Ilych*, two narratives that can hone empathy skills through their illumination of the illness and death experiences of two men and the resulting complexities, emotions, fears, and personal transformations. Medical ethics, importantly, involves an understanding of, and consideration of, the patient's experience. Hence, many pieces can illuminate the role of empathy within medical ethics. For instance, Charon et al. (1995) also suggested Ernest Hemingway's *Indian Camp*. This striking piece addresses the interplay of empathy and ethics as the main character, a young boy, watches his father's detached, unemotional practice of medicine, even in the midst of the pain and cries of his patients. Wear and Nixon (2002) suggested Arthur Ginsberg's *Line Drive*, Rafael Campos' *Like a Prayer*, and Dannie Abse's *Case History* as tools for the medical classroom. These pieces also examine the humanism of medicine and its ethical implications, illustrating the tension between the emotional reactions that physicians may experience in response to their patients, such as disgust, anger, or indifference, and the humanistic/nurturing role of the doctor (Wear & Nixon, 2002). A. H. Jones (1999) asserted that numerous pieces written by Williams Carlos Williams and Richard Selzer are well known and commonly taught in medical schools to hone medical ethics. For reflection on the role of physician and the possible positive implications for both the patient and the doctor, Charon et al. (1995) suggested Henry James' *The Middle Years*. Other literature cited as useful for narrative medicine courses includes: texts by Anton Chekhov; novels by John Berger and William Maxwell; poems by Walt Whitman; the short story, "Corinne," by Mme. de Stael; Virginia Woolf's essay, "On Being Ill"; Albert Camus' novel, *The Plague*; Thomas Mann's novel, *The Magic Mountain* (Smith, 2003); and Franz Kafka's *The Trial* (cited by Broyard, 1992). One of the most comprehensive analyses of literature dealing with illness is Howard Brody's (2003) *Stories of Sickness*.

Narrative literature that could be helpful to medical practitioners also exists in the intercultural context; notable is Anne Fadiman's (1998), *The Spirit Catches You and You Fall Down*. Although this volume provides an actual case history of a Hmong child and her collision with Western medicine, it nonetheless presents a compelling story that describes the complex interaction between health care and culture. Likely, additional stories, fictive and otherwise, illustrate intercultural health care and could be useful components of narrative medicine pedagogy. Two of the most compelling recent narrative accounts of patients' stories of death and dying include the Pulitzer Prize winning drama, "Wit" by Margaret Edson and the recent, excellent televised documentary series by journalist, Bill Moyers, "On Our Own terms: Moyers on Dying." As Ragan, Wittenberg, and Hall (2003) explained, the patients in these two works are eloquent spokespersons for the benefits of palliative care.

## CODA

The burgeoning humanities movement in medical school education that includes narrative medicine certainly offers hopeful means of extending and promulgating a biopsychosocial approach to medicine, one that remains compatible with the values that most social science researchers bring to the health care context. However, as communication scholars, we question whether, in fact, an education in the best-told stories of death and dying will really engender a more empathic and less distant physician. Will reading and analyzing the fictive stories of Leo Tolstoy and William Carlos Williams, for example, facilitate improved listening skills when doctors are daily hearing the disfluent, uneducated, and sometimes incoherent voices of their real patients? As Rita Charon questions in a recent interview: "How many times does a patient try to tell a doctor what happened in a sickness, and the doctor interrupts with, 'What was the pain like, sharp or dull?,' preventing the patient from unfolding the account, and losing diagnostic accuracy, losing a context?" (cited in D. Smith, 2003, para. 28).

Sharf (1990) asked whether the narratives co-created by doctors and patients can always "fulfill the criteria of a good story for the other" (p. 227). In a medical story she analyzes, in which the physician is a 28-year-old White male, and the patient a 48-year-old Black male, neither produces "sufficient coherence and fidelity to gain the imaginative involvement, let alone active cooperation, of the listener" (p. 277). Real patients do not always speak about their pain and suffering and fears of dying with the eloquence of Anatole Broyard (1992) or the professor of literature in "Wit," or even the actual patients interviewed by Bill Moyers in his documentary on dying on our own terms. Doctors notoriously interrupt, steer the medical interview toward the biological with which they are more comfortable, and eschew the emotional outpourings of their patients.

One of the problems in teaching physicians about narratives involves teaching them to be dialogic communicators. Physicians must be taught not only about the value of patients' narratives for developing their empathic and moral characters; more critically, they must also internalize the notion that stories are co-constructed by both patient and physician. In the story cited by Sharf (1990), the White physician does not collaborate with his Black patient in a way that produces a meaningful account of his patient's suffering; instead he speaks with the monologic *voice of medicine* (Mishler, 1984), insistent on the biological facts of the story and oblivious to the lived experience of his patient. In view of medical-school education, which largely instructs future doctors in ways that encourage and even reward authoritative, monologic modes of communication, the narrative movement in medicine—and its concomitant emphasis on dialogue—can be seen as antithetical to the dominant instructional paradigm.

How, then, can doctors learn to dialogue with their patients, to become co-authors of their patients' stories without imposing their own biomedical agendas that subvert and distort the voice of the lifeworld? (Mishler, 1984). Can narrative analysis taught in medical humanities courses change this pattern? Do the narrative and empathic skills honed both by reading and writing medical narratives translate to real doctor–patient interactions? Possibly, the practice at some medical schools of asking students to write about illness from their patients' perspectives or requiring them "to write narratives about the imagined life of their 'first patient,' the anatomy cadaver" (Hunter et al., 1995, p. 790) can facilitate the transfer of narrative analytic skills to clinic and hospital settings. Dr. Rita Charon, Professor of Clinical Medicine at Colombia University's College of Physicians and Surgeons (who holds both an M.D. and a PhD in English and comparative literature and who co-edits the journal, *Literature and Medicine*) may have experienced some success in training future physicians to become more dialogic in their communication with patients. For example, in a study recently conducted by Charon and her colleagues, cited in the February 13, 2004 issue of *The Chronicle of Higher Education* (Mangan, 2004), Charon found that students who wrote stories about their patients in their third year clinical experiences "were judged by faculty members to have better relationships with their patients and to be better at interviewing them" (p. A48).

Other studies of literature and medicine courses have found similar conclusions. In Welch's (2000) ethnography of medical students enrolled in a (required) medicine and literature course, she argued that the study of literature prompted the students to view medicine as "an interpretive, personal, and idiosyncratic activity rather than as a stagnant diagnosis-based process" (p. 311). Additionally, Lancaster, Hart, and Gardner (2002) found in their study of a 4-week course in medicine and literature that the students felt they had gained new insights into illness, understanding, and empathy. Additionally, they perceived themselves to have honed clinically relevant skills, such as communication, analysis, presentation, and ethics.

Finally, the Maine Humanities Council program entitled "Humanities at the Heart of Health Care" offers evidence for the potential of the study of literature and medicine as well. Meeting once a month from January through June, doctors, nurses, and other health care professionals discuss literature and its applications to medicine and, specifically, their jobs. Victoria Bonebakker, associate director of the program states, "I've been amazed that the doctors, nurses, and other professionals tell me that they find more satisfaction in their work ... Doctors say they listen more and take more time with their patients" (L. Rogers, 2002, para. 16). Notably, physicians are not the only ones telling her that the study of literature in her program has changed their approach to medicine—so too have nurses, receptionists, and trustees. This program has found such success, that in 2003, similar programs were set to be launched in Massachusetts, New Hampshire, Rhode Island, Vermont, North Carolina, Utah, and Illinois.

Although the results of several studies have ascertained the positive influence of narrative practices on students, physicians, and patients (Charon, 2001b), much research remains to be done in order to assess, empirically and longitudinally, the efficacy of narrative medicine. Whether patients also would deem those physicians trained in narrative medicine as having "better relationships" with their storytelling patients, as listening better, or as having more-developed clinical skills is yet to be determined.

We, nonetheless, remain optimistic that the stories told and written by and about dying patients can enlighten end-of-life care. As Broyard (1992) attests: "To die is to be no longer human, to be dehumanized— and I think that language, speech, stories, or narratives are the most effective ways to keep our humanity alive. To remain silent is literally to close down the shop of one's humanity" (p. 20).

Physician Arthur Kleinman, as cited by Brody (2003), recounted the story of Gordon Stuart, a 33-year-old writer dying of cancer. Under hospice care at home and right before his death, Stuart tells his physician:

> All that nonsense that's written about stages of dying, as if there were complete transitions—rooms that you enter, walk through, then leave behind for good. What rot. The anger, the shock, the unbelievableness, the grief—they are part of each day. And in no particular order, either. Who says you work your way eventually to acceptance—I don't accept it! Today I can't accept it. Yesterday I did partly. Saturday, I was there: kind of in a trance, waiting, ready to die. But not now. (p. 147)

Yet, Stuart's story later relates his acceptance of his death; he speaks of the importance of being at home in his own garden and reflects on the meaning of being a writer and facing death. After Stuart's death, his family physician wrote:

> Gordon died a good death. He was clear right up to the end. He had fortitude and character and died as he lived, very much his own person. He was no less angry, not accepting at the end, but he kept his sense of irony,

his way with words. He seemed to grow into whom he wanted to be. His death confirmed his life. He was a model for me. I would wish to do the same for my own death. (Kleinman, 1988, p. 149)

Brody (2003) asserted that healing obtains for both patient and physician through the narrative process:

[W]hen the sufferer tells the story of his sickness to the community, and the community listens ... the sufferer feels healed to the extent that he has attached meaning to his experience with his words and his story and to the extent that the act of telling has reconnected him to his fellow human beings. The community is healed to the extent that they see a fellow person coping with illness and suffering and think that when their time comes, they, too, can find ways to cope and perhaps even to flourish despite illness and approaching death. (p. 113)

Particularly in the practice of palliative medicine, we believe that stories facilitate this "healing" in that we participate as fellow sufferers of the (finite) human condition. Whether listening to the stories of fictive patients and doctors in television's popular *ER* or *Scrubs* (or in those older television favorites that many of us grew up with—*Marcus Welby, Trapper John, M*A*S*H, Chicago Hope, Ben Casey, Dr. Kildare*, to name a few), or of real patients in Bill Moyers' celebrated documentary on death and dying, "On Our Own Terms," or those of actual patients whose stories are not edited for coherence and lucidity, physicians in training are socialized in the patient stories of our culture. As E. L. Rothman (1999) discussed in her reflections about her Harvard Medical School education:

*ER* was not just another popular TV show. It was the experience of watching physicians, residents, and medical students deal with detailed medical information against a backdrop of complicated personal situations and ethical issues. It was like watching seven or eight live-action tutorial cases in an hour. (p. 25)

Whether formally trained in narrative medicine and/or informally trained as members of the culture, physicians who attend to patients' stories participate vicariously in their suffering and in their coping as they face illness and death. This potential for healing, for coping, and perhaps even for flourishing in the face of death holds the most hope from the teaching of narrative medicine in palliative-care education.

# 13

## Contesting Narratives of Workplace Maternity

∾

**Patrice M. Buzzanell**
*Purdue University*

**Laura L. Ellingson**
*Santa Clara University*

*I thought that [my supervisors] would more or less help [when I was pregnant] and not really so much [give] special privileges, but they would be a little bit more understanding; but instead it was more like they were out to get you.*
—"Tara," photo technician at a national retailer

There are a number of competing narratives that accompany maternity in the workplace. Most stories are gendered contrasts to an entrepreneurial master narrative that assumes wellness and paid-work prioritization. We situate discourses and practices of workers, paid work, and wellness within contemporary organizational imperatives, and then argue that maternity in the workplace will continue to be associated with deviance, sexuality, the feminine, unreliability, illness, and disability unless organizational and health communication researchers construct multiple creative narratives about workplace pregnancy and maternity leave that decenter the master narrative.

A case study of Tara, who has pregnancy-related complications, illustrates how the master narrative justifies supervisory responses that are physically and emotionally harmful to her. Tara's story was recorded when she was interviewed about her pregnancy and maternity leave for a larger project on maternity leaves. However, her interview

277

becomes an opportunity to instruct others about what could happen when women who are pregnant and who rely on their jobs to support themselves and their families are faced with medical problems and unsympathetic bosses. Neither notes from doctors, customers' complaints, nor commentary from herself to her boss change the situation. She appears to be a lone voice in her company—and there seems to be no way to handle the complications and routine inconveniences of pregnancy. She finds comfort only in some managers and in co-workers who offer assistance.

Tara's story embodies a different narrative of pregnancy and work from that which is typically published in organizational and communication journals. Most of the academic work on maternity and maternity leave describes women who are well paid and able to negotiate roles and needs to some extent (e.g., Ashcraft, 1999; Miller, Jablin, Casey, Lamphear-Van Horn, & Ethington, 1996). In addition, most scholars assume that women feel well and can work until the last minute before delivery (e.g., J. Martin, 1990), and describe women who are powerful contributors to decision making or founders and owners of companies (e.g., Ashcraft, 1999). Tara's narrative gives voice to lower-paid, marginalized women whose pregnancies are complicated and whose inability to engage in unimpeded labor incur negative repercussions in the workplace.

We begin by exploring the myth of the ideal organizational worker and describing the master narrative of pregnancy that permeates contemporary workplaces. We then offer an analysis of Tara's narrative, demonstrating the impossibility of fitting her experiences within the dominant narrative that her organization provides. Using Minow's (1990) theory on the social construction of difference, we explore how the organization's narrative positions Tara's embodiment as problematic, while obscuring its own agency and accountability. Finally, we discuss the potential for narratives such as Tara's to disrupt dominant narratives of difference in organizations.

## IDEAL AND PREGNANT WORKERS

This section first discusses how our analysis is situated within organizational storytelling research, then establishes the narrative of the ideal, entrepreneurial worker so that images of pregnant women can be contrasted. Many narratives of maternity in the workplace feature the pregnant executive (career narrative in which pregnancy is a concern for advancement and for changing organizational cultures but in which wellness is assumed); the pregnant or potentially pregnant worker (reproductive narrative, fulfillment of sex and capitalist role to produce future workers); and maternity as disability (medical leave and organizational policies construct pregnancy and postpregnancy as disability, narratives that depict women as not male and "ill").

## Organizational Storytelling

Mumby (2004) and Czarniawska and Gagliardi (2003) noted that organizational storytelling research over the last couple of decades positions narrative as a central organizing process by which members make sense of their experiences. Although most narrative work is interpretive in that it highlights how societal and organizational members intersubjectively create shared understandings of their experiences, critical and postmodern scholars uncover and record (in various forms) how these collective meanings are shaped by and shape certain interests and identities in particular contexts (Boje, 2001; Czarniawska, 1998). In this political view, narratives (re)produce, reveal, and offer opportunities to resist taken-for-granted social realities and power relations. As such, storytelling displays ongoing struggles between dominant and dominated groups to fix meaning and influence what people envision is possible and not even part of everyday conscious thought, identity constructions, and action (see Mumby, 1987, 1988, 1993).

Storytelling embodies these struggles and tensions, and narratives become sites of control and resistance that have real psychic and material consequences as different group members attempt to both reinforce master cultural narratives (e.g., entrepreneurial worker, modernity, societal scripts, heterosexuality, White privilege) and construct compelling counternarratives (Boje, 1991; Lindemann Nelson, 2001; Mumby, 2004). It is this sense of opportunity to refashion narratives and engage in subversive storytelling that is so engaging and useful about organizational narratives. As Czarniawska (1998) suggested, narratives are "both inscriptions of past performances and scripts and staging instructions for future performance" (p. 20). These future performances hold the potential to engage in narrative repair by which "the person could attain, regain, or extend her freedom of moral agency" (Lindemann Nelson, 2001, p. 150). It is this kind of story—one that rewrites institutionalized narratives of ideal entrepreneurial and pregnant workers—with which we conclude.

## Master Narrative of the Ideal Entrepreneurial Worker

The ideal worker is the main character in the master narrative of wellness in the workplace and the obscured norm against which all deviant worker bodies are compared and found wanting. The ideal worker is dedicated to paid work in terms of time and energy allocation. This worker is the employee who is always fit, energetic, even tempered, and productive (Nadesan & Trethewey, 2000)—except when the worker is aging visibly (Trethewey, 2001), ill and must self-medicate (Deetz, 1995), or cannot control her own leaky, emotional, protruding, and unprofessional body despite efforts to discipline herself and fit the male norm (Trethewey, 2000). The ideal (male) body supposedly does not undergo daily, monthly, or age-related changes, such as hormonal shifts, menstruation, and menopause (although evidence for masculine cycles exists; see Lorber, 1994).

The ideal worker not only demands the appearance of youth and of high productivity 24/7/365, but also prioritizes wage work over family, friends, health, religion, and leisure. Paid work and adherence to corporate norms govern decision premises and appropriate roles of workers as consumers and supporters of the corporate imperative (Scott & Hart, 1989). The ideal worker spends time at work, thinks about work when not in the office, and displays loyalty and organizational commitment through presence; that is, being available when projects are being completed (Bailyn, 1993; Perlow, 1998). The ideal worker may also find the workplace more relationally friendly than home (Hochschild, 1997). In short, the ideal worker is young, male, committed to employment and work, and fit.

## Pregnant Workers

In contrast to the dominant narrative script of the perpetually "fit" entrepreneurial worker, stories of maternity pose deviant conditions. Pregnancy marks women as "other" (not men) and connotes notions of unreliability and unpredictability in ways that people—even those who have been colleagues for years—may not understand fully (e.g., Mock & Bruno, 1994). The pregnant worker obviously has other things in her life besides work. She has become sexualized (through the causes of her condition) and curiously desexualized (as she becomes "mother"). She no longer can be counted on for total dedication to projects because of potential or real work–family tensions. As a result, the person who may most question the pregnant worker's dedication and reliability is the supervisor. In hierarchical organizations, it is the boss who must make sure that work is covered, projects are delivered, promotables are advanced, and so on. In self-designing teams, it is the co-workers and team leaders who construct generative forms of control that insure work completion and normative behavior (Barker, 1999).

Besides embodiment of deviance in the physical manifestations of pregnancy, other narratives about maternity associate pregnancy and work–family concerns with career challenges (Schwartz, 1989, 1992), reproductive workers (i.e., valuing mothers and children as breeders of future workforce participants and as future workers, respectively; Lorber 1994), and disability (Lorber, 1994; Tavris, 1992). With regard to career challenges, the dominant maternity narrative assumes that the woman (often an executive) continues with her work unconstrained by hormonal changes, fatigue, increasing weight, and other possible pregnancy-related conditions. She even schedules Caesarian delivery dates around project deadlines (J. Martin, 1990). Despite her prior status as an ideal worker who happens to be female, her pregnancy calls into question her reliability and her loyalty (Mock & Bruno, 1994; Sheppard, 1989). As colleagues try to ascertain how her pregnancy and future mother status will affect her work abilities, they fail to recognize the ways their organizational cultures are not family friendly. "Mommy" tracks or career delays and dead-ends are real possibilities for these pregnant executives (Schwartz, 1989). In this story plot, the pregnant employee has tailored outfits, seems energetic and perfectly healthy (with no complications), and wears her pregnancy as a temporary state that changes little in the workplace and from which she emerges as the same dedicated worker as before her maternity leave.

Reproductive workers are those who fulfill their capitalist roles as bearers of future workers but also those who have few options to negotiate roles, benefits, maternity leaves, and other issues related to pregnancy, maternity leaves, and returns to work. With increased technology in the workplace and less need for human laborers (Rifkin, 1995), the worth of women's reproductive capabilities and of their offspring as future workers means that there may be less investment in the safety of pregnant women and neonatal care (Lorber, 1994). Where childbearing women and their children are less valued by society, organizational policies, everyday procedures, and ordinary interactions may not safeguard them. Recent reports indicate that bosses are lowering the amount of parental leaves and are terminating employees on leave (Shellenbarger, 2003) despite Family Medical Leave Act (FMLA) guarantees of jobs under certain conditions.[1]

Notwithstanding governmental and organizational guarantees of unpaid leaves with assurances that there will be jobs upon the individual's return to paid work, those who take leaves may suffer penalties. Research indicates that some women incur wage decreases (, 1999). Race/ethnicity, sexual–social orientation, and class biases may influence women's use of the FMLA insofar as women who are poor and non-White, in particular, lack the resources and support to take unpaid maternity leaves (Gerstel & McGonagle, 1999). For instance, Buzzanell et al. (2003) found that pink-collar women told a fairly uniform narrative about needing to get back to work because of finances, being grateful for anything that is done, and being pleased that they are not forgotten while on maternity leave (without recognizing the extent to which they are controlled by phone calls and notes from bosses asking them how they are doing and when they will return to their employment).

Finally, narratives about maternity as a negative medical condition are perpetuated by policies and procedures that classify maternity leaves as disability leaves. In general, the logic of "disability" treats maternity as an illness or a sickness. In maternity leave, viewing disability as a medical issue "emphasizes the dichotomy between the abnormal (person with disabilities) and the normal (person without disabilities)" (Coopman, 2003, p. 345).[2] This bifurcation is a particularly irritating point of contention among feminists who argue that pregnancy is a natural state for women. Pregnant workers become "others" by their distinctions from "normal" women as well as from male workers. Female workers can be identified by their pregnant or nonpregnant state and, when pregnant, presumably become dependent on others for their everyday functioning (Coopman, 2003). *Maternity as a medical disability* is oppressive because the label involves social restrictions, biases against women in this condition, indications that pregnancy is "unnatural," and restricted access to public spaces (in this case, to the workplace, because disabled persons are, by definition, unable to work or function in a normal life). The use of the term *disability* in leave policies enables accommodation to women's varied experiences with pregnancy at the price of adhering to the male norm "that construes pregnancy as a *di*sability rather than, say, as an additional ability" (Tavris, 1992, p. 118). The term fails to displace the current incompatibility of pregnancy and the workplace and fails to acknowledge that full recovery from childbirth can be nonroutine and unpredictable (Hyde, Essex, Clark, Klein, & Byrd, 1996; E. Martin, 2001).

The equation of pregnancy with disability is related to feminist equality-sameness debates (Tavris, 1992). Fighting blatant discrimination, liberal feminists emphasize that pregnant women are capable of working just like anyone else. Such equality arguments position pregnant women as men with temporarily disabled bodies: "According to equal-rights advocates, pregnancy should be treated like any disability that might cause workers of either sex to lose a few days' or a few months' work" (Tavris, 1992, p. 117). The rhetoric of "sameness," while effective in passing legislation (e.g., the Pregnancy Discrimination Act; see Equal Employment Opportunity Commission [EEOC], 2003), enables and constrains. With the standard for equality established on the basis of treating everyone in the same manner, no accommodation of difference is required. Cultural or structural feminism, on the other hand, bases its call in acknowledgment of fundamental differences between the sexes and promotes a discourse of equity based upon respect and valuing of differences. From this lens, women's roles then do not need to be redefined or challenged as much as they need to be valued and appreciated (Wood, 2003). Cultural feminist arguments suggest that "it is ridiculous, demeaning, and antiwoman to ignore the special condition of pregnancy" (Tavris, 1992, p. 118) when forming laws and policies.

The opening up of a space for pregnancy as a valued state requiring accommodation is complicated further by the legal denial of the Americans with Disabilities Act (ADA) disability status for pregnancy (see EEOC, 2000). Disempowered pregnant women find little discursive assistance in their quest for accommodation in formal leave policies, equal opportunity laws, pregnancy discrimination legislation, or the ADA. Organizational leave policies, drafted or modified after the passage of the FMLA, ordinarily define pregnancy leave as covered by short-term disability insurance: "Title VII requires the employer to treat pregnancy and related conditions the same as non-pregnancy [serious medical] conditions" (EEOC, 2000), as "temporary disabilities." Yet, the ADA does not consider pregnancy to be a disability: "Other 'serious health conditions' may not be ADA disabilities, for example, pregnancy ... This is because the condition is not an impairment (e.g., pregnancy)" (EEOC, 2000). So pregnancy is to be treated as a (temporary) disability by an organization, but it is not an ADA disability; moreover, it is labeled a *serious condition*, but not an impairment.

In addition to the confusion resulting from such subtle distinctions and multiple conceptualizations of the term *disabilities* inherent in these policies, the medical definition of pregnancy remains uncontested. A biomedical definition of pregnancy as an abnormal, pathological, "serious" medical condition requiring physicians' technological interventions underlies these definitions (Nelson, 1996; Pollock, 1999; Rothman, 1991; Sterk, 1996; Sterk, Hay, Kehoe, Ratcliffe, & VandeVusse, 2002).[3] Pregnancy is thus a serious medical condition to be minimized, or ideally, ignored by the organization, but which does not require (ADA) accommodation.

## Summary

The primary cultural narrative of the workplace is the story of efficient, dedicated workers who are never sick or, if they succumb to a minor illness, do not let their illness hamper their performance and professional demeanor. Because wellness is taken for granted and work is prioritized over all other life events and circumstances, illness is a distraction, is not considered worthy of discussion, and is silenced. Illness simply does not exist in most workplace narratives—or, when it does, it is treated as unusual or a necessary evil—"time off work" (sick days and maternity leave), disability (including pregnancy, maternity leaves, and ADA conditions), and violations of safety regulations (work-related injuries and deaths, OSHA). There are numerous stories that can be told of workplace pregnancy but most position the female worker as "other," or different from the norm. Rarely are there narratives told in the words of women who fought for accommodations to their pregnancy-related medical conditions. In these cases, pregnancy is not just an illness or disability but is seen as an employment liability. Pregnancy as a serious medical condition removes this natural process from the realm of the normal and offers no script for handling individual women's cases.

## THE STORY OF "TARA"

### Synopsis of Tara's Case

The case study interview features a White, middle-class, married woman who has some college credits and who works as a photo technician in a retail company in the midwestern United States. Tara was employed for 2.5 years at her company when she experienced her pregnancy and maternity leave in 1994, one year after the FMLA took effect and 16 years after the Persons with Disabilities Act was passed into law. Prior to this pregnancy, she had one miscarriage. Although it was a couple of years since she lived through her pregnancy and maternity leave, her account is filled with vivid language, concrete details, and emotion. Indeed, women's stories of pregnancy, birthing, and the context surrounding these events remain accurate over long periods of time, as Sterk et al. (2002) reported in their research on women's stories of birthing assumptions, practices, and attempts to create change in medical and private procedures.

Shortly into her interview, Tara talks about the differences between what she expected or was told about maternity leaves and what actually happened when she was pregnant. It appears as though there was no routine way to treat pregnancy, and no regular way to circulate information despite her mention of a maternity leave packet and a toll-free number. Tara seems to have been misinformed, misled, or was confused about the amount of time she could take off from paid work, her payment (or lack thereof) during her leave, and her insurance. She thought that the procedures would operate more smoothly:

> Yeah, I thought that when you took a maternity leave that your company basically would understand—they would be, you know, really supportive. Um, that they would try to understand and help you the way that they could. I thought that was designed to help you and not the company that it was like a benefit that the company provided. But, when I did apply, ex-

cuse me, for my maternity leave um I had a very hard time with them losing my file then losing my doctor's notes, you know, and everything else.... I had to carry very heavy furniture that I was not supposed to be carrying and it wasn't what I thought it was gonna be because I perceived it in a different way than they told me, or they led me to believe, because they never really told me anything.

From the beginning of this pregnancy, nothing was easy for Tara. Despite her past miscarriage, her ongoing problems with asthma and toxemia, and her notes from her doctor about what she should and should not be doing, Tara found that her supervisors would not accommodate her requests to go to the bathroom or get a drink of water ("I got written up for it [going to the bathroom]—for leaving without notifying anybody"), to obtain assistance in carrying heavy objects, or to leave work ("Another time I had fallen and I started spotting and I asked if I could go home and they would not let me go home"). She found inconsistency in how policies were applied and how much help people obtained from management. Despite all of these problems, Tara reported high job satisfaction and feelings of job security both before and after her maternity leave. However, she also reported feeling discouraged about her employment and advancement opportunities both before and after her maternity leave. Tara described her perceptions: "it seems like they don't keep you in mind for like advancement in the company now, because they think that you wouldn't be able to now because you have a baby ..."

## Problematizing Tara's Narrative

Workplace pregnancy and maternity leave are nonnormative events in the masculine public arena. As a result, there are few coherent cultural narratives of working while also being pregnant. Organizational members do not hear about how women work, what they feel, how they accommodate their physical changes, and how they may change their attitudes toward work–family and other issues as well as to work space and duties while pregnant over the course of their lifetimes. Moreover, variations exist in what it means to be woman, to be pregnant, to be a worker, and to take a maternity leave (see E. Martin, 2001). These differences exist within and across women and organizational contexts in ways that intersect with race, class, sexuality, and other differences (see Ashcraft & Mumby, 2004). Even individuals within particular organizational cultures can have different perceptions and enactments of their roles (e.g., "employee" or "professional"), their expectations for treatment (e.g., accommodations, or no accommodations, to pregnancy), and their work–family orientations (e.g., with varied prioritizations of work, career, family, self, volunteer activities, or leisure).

In our specific case, Tara's pregnant body cannot be the ideal worker body; it cannot be ignored, despite attempts by her supervisor to do so (as a representative of her organization). Her pregnancy cannot be treated "like other serious medical conditions" because it is not like them. Tara's pregnancy involved a dynamic flux in physical conditions. The ideal worker body sets a single standard that employees either meet or do not meet, and Tara's body refused to settle into a single category based on the dichotomy of being either well or ill.

## Re/Constructing Pregnancy as Difference

A cultural narrative challenging negative conceptualizations of pregnancy as a serious medical condition that is disabling, while still acknowledging the need that many pregnant women have for flexibility and accommodation, would have to challenge the pervasive healthy–ill dichotomy. The first step in resisting the well–ill bifurcation is to advance the point that all bodies vary—not just women's, and not just pregnant women. According to Grosz (1999), "Feminists have stressed that the generic category '*the* body' is a masculinist illusion. There are only concrete bodies, bodies in the plural, bodies with a specific sex and color" (p. 270; italics in original).

Researchers must decenter the ideal worker body by challenging the biomedical healthy–ill notion that pervades contemporary Western culture. Pregnancy is not a health emergency, but it is sometimes accompanied by medically defined symptoms and physical limitations. With birth, it does require accommodation for recovery. If researchers reframe the well–sick dichotomy as a dynamic continuum, there would be a great many more choices for how to deal with bodily variations in the workplace.

What would a cultural narrative of variation as normative look like? A narrative that radically alters definitions of "normal" is necessary (for counternarrative construction, see Lindemann Nelson, 2001). Minow's (1990) articulation of the five assumptions of labeling some things as *different* and some as *normal* provides a useful framework for considering the changes needed to alter the story of pregnancy as difference and Tara's story of workplace pregnancy. As we discuss each assumption about difference, we also relate each assumption to the dominant narrative of workplace pregnancy and suggest how a counternarrative could be constructed. Through this counternarrative, we question unstated norms and reframe pregnancy as one of many embodied states that workers experience.

First, Minow (1990) contended that "we often assume that 'differences' are intrinsic, rather than viewing them as expressions of comparisons between people on the basis of particular traits" (p. 50). In the organizational narrative of pregnancy, Tara's pregnancy is specific to her body and her self; the embodied trait is marked as hers alone, and the state of being nonpregnant is left unmarked as normative. In her story of workplace pregnancy, Tara announces her pregnancy to her co-workers as soon as she finds out, before her condition is physically evident: "I called from [offsite training location] and told people that I worked with in the [photo] lab that I was going to be a mommy ... I was, what, five or six weeks when I found out." Because of bleeding, Tara missed work to undergo ultrasound testing, a fact that was common knowledge among her co-workers and supervisors: "So everyone kinda knew then [after the tests] that I was [pregnant], and I didn't really have much of a choice" about revealing the pregnancy to management. While Tara's body is marked by her own admission (soon to be followed by visible evidence of the pregnancy), the other workers retain the privilege of having their bodies unmarked (Thomson, 1997). The marked body does not disappear after Tara gives birth to her baby and returns to work. Speaking of her supervisor's reactions immediately on returning to paid work from her pregnancy leave, Tara said, "They don't look at you the same way, it's kinda like you're almost starting over or like you have a disease ...."

In a counternarrative of pregnancy, all bodies must be viewed as having embodied traits (Grosz, 1999), and those traits must be considered in relationship to others' bodies. Thus, Tara's (currently pregnant) body should be considered in comparison to others' bodies (and their capabilities) instead of comparing Tara to the norm of a (nonexistent) nameless, abstract, disembodied, ideal worker. For example, other workers are limited by asthma, some are unable to lift heavy objects due to back problems, others have less muscle strength than others. Moreover, nondisabled employees are not superhuman; they too have specific height, weight, and muscle-tone capabilities. These traits should serve as points of comparison for pregnant workers, not a nonexistent perfect body. New narratives of pregnancy include many characters (not just Tara and those labeled disabled by companies) and describe both their limitations and their abilities.

Second, Minow (1990) argued "We typically adopt an unstated point of reference when assessing others. It is from the point of reference of this norm that we determine who is different and who is normal" (p. 51). Tara's bureaucratic structure is so obscured that she cannot even contact the appropriate person to arrange her leave, despite multiple calls to an out-of-state home office:

I thought someone would have come and told me ... these are your options, you know—meaning insurance wise and maternity leave wise,
though. There are your options, but instead I had to go to them ... I mean
literally *chase them down*. You know, they never had time just to sit
down one on one, answer questions. They *wouldn't* answer questions.
They'd make you call down, you know, down to [the home office] and everything else. They would never give you a straight answer about anything ... Every time I'd call and say, you know, "well, I called a few minutes
ago and I talked to so and so, they told me this, but I don't really understand this part." "Well they shouldn't have really told you that because
that's not true, this is how it works" ... I could never get a straight answer
from anybody.

Neither the organization as an entity nor any specific person takes responsibility for the judgment of Tara's condition. No one takes responsibility for providing accurate and complete information about that
judgment and its consequences for her working conditions and leave.

As case analysts, we do not know if the author of the hard-to-locate
policy is or has been pregnant, has any medical training related to the
determination of health status and ability to work, is aware of working
conditions in Tara's job, and so on. The unstated norm of nonpregnant
bodies simply exists, and the exception to normalcy for which Tara
seeks approval is handed down from nowhere.

Thus, the current organizational narrative of pregnancy is missing
key characters. Tara is the protagonist with her needs and requests, but
the antagonist remains obscured, acting behind the scenes in ways that
have real ramifications for Tara and her fetus, but not showing a face.

Specifying the key players in the negotiation is a first step to constructing a counternarrative of pregnancy. Individuals in a new narrative would articulate and assume responsibility for their decisions and
the consequences of those decisions for others.

Those key characters must also be understood as not being neutral.
Minow (1990) described the third cultural assumption of difference
as, "We treat the person doing the seeing or judging as without perspective, rather than as inevitably seeing and judging from a particular situated perspective" (p. 52). The human resources (HR) specialists and
Tara's supervisors have as their primary goal the perpetuation and financial success of the organization. Tara's supervisors never told her
that her discomfort, and even serious symptoms, were judged unim-
portant relative to the needs of the organization; neither was she told
that she and her fetus were expendable pawns in a huge capitalistic enterprise. The organization judged that it had nothing to gain from
Tara's pregnancy except the possibility of a long-term payoff of a future
cheap laborer. Her short-term productivity is endangered by the pregnancy, however, and child care needs could further interfere with her

productivity in the near future. These judgments appear to underlie the perspective of those in power and their callous, even dangerous, treatment of Tara, but they are never named. In Tara's story, she perceives that the organization is actively working against her:

> They more or less were making me do things that I shouldn't or thought that no pregnant person should be doing. You know, and when you asked them, you know, please try not to do this ... [I felt] like they were looking for little things that you did wrong, you know, to yell at you or maybe fire you for, you know they can't fire you because you're pregnant.... I thought that ... they would be a bit more understanding; but instead it was more like they were out to get you.

Tara's perception that her supervisors were actively looking for ways to find fault with her reveals an organization that is a threat to her safety. She has learned from her experience to anticipate poor treatment and violation of her rights in favor of advancing the organization's goals.

A revolutionized narrative of workplace pregnancy necessitates dialogue among all levels of workers, including HR specialists. Organizational goals must be named and brought to the stakeholders' table. No one could argue from "the god trick of seeing everything from nowhere" (Haraway, 1988, p. 581), but would have to name their specific standpoints and stakes in the organizational decisions made about pregnancy and maternity leaves. A new story of pregnancy must include character motivation on the part of key organizational policymakers and supervisory decisions regarding pregnant employees' assigned tasks and restrictions.

In addition to the obscuring of the organization and its key players from the story, the organizational narrative of pregnancy casts Tara in a virtually silent role. Minow (1990) explained that in determining and labeling *difference*, a fourth assumption is that "the perspectives of those being judged are irrelevant or are already taken into account through the perspective of the judge" (p. 52). The organization did not ask Tara for her input or feedback. She reports having to "literally chase down" supervisors to be heard. Despite repeated requests for help with her pregnancy symptoms and leave, she was denied explanations. She was not even allowed to contact HR professionals during working hours or at the company's expense, further silencing her through economic disincentives ("I had like a $200 and something dollar phone bill that month, because I had to keep calling [the home office] to find out things"). Tara had few discursive resources with which to counteract the written reprimand she received for leaving her position to use the bathroom without first getting permission. Her frustration at her silencing comes through in the advice she offers to other pregnant women at the conclusion of her story:

Make sure that you understand how long you're gonna get for [maternity leave]. You know, make sure you know, most probably, the most important thing is make sure that you understand your rights, you know being pregnant, you, while you're at work and when you come back, you know, that they cannot demote you. That they cannot take your position unless you're gone for over a year ... If you're back within a year they have to guarantee you the same pay ... Make sure you let the place that you work know and you understand everything that you're supposed to get so they can't more or less intimidate you ...

Tara positions herself (and those to whom she is offering advice) in an adversarial position vis-à-vis the organization where they must insist on being heard. Disappointed in her treatment by her organization, Tara imagines an audience to hear her and speaks directly to this audience: "Make sure you ..." Given her low status on the organizational hierarchy, Tara's lack of voice is considered irrelevant; her thoughts and experiences on being pregnant do not need to be understood in order for the organization to implement and enforce its policies.

Deconstructing the portrayal of pregnancy as *difference* involves enabling workers to have their voices heard in the formation of pregnancy and maternity policies. Moreover, the silencing of pregnant women such as Tara in day-to-day work also must end. Tara must be able to voice her concerns to responsive supervisors; clearly the supervisors who would not excuse Tara from lifting and wrote her up for leaving her post to go to the bathroom were not listening to Tara's explanation of her pregnancy. In a new narrative, embodied workers—pregnant or otherwise—engage in dialogue with each other and with supervisors to voice their concerns, and accommodations are negotiated.

Tara's lack of voice is unproblematic to the organization because it operates on the premise that the status quo is inevitable: "Finally, there is an assumption that the existing social and political arrangements are natural and neutral" (Minow, 1990, p. 52). Capitalism and the maltreatment of workers such as Tara form the background of the organizational narrative of pregnancy as *difference.* Hierarchy, exploitation, and placing the needs of the organization ahead of those of the workers serves as the unscrutinized context in which Tara's pregnancy is judged to be a problem. Her capacity for reproduction has been labeled as deviant because it serves particular social orders to do so; the exclusion of pregnant women from the category of *normal* naturalizes and perpetuates masculine systems of power. The focus of the "problem" in the cultural story of pregnancy is on the woman; it is not on the inflexible, sexist, hierarchical configuration of workplaces.

In Tara's narrative of working while pregnant, her lack of power and inability to construct (with her co-workers and/or managers) an alternative story in which she could enact agency clearly are evident. She cut out the soles of her shoes because she could not push her swollen feet into them. She stood for long hours because there was no recognition that standing could cause problems for her and her unborn child. She lifted and carried heavy objects knowing full well that she should not be doing so. She stayed at work when she was spotting because she was told that she could not leave. While individual managers might notice her distress and tell her to go home and rest, other managers went so far as to write her up for going to the bathroom. Thus Tara adapted, complied with her boss's orders, accepted assistance from co-workers, took risks, and forged a space for her pregnant body at work, whereas the organization made few accommodations and garnered profits from her work.

The corporatization of the United States economy is neither natural nor neutral; it came about in response to specific historical events and in service of the privileging of certain socially powerful groups. The pervasiveness of worker exploitation does not make it inevitable, natural, normal, or morally acceptable. Yet the system in which Tara is caught remains completely unquestioned and unchallenged as "the way it is" in the narrative of workplace pregnancy. The axiom of the powerful organization and the powerless employee frames Tara's story of pregnancy, but its presence is obscured as the natural order of the world, and hence completely unstated (Minow, 1990). Moreover, Tara's story poignantly illustrates that many workplaces in this country continue to be incompatible with women's reproductive roles (E. Martin, 2001).

In summary, the master narrative constructs pregnancy as specific to individual women's unruly (different, inferior) bodies. The organizational definition of pregnancy as aberrant and simultaneously ignorable or irrelevant reinforces the power and privilege of high-ranking organizational decision makers by reifying an ideal worker body that does not exist. Organizational power, perpetuation of inequalities, and the absence of responsible, accountable policy makers are all normalized in the master narrative, while pregnant women are silenced. Alternatively, a transformed narrative of pregnancy presents bodily variation and fluctuation as normative; gives voice to pregnant (and other marginalized) workers; positions specific powerful individuals within an organization as the source of erroneous, oppressive norms and the policies based on these norms (as opposed to vague conceptualizations of the organization as an entity); and explores the ways in which systems of power (capitalism, elitism, masculinity) are perpetuated by the master narrative of workplace pregnancy. Furthermore, moral and ethical consideration of capitalism and its practices forms an integral aspect of a new narrative of workplace pregnancy. A feminist narrative of pregnancy as a normal part of the workplace (or indeed, of *any* place) highlights the power relations between Tara and her supervisors, showing how they benefit directly from her marginalization and disempowerment.

## DISCUSSION

Tara's experience reflects the pervasive master narrative of pregnancy in workplaces and the harms inherent in this approach to accommodating pregnancy. In organizations' haste to protect women's rights to work and treat them as equals to men, there has not been much discourse on what considerations may need to be made for pregnant women. These conditions operate as dialectical processes that can change momentarily and that mean different things for different women (and men) over the course of days and/or lifetimes. For some women, pregnancy is a bodily change that does not hamper work performance. For others, pregnancy involves illness—being sick, struggling with symptoms—and yet supervisors, co-workers, and HR policy makers do not know how to accommodate such experiences.

Moreover, the implications of Tara's and other pregnant women's stories not only are similar to the construction of difference in workers needing accommodation under ADA regulations, but also in organizational efforts to value racial, ethnic, and cultural diversity; in workers' resistance to hostile climates, sexual harassment, and gender-based discrimination (i.e., glass ceiling and walls), and in-groups trying to improve working conditions for employees in low-paid, low-status positions. In each case, the norm is narratively obscured as neutral, inevitable, and natural, instead of the result of specific historical events, and the difference, or problem, is located in the narrative's protagonist (see Lindemann Nelson, 2001). Furthermore, there is no connection in the story between the person's problem and the social and political power arrangements that benefit from the continued oppression of the individual and her/his abnormal body. Without these connections, personal stories remain nested within taken-for-granted master narratives of the workplace (e.g., gender, ability, wellness/illness, and entrepreneurial workers) and are, thus, resistant to change (Lindemann Nelson, 2001; Somers, 1994).

The primary narrative that must be advanced to pave the way for greater equity is the inevitability of bodily variation. Narratives must reinforce the dynamic state of real bodies and resist the invocation of the nonexistent ideal body. Stories must reflect the fact that bodies are produced through discourse and do not have materiality totally apart from these discourses: "There is no reference to a pure body which is not at the same time a further formation of that body" (Butler, 1999, p. 240). Our cultural constructions of the meanings behind bodily variations are formed through language, and they can be altered the same way. Tara's and other marginalized workers' stories must be told for awareness and retold in counternarratives until they impact cultural and organizational delusions of ideal bodies and perpetuation of the sick–well dichotomy.

# NOTES

1. The FMLA guarantees jobs and leaves under the following conditions: people employed for more than 12 months (or 1,250 hours) in companies with at least 50 employees within 75 miles of their worksite can take up to 12 weeks unpaid leave per year. Without losing their jobs, these workers can take that leave to care for newborn or newly adopted children, for seriously ill spouses, children, or parents, or to recover from their own serious health conditions, including pregnancy. Serious illnesses and health conditions are defined as those requiring at least one night in the hospital or continuing treatment by a health care provider (Gerstel & McGonagle, 1999, p. 510; see also U.S. Department of Labor, 2003).

   As noted, the FMLA applies only to organizations employing more than 50 people. Women make up the majority of employees in small businesses, leaving many pregnant women vulnerable to the whims of small business employers.

2. Adapting Putnam, Phillips, and Chapman's (1996) metaphors that guide organizational communication research and thinking, Coopman (2003) described several approaches for disability through which researchers and practitioners have defined disability and have drawn implications: conduit/medical problem; lens/cognition; performance/in culture; symbol/as culture; voice/politics; and discourse/community. Although disability as conduit/medical problem is used in our text, a second approach outlined by Coopman (2003) also is relevant to our arguments. Maternity viewed through the voice/politics lens centers on the social construction of disability as a process that legitimates social relations, acknowledges the human body as a symbol that carries messages with implications in all life spheres, and deconstructs the everyday marginalization of people with disabilities to provide directions for empowerment. Extending Coopman's discussion, in the case of female workers maternity becomes politicized because it draws attention to the sexual nature of workers and the ways women's varied identities may deviate from that of "worker" (see also J. Martin, 1990).

3. There has been much controversy in feminist circles over whether conditions such as pregnancy, childbirth, and menopause are medical or nonmedical. On one hand, medicalizing a condition can legitimate it as a bona fide problem, entitle people to legal and economic benefits, and free them from certain obligations. But it also creates an identity as "ill" and "deviant." More importantly, the process works within the definitional framework of extant master narratives and is difficult to challenge (Lindemann Nelson,

2001). On the other hand, refusing medicalization means that the person is considered "well" and thus must perform and enact all the expected behaviors of that status. The either/or dichotomy refuses the complex identities and needs of women like Tara.

# 14

## Wholeness in a Breaking World:
## Narratives as Sustenance for Peace

ॐ

**Magdalyn Z. Miller**
*National University of Cajamarca*

**Patricia Geist Martin**
*San Diego State University*

**Kristen Cannon Beatty**
*Art Institute of California-San Diego*

*An eye for an eye makes the whole world blind.*

—M. Gandhi

On a cool San Diego night in January of 1995, Tariq Khamisa, a 20-year-old college student, was delivering pizzas for a local restaurant when four teenage gang members surrounded him and demanded the pizza. Tariq refused and tried to get in his car to drive away. As he attempted to leave, the 18-year-old gang leader, Antoine Pittman, ordered 14-year-old Tony Hicks to shoot Tariq with a nine millimeter handgun. As Tariq tried desperately to flee for his life, Antoine shouted, "Bust him, Bone, bust him." Tony obeyed.

A single shot from the 9mm handgun exploded in the night air. Tariq Khamisa lay dead in the front seat of his car. The killer: eighth grader Tony Hicks.... The last words Tariq uttered in his life were, "Help me, No! No!" The shot, through a rolled-up window, into a moving car, from the hand of a young inexperienced gunman, could have gone anywhere. It could have missed completely. It could have inflicted an insignificant wound. But it didn't. It penetrated Tariq's shoulder, and continued through his left lung, then his heart, then his right lung. The car shuddered to a stop. The Black Mob ran down the street and disappeared. They were seen by a man walking his dog, who would later report what he saw to the investigating police. In the Volkswagen, the pizzas and Tariq's body grew cold in the January night air. In his pocket, the delivery slip showed the amount due for the order: $27.24. (Khamisa, 2002, pp. i, 34)

Under a new law, Proposition 21, in effect only 3 weeks prior to Tariq's murder, Tony Hicks became the youngest person ever indicted as an adult for murder in the State of California. The immediate response of Azim Khamisa, Tariq's father, on learning of his son's murder, defied the usual emplotment of revenge and retribution. Azim's actions and words in the aftermath of this tragedy serve as an inspiration and a call to action—Azim believes that on that tragic night, two families and our society lost two sons: one forever and one to the prison system. Azim stated through his grief:

From the onset, I saw victims on both ends of the gun. I will mourn Tariq's death for the rest of my life. Now, however, my grief has been transformed into a powerful commitment to change. Change is urgently needed in a society where children kill children. (Tariq Khamisa Foundation, 2003)

While the state of California focused primarily on the criminal action that resulted in Tariq's death, Azim Khamisa sought to honor his son's life and find meaning in his death. Amidst his intense, private grieving process, Azim honored his son's life by establishing the Tariq Khamisa Foundation (TKF). In October 1995, with Deputy District Attorney Peter Deddeh, Azim met with Tony Hicks' grandfather and guardian, Ples Felix. The two men formed an extraordinary bond, and Azim invited Ples to speak at the second foundation meeting in order to meet the Khamisa family members and to join the foundation in the quest to save other families from the tragic loss of their children. This remarkable act and relationship gave birth to TKF's work and mission to "stop children from killing children, to break the cycle of youth violence by inspiring nonviolent choices and planting seeds of hope for our future" (Tariq Khamisa Foundation, 2003).

Prevention of violence and trauma of all sorts remain central concerns of public health specialists. Yet single, one-shot, monologic mediated messages often have little or no effect. Health communicators must engage in long-term educational, persuasive and supportive efforts in communities, seeking to replace unhealthy choices (e.g., aggression and violence), with choices that are health-enhancing and life-affirming. The TKF story unfolds as a narrative case study of how, in one instance, health organizers work to promote healthy and nonviolent behaviors in a community of young people. The TKF story, as a constellation of interrelated stories, is at once powerful and haunting, and participants' narratives inspire the human spirit and leave the reader with hope.

The inception of TKF, followed by 8 years of dedicated work by TKF to serve at-risk youth, brings us to the present moment. The shared journey of TKF's work and our life-changing experiences with this foundation are best told through narratives. This chapter honors the work of TKF—the programs it offers and the students it inspires.

We begin by discussing the vulnerability of our youth to risk-taking behaviors such as violence, and offer a narrative approach as a vital vehicle for engaging students' emotions, constructing agency, creating community connections, and in doing the work of preventing violence and enacting peace. We describe TKF's nonviolence programs, critically reflecting on the functions of narrative for pedagogies of peace. The heart of our chapter is the first-person narrative of one author's (Maggie) journey teaching peace. We invite you to experience what Maggie and her students learn, struggle through, and practice. We hope you witness the celebrations and dilemmas of the process of teaching and learning peace in an alternative organizing format. Finally, we offer conclusions that reinforce the value of narrative work for public health communication and organizing for social change.

## YOUTH VULNERABILITY AND VIOLENCE

DiClemente, Hansen, and Ponton (1996) described adolescence as a developmental period of "accelerating physical, psychological, sociocultural, and cognitive development, often characterized by confronting and surmounting a myriad of challenges and establishing a sense of self-identity and autonomy" (p. ix). Adolescence unfolds as a time of change, self-consciousness, and identity construction (Tiggemann & Pennington, 1990). What happens during adolescence "is to a large extent defined by the culture in which one lives, by the expectations society places on its young" (Robbins, 1998, p. 47). During adolescence, young people's communication often shifts more exclusively to their friends, and communication with others becomes restricted as young people grapple with a range of developments: Becoming more independent, making sense of the profound physical changes, becoming more interested in the opposite sex, trying out new behaviors, and trying on new identities (Robbins, 1998).

Youth violence is a high-visibility, high-priority concern in every sector of U.S. society. No community—whether affluent or poor, urban, suburban, or rural—remains immune from the devastating effects of youth violence (National Center For Juvenile Justice, 1999). Youth homicide and suicide are higher in the United States than in any of the 26 wealthiest nations. In fact, the homicide rate for 15- to 24-year-old males in the United States is 10 times higher than in Canada, and 28 times higher than in France or Germany (Office of Juvenile Justice and Delinquency Prevention, 2001).

Adolescents engage in narrative work to reconcile their contradictory feelings, balance what happens to them with what they hoped would happen and what they have learned is "supposed to happen," grapple with their sense of loss of childhood, and maintain a continuity of self in the face of physiological, cognitive, and emotional change (Levy-Warren, 1996; K. A. Martin, 1996).

## REFLECTING REALITIES: THE FUNCTIONS OF NARRATIVE IN TEACHING PEACE

Narratives serve as the primary means by which we negotiate the demanding moments of our personal lives and our changing identities (Hanne, 1994). Through stories, we explain, exemplify, recount, and account for our decisions (Fisher, 1987). We envision narratives as constructions we craft for ourselves and with others to make sense of our lives (see also Bruner, 1987; White, 1981).

Implicit in storytelling are the "underlying values, such as desire for information, personal control, recognition of individuality, or enjoyable quality of life" (Sharf & Vanderford, 2003, p. 15). A narrative approach allows us to understand the significance and meaning of the stories told, and the ways they function for the storyteller and for us as interpreters of their stories. Sharf and Vanderford (2003) offered five functions of narrative that guide our analysis of the stories told in and through the experiencing of PeaceWorks. We see vividly how individuals use narratives to: (a) engage in sense-making, (b) assert control, (c) transform identity, (d) warrant decisions, and (e) build community. Narratives function as *sensemaking*, creating meaning of random events, people, and action (Sharf & Vanderford, 2003). Narratives function to reassert some *control* in the midst of loss, where people are wounded, not just in body but in voice. Narratives function to *transform and reshape identity*. Narratives function to reveal values or *reasons for taking action*. Narratives function to *build community* by allowing individuals to support one another, raise public awareness, and advocate for change.

Narratives have been a long favored route for teaching moral and ethical behavior. In narratives, fact or fiction, we envision and embody both positive and negative behaviors, and reflect on short- and long-term behavioral consequences—for individuals, groups, societies, environments, and our world both in the present and the future. Engaging a narrative necessarily places the reader/listener in a position of moral reflection. Constructing and sharing a narrative becomes a morally reflective act, one that invites the reader/listener to share one's thoughts, emotions, relationships, and actions at that moment in time (Brody, 1987, 1992; Coles, 1989; Polkinghorne, 1988; Rabinow & Sullivan, 1987). At their best, narratives can be open-ended resources, sources of healing and comfort, spiritual maturation, privileged moments of self-change, epiphanies, turning points, and lessons to live by.

These narrative lessons may, then, play a fundamental role in social movements, and the activities of organizations that do the work of movements. Individual, familial, and community narratives are used as strategic resources for social change (e.g., Mothers Against Drunk Drivers (MADD), the Amber Alert System, and Take Back the Night). For example, the story of one family's tragic experiences of loss due to drunk drinking served as an impetus to MADD, and over 10 years later, we have tougher penalties and greater enforcement of drunk-driving legislation. Indeed, in many lobbying efforts of the United States Public Health System and private medical foundations, it is almost obligatory to include personal narratives of individuals and/or families dealing with the featured illness/loss.

Interestingly, critics of social-movement theory argue that the study of social movements is limited too often to materialist approaches that emphasize political economy and resource mobilization (e.g., Hart, 1992; Jacobs, 2002). Hart coined the term *mobilizing narratives* to highlight the fundamental role of narrative in creating collective identities for social movement organizations. Jacobs (2002) argued:

> Because narrative is so basic to the formation of identity, it is an essential resource for social movements. In order to mobilize actual and potential members into a committed and coherent movement, cultural entrepreneurs generate a set of collective narratives that situate the group in time and place. These collective narratives tend to be most effective when they are flexible enough to integrate a diverse set of life histories, when they tell a story of agency and ultimate success, and when they are able to effectively block or demobilize other competing (and potentially antagonistic) group identities. (p. 222)

The story co-constructed by Azim Khamisa and Ples Felix serves as a mobilizing narrative for TKF and its goal of hope and wholeness in a broken world. The TKF mobilizing narrative consists of relationships among characters who defy the traditional hero-versus-villain roles so often portrayed in stories that typically arrange relationships between individuals in terms of contrast or tension. Indeed, both Tariq and Tony are cast as victims of sorts of a broader, broken system.

## INSPIRING NONVIOLENCE: THE TKF PROGRAMS

Since TKF's inception, millions of youth nationwide have been exposed to the TKF story. TKF inspires nonviolent choices through educational programs serving 4th- through 8th-grade students in schools considered most at risk for violence. TKF has reached over 50,000 students in 120 schools in San Diego County with violence prevention programs that focus on utilizing the "power of forgiveness" to break the cycle of violence. The comprehensive program structure includes the Violence Impact Forum® (VIF), which is a high impact, interactive student assembly that tells the TKF story, the consequences of violence, and the reality of gangs, guns, and prison life. A panel of guest speakers, including former gang members, Azim Khamisa, and Ples Felix, encourage students to make peaceful choices and resist negative peer pressure. TKF PeaceWorks, a classroom-based, 16-week program designed for 6th- and 7th-grade students, reinforces the key messages of the VIF assembly. The highly experiential curriculum (developed in 50-minute units) teaches students to become peacemakers by focusing on topics including empathy, positive choice making, forgiveness, and envisioning wonderful dreams.

During the fall of 2002, the newly developed *TKF PeaceWorks* curriculum was piloted with the hopes of instilling positive behavioral change and providing a trusting classroom environment for students to express themselves. The program was piloted at Kroc Middle School in San Diego, California, involving 17 classrooms and approximately 575 seventh-grade students. Five individuals were trained to become PeaceWorks Program Facilitators to teach the weekly classes for 16 weeks. At the completion of the 16-week program, the *TKF PeaceWorks* graduates engaged in a special graduation ceremony to celebrate their achievements and to honor them as peacemakers. Students also displayed the various projects they worked on during the program, such as peace artwork and forgiveness books.

## CONNECTING THROUGH PEACE: THE STORIES WE HAVE SHARED

Who are we? What are our connections to Tariq, Tony, and the amazing TKF story? How has the experience of working with TKF and PeaceWorks changed us, and how have we changed others by virtue of our experience?

I (Maggie) am the Program Director at TKF and have been an active program staff member for 4 years. My passion as Program Director is recharged everyday in my work as I have the opportunity to put peace into action with young people. Something amazing happens for me each time I observe the faces of the young people in our programs as they encounter Ples Felix and Azim Khamisa sitting next to one another: "This man's grandson killed this man's son, yet they are sitting here together." I remember the first time I saw these two men in 1999, struggling as a wounded woman to come to forgiveness in my own heart from the life of abuse I suffered as a young girl throughout my adolescence. I knew I had to be part of this organization, ignited by my favorite words of Gandhi, to "be the change I wish to see in the world."

I (Patricia) felt a deep connection to the message of TKF from the moment I learned about TKF. I did NOT know, however, that I would constantly be moved to tears of joy and sadness as I gathered and analyzed data and wrote up the results of the PeaceWorks evaluation (Dozier, 2003; Geist-Martin et al., 2003). This project has been life-changing, not only in my commitment to TKF, but also in finding ways to volunteer my time to the multiple and complex causes represented in a program such as PeaceWorks. I know that any person who comes in contact with the people of TKF, the message of TKF, and the students of TKF will be inspired and hopeful as well.

I (Kristen) became involved with TKF to assist with the qualitative evaluation of PeaceWorks. I was immersed in every aspect of the study (e.g., study design, data collection, data analysis, and report writing), co-authoring the final report. As I observed the program in action, I witnessed how each facilitator served as one of the rare examples of peace and compassion to which many of these students were exposed. The facilitators' role-modeling was challenged by the multitude of negative messages in students' lives, emanating from home, neighborhoods, school, and the media. This is why I believe in PeaceWorks. At the time of this writing, 8 months after the pilot program ended, I am now a PeaceWorks facilitator. So far I've seen success, I've seen heartache, and I am constantly reminded of the need for these teachings.

## CONTEMPLATING QUESTIONS: ONE WOMAN'S STORY

The central questions we pose in this chapter include: What individual functions (e.g., therapeutic goals for the Khamisa and Felix families, reenvisioning of futures for student participants) and collective functions (e.g., collective identity construction, resource mobilization, social change) are served by the web of storytelling that emerges from the co-constructed Khamisa–Felix story? How do students (e.g., voices of our participants) and staff of TKF (e.g., Maggie) identify with the mobilizing narrative, altering and embodying it in the differentiated contexts of their daily lives and to varying ends? How are the morals of the mobilizing narrative (e.g., compassion, forgiveness) woven into the curriculum and structure of TKF interventions? How do participants' experience/enact similar emplotments in their own storying of their lives and their TKF experience? (e.g., the story of forgiveness to come). How are teaching/learning reenvisioned through the mobilizing narrative of TKF? (e.g., deliberation, recognition, and reclamation).

Specifically, the narratives embody the experiences of students and one teacher (Maggie) of the TKF PeaceWorks program. Students' experiences are described through Maggie's narratives, which include the poetry students write and submit to her in class, the conversations Maggie has with students in the classroom, and Maggie's reflections on the dilemmas of teaching peace. Throughout this text, you will read Maggie's ruminations from the unique space she had as a facilitator during the pilot phase of PeaceWorks; she acted as a liaison between TKF, Kroc Middle School, and the San Diego State University (SDSU) Evaluation Team. Their words, taken to heart, reveal that we have much to learn about teaching and modeling peace. They also demonstrate the varied and complex functions of narrative.

## NARRATING REVELATIONS:
## CREATING WHOLENESS IN A BREAKING WORLD

*What I See*
*I see violence in this world as well as hate.*
*The Earth is covered in a violent mist of black and white.*
*The light tries to overcome the darkness*
                *but it is swallowed up like it is sinking.*
*The bright light called hope is slowly disappearing in a pool of darkness*
*called despair.*
*As hope begins to fade the darkness ...*
*the darkness suddenly disappears as HOPE remembers what it is*
*supposed to do.*
*Hope is what helps you through the darkness.*
*Hope never loses to the darkness of despair.*

*—Cynthia, 7th grade*

\*      \*      \*

*Maggie's reflections from today's class*

The room is cool, the heater blows in the corner. Kids sit in different chairs and on the floor in front of their desks. "It smells like an old person and fish in here!" I find myself leaning toward my clothes, worrying that I am the one who smells like an old person (or maybe it's my patchouli?). "Why you wearing a raincoat Mags?" a boy asks, his hair an afro with a blue pick sticking out of the side of his bushy hair. He is looking right at me, head cocked sideways looking intently with squinty eyes and a half-open mouth. "YOU should know by now I dress differently, but this is the way I am comfortable." I answer confidently, but suddenly I am internally embarrassed by my long brown coat that used to be someone else's short dress. "Yeah, she's different" remarks Brian. "Definitely different" someone else repeats and almost chimes in at the same time. The heat is flying out of the vent in the ceiling and seems to be hitting me in the face, drying my eyes. My face feels like red looks.

Our guest speaker, Javier, enters. Javier is an ex-gang member who served as an "enforcer" in his South Bay San Diego gang until he was shot while on one of his "jobs" to get the money or to kill the man who bought mass quantities of drugs from him and didn't "pay up." Javier speaks to the kids with his glasses pushed up on the top of his head, exposing the reality of his blindness with them as his white eyes roll back into his head. He speaks slowly, the hot air turns off above him just in time for the kids to hear him speak. "When it came down to it, my so-called 'homies' weren't there for me." Ramen is watching wide-eyed, red shirt, new fresh braids pressing closely to his head. Ryan raises his hand and Rosemary calls on him, Ryan speaks firmly "You know how you got shot from that gun? Well I got a bullet from a 9mm on my necklace and I have a 9mm at home." He pulls his shiny silver chain from under his shirt and there is a shiny silver bullet hanging there against his skin. The kids are whispering, some murmuring slightly, some staring. For a moment I see a smirk on Ryan's face: *He is cool, this is power, he is the king. And some of the kids are afraid ... and getting noticed is better than being unnoticed.*

Isn't that the story? BEING NOTICED in a world that doesn't really notice. I used to do all kinds of "singing and dancing" just so my own Dad wouldn't have time to beat me to the floor, just so SOMEONE would notice I was alive and say I was important. It was the only way I felt like I could survive growing up.

The class is walking out the door and about ten of the boys stop to talk with Javier. They have hands of all colors and sizes touching Javier's face where the shells of 14 bullet cases sit under his skin. They are silent and in awe mostly, with an occasional "Does it hurt man?" And I watch Javier give them his gift—by allowing them to learn from his tragedy and his bad personal choices to be an "enforcer" in a gang. He allows these wondering souls to break all his personal barriers and touch his face with their hands. "Wow man, I can't believe how much this must have hurt!" Rafael remarks loudly. Eric is a boy who watches Javier intently as he touches his face and feels the bullets, Eric's mouth is partially opened in amazement, he is always quiet in his dark-blue windbreaker and asks Javier "What did it feel like to get shot?" Eric has NEVER wanted to talk before and HASN'T talked before. But he is intent on speaking to Javier. I tell him, "I'll write you a late pass, Eric" as he continues to talk with Javier....

Meanwhile Ryan walks past me, I ask Ryan about the bullet around his neck, interested and compassionate as possible. "What does your bullet mean to you? What does it represent? Why is important to you to wear it?" *I don't want to lose this kid, I have watched him carefully open up since week one when he yelled out "Forgiveness sucks!" He is open to me, he just wants to mean something, SOMETHING ... I am thinking about what that feels like.* Ryan holds the bullet out toward me proudly, "I have no gage and no gun powder or stuff like that so don't worry, but we do have a gun." *I am thinking I don't know what "tools" you need to shoot someone.* Ryan is walking out now, past me, and I try my best to show interest and give him respect so I don't lose him. "Hey Ryan," he is walking out the door now ... "can we talk about your bullet more next week after class, just you and me?" He nods, "Sure, OK. ..." and closes the door to Bungalow 7, my grounds for teaching and learning.

*     *     *

*In My Eyes*
*When I look around I see people who seem peaceful and happy.*
*But really inside they might feel crappy.*
*They try to hide the bad and bring out the good.*
*To me life is misunderstood.*
*People ask, "What are you?"*
*Are you a gansta, a punk, a skater?*
*But you really want to say, "I'm ME, now go away and let me be."*
*Around us, we see good and bad things ... fights, friends, violence, and*
*  family.*
*Sometimes I just wanna hide and forget my life and be in a dark alley.*
*That is what I see in my eyes.*

—Jenice, 7th grade

*     *     *

*Building Bridges*
*I just LOST it.*
*funny paradoxes of life*
*my kids say I am "the nicest teacher they've ever had"*
*but they're used to "street teachers"*
*          breaking them down.*
*I ask how come you have to further break the b ro k en?*

*how come you can't build someone a bridge*
*and let them cross?*
*they see me hurting I think*
*my eyes fighting stinging tears*
*how I wish so much for them*
*in a world that highlights so little*
*i sit silent heart SWOLLEN*
*some of our best lessons are unspoken*
*funny paradoxes of life,*
*not so funny at all.*

\* \* \*

Third hour nightmare. Full moon craziness? Maybe that and a little something called puberty, called LIFE, called "don't know what to do with yourself" in a world that offers a limited menu of fast food options for your future:

"Sit down!"
"Go back to your seat!"
"Be quiet."
"Shut Up."
"Later."
... we teachers might as well say, "Shut up, I'm NOT interested in you."

\* \* \*

Voices from teachers who ask and inquire and wonder and wallow about attitude and being "rude." Maybe our children are nothing but ventriloquists speaking what they hear. Is this the job of teaching? Should we start with a fresh voice? How do we alleviate the crackling walls of our institutions?

What got to me today, I am unsure of. I have ALWAYS been the kind of person who pushes through suffering and difficult times, who keeps on going despite hardship. I have always made it my motto to push myself, sometimes too hard I suppose. But today, I simply could not keep it together. I watched these kids in third period be the craziest I have ever seen them, out of control, kids crawling on chairs, throwing paper balls, looking at photos, titling on chairs precariously, crawling on the floor DESPITE consistent directions to chill out on these things and with increasing consistency in my voice.

Then my first classroom fight breaks out—or almost. O'Ryan gets pissed off because Julio knocks him with his backpack, now O'Ryan is towering over Julio with his chest sticking out powerfully and proudly, nostrils flaring, his lips tight and eyes white and wide against his black skin (I see him donning his colorful feathers for the young ladies in the room ...) "Yo, you don't ever hit me with no back pack, you FUCKER." With that announcement, O'Ryan shoves Julio into the wall with both hands against his chest and Julio pops his face out of his navy blue sweatshirt with kind of a startled look. Suddenly, the realization hits me that these two are gonna go at it and I instinctively step between them. the testosterone is PALPABLE and I smell their anger, young sweat and B.O. and pride all mixed together and I am now in the midst of the firing range.

"Chill out you guys, just chill!" I say calmly as I can. I have my hands up and out against each of them. O'Ryan is pushing against my hand with pressure and Julio looks afraid in the face of this fight but seems to maintain a smart-ass smirk for looks. I think the other kids are watching us as most of them have filtered into the room, but I am concentrating on holding these two apart.

"Stop NOW," I say it clearly looking at both of them. "Don't get yourselves in any trouble here. You are fighting over a backpack and bumping skin and some invisible pride, it's not worth it. I know you're both pissed, I've felt that way before. Why don't both of you put your hoods up and hold your anger inside of them till you can come out. It always makes me feel better." They both look at me like I am crazy. I am thinking of how they want to beat each other's asses to a pulp and I keep letting beams of goodness come out of my heart, knowing that I have the best tool of all—love. Sounds corny, works for me.

O'Ryan pulls his thick black hood over his head, surrounding his head and face, his anger collected within. They both subside and back away slowly, now cognizant of their classmates watching them. I disparage myself to break the tension, I don't know what else to do? "Hey dudes, I am old and out of shape, I can't be breaking up fights too often, so now we have something interesting to talk about today since I was gonna teach you all how to chill out today." This crazy energy created by them and (whatever else/EVERYTHING else) is contagious to the rest of the class.

I spend 5 minutes going around the room letting them share "what makes me mad" (without using specific names of classmates), but it doesn't matter what I do, what I ask, they are WILD. They don't give a shit, they are bound to eat me up and spit me out, I can feel my frustration mounting, and then I feel incredibly bummed out!

I sit down silently on a chair near the whiteboard and watch them talk for a minute, they don't notice me as a group for a couple minutes. I stop talking, some kids notice me right away and some start in with "SSSSHHHH!" and "Quiet!" until eventually it is quiet. They are all looking at me now, my heart is literally on the outside of my shirt (and probably looks all shredded up and pinned back together again by now, and they KNOW).

I start in, quietly and slowly, because I feel like I am gonna cry and I am not gonna unload my baggage on them. "I feel really bummed out right now you guys. I keep trying to teach you and to have your respect, the same respect I give to all of you, and I am getting nothing back from you. I want you to know I come here because I want to be here, my regular job takes up a lot of my time, but I look forward to coming here and being with all of you, I like all of you. But I can't keep begging for your respect, you should give respect to people that give it to you in your life. So for the rest of the time here today, why don't you all do whatever you want as long as it fits in with your school rules and is appropriate. I feel like I am wasting your time and I don't wanna do that if you don't wanna learn. I will be OK, just so you know that, I will be back in my peaceful stride soon enough, but that doesn't take away that I feel sad."

They all look at me for a moment, none of them quite knowing what to do, and then some of them start in with their "other business." As they begin to talk among themselves and some still stare at me, I start writing the first line of the poem I started this entry with in my notebook.

"Are you writing down our names to tell on us?" Someone asks, heads pop up, and others listen for the answer because it is their "grade."

"No, actually I am just writing down how I feel bummed out. Writing is something I do when I want to cool my anger or want to express what's going on inside of me." I see some surprised faces, some kids watch me and others carry on.

"Ernesto wants your phone number Miss Mags." Rene looks up laughing and now has obviously annoyed and embarrassed Ernesto. I don't even entertain the comment, I look up feeling bummed, probably looking really bummed, and return to my work in my notebook. Laughter subsides for Rene's comment, it's getting quieter still in this classroom even though I gave them free reign. They seem to not dig that I am "done" with them even though there are 15 minutes left in the class.

Dominique, a kid who got kicked out of another class and out into mine (we bonded last week), seems to notice that I am feeling really down (I think). He tries to start conversation with me while I write. "My mom makes hippie purses like the one you have Mags."

I answer, "Oh, that's cool Dominique, I bet you I would love them and maybe even buy one if I got to see them, if she sells them." I return to writing, I feel my face is flushed and my eyes are glassy because I am so disappointed, in myself and everything. Dominique, Kiendra, and Marissa all sit near one another. Here are three kids I have personally reached out to in the last 6 weeks in some way, I have spent time lifting each of them up in some way and hope that I made each of them feel cared for at some point. They seem to watch me now, I sense they are concerned with my disappointment and apparent sadness.

Dominique says, "Well, what were you gonna teach us today Mags?" "I was gonna teach you how to chill out when you feel mad," I say quietly, I am still fighting back my tears from welling up. Kiendra responds, "Can you tell us how to do that Mags, I wanna know how to do that?" Marissa nods next to her in agreement. "What happened today you guys? What kind of teacher do you think I am in your opinion?" I ask them, now awaiting their answer, God knows what they'll say. "You're the nicest teacher we've ever had. We're used to street teachers bringing us down and being tough with us like street folks," Kiendra says.

WOW. What an answer. I gather my thoughts quickly about all that I have been thinking about in regard to education this semester. "So, do you think my job is to break you down or to make you better and build you bridges to cross?" "Build bridges," Thomas adds in now joining the conversation "I think your way is best." "If my way is BEST, then how come I'm not teaching you anything right now?" "You are," Dominique says. "What am I teaching you then?" I inquire. "That we don't need to get broken down," he answers.

That kid just filled me up with more life than he could ever know. I feel tears welling up in my eyes. I am so pissed that I beat myself up in my head, what is "successful" teaching anyhow? I'm pissed that learning means getting beaten down in the first place, I'm bummed. But these kids, these beautiful little kids got my goat and gave me the lesson today. And here sit three kids from the "hood" in Southeast San Diego, all who have spoken to me about their spaces of anger and distance and hurt and violence and emptiness in their lives, and they are now building me up and giving me life.

Paradoxes abound, lessons learned, another breath, another day, I never realized the kinds of gifts I would be getting teaching peace.

\*   \*   \*

We see in both the students' poetry and Maggie's experiences in the classroom that students' narratives clearly function to tell the stories of their individual and collective experiences. Their words tell us of their own individual experiences (e.g., that there is hope in the face of despair, that forgiveness sucks, that peace is inside) but at the same time we can see how they collectively speak in unison of the emptiness and violence that surrounds them (e.g., wanting to be noticed, to mean something, to experience learning that builds them up, not breaks them down).

We also see in these narratives that students are identifying with TKF's mobilizing narrative of hope and wholeness in a broken world. In just a 1-hour classroom lesson, former gang member Javier may be viewed simply as a villain who becomes a hero. But the words of Maggie and the students here show that he is much more. The morals of the mobilizing narrative are vividly displayed in Javier's narrative—his forgiveness of himself and others for the past, but also in his compassion for the students, offering them intimate understanding of what pain lies beneath the surface of his face. The students' responses here and again in the classroom chaos that breaks Maggie down reveal how students clearly are beginning to identify with the mobilizing narrative—they too show hope and compassion. But even more, we see clearly in this final scene a narrative that reenvisions teaching and learning. The students teach Maggie that not only do they "get" what she is trying to teach, but they too can teach her what her form of teaching means to them—she embodies, models, and truly gives the gift of compassion.

\*    \*    \*

*Peace*
Peace.
What a beautiful word
Like the white dove in the sky
When you don't feel any pain
Everything is at a comfortable silence
There is not war, there are no weapons
Where there are angels
Where deep inside, when you feel angry
Deep inside, peace still lies
You just have to look deep inside
To find it.

*—Cynthia, 7th grade*

\*    \*    \*

*Writing forgiveness*
Today in class we ended PeaceWorks with a lesson on forgiveness. It was a perfect way to end, perfect coming together of the ways to practice peace. We spoke about how forgiveness entails your decision to say that you are NO LONGER willing to carry around the pain and anger related to something that hurt you. I wanted to make sure they heard that part about working toward letting pain go ... I said it again and again in different ways that I could. To understand that they will experi-

ence pain, suffering, anger, regret, hurt, betrayal, and so on in their lives. BUT TO UNDERSTAND THAT THE PROCESS OF LETTING ANY NEGATIVITY OUT OF THEIR HEARTS HAD TO COME FROM THEM. I spent some time sharing with them part of who I am—about the forgiveness in my own life toward my dad for what/who he made me believe I was through his beatings and words. I told them the truth straight up as I have asked them to tell me the truth for the past 16 weeks. After we spoke, all the students wrote on a piece of paper one intention of forgiveness in their lives, folded it up, and put it into the forgiveness box. All of the 7th grade PeaceWorks students' letters will be put together and given back to Kroc at their PeaceWorks graduation in one, large forgiveness box. I will not forget the power of today as a human, as a teacher, as a learner. Every moment has been a lesson in growing a humble heart and extending heart in the face of their sufferings, EVEN when they are unkind. I believe that is part of what LOVE is, extending compassion through all sufferings, however long that takes someone.

*    *    *

*Forgiveness is very hard sometimes and sometimes you feel like you can't forgive, but I think it is better to forgive, before inside it eats you up from inside your heart. I can relate to this. It has been hard to forgive my girlfriend cuz' she cheated on me with my friend (or my x-friend cuz' he did it too). This happened last week on 1-27-03, it was a Monday and I said to my girl [friend] that I forgive her and got back with her after a week. It was hard because after all I still feel anger about what they both did and I just want to fight my friend, but I know that won't solve anything, cuz' what happened, happened. I try to think about the future with my girlfriend and that makes me happier. Maggie, thank you for being here for all of us and for taking all the crap I gave you. Also, I wanted to say that I am sorry for sometimes being an ass.*
*Take care and love always.*

—Adrian, 7th grade

*    *    *

Adrian wrote this letter in class today—he stayed after to finish it. After the classroom was empty, he walked up to me and handed me his letter instead of throwing it anonymously into the box where all the other students placed their letters. He looked at me with the same smirk I have witnessed all semester, handed me the letter, and said, "I want you to read this Mags. Read it when I am gone since I am kind of shy about it. I'm gonna miss you." He gave me a hug and I told him, "I won't forget you Adrian, you're gonna have a wonderful life, just keep it in your heart that you are wonderful, don't forget that ever. I'm gonna miss you too." I read the note after he walked out, thinking back on the many moments I spent with Adrian, thinking of the ways I hope he won't forget what I tried to give to him and thinking of the ways he taught me and how I won't forget him.

\*   \*   \*

Dear Auntie,
I do forgive you for physically abusing me and verbally abusing me at one of the worst times in my life ever possible—after my mom died. I forgive you for putting my mom down because of the stuff she did before she was saved from this place. I forgive you for forcing me to eat and every time I couldn't eat a bite for whipping me with a belt. I forgive you for telling me I was dumb and ugly and that no one loved me and my mom left me because of that. I forgive you for making it so that every time my best friend in the whole world, my sister, goes to touch me or hug me I flinch and put my hands over my arms or face. I forgive you for making my life hell. I forgive you but I'll never respect you or love you or consider you my auntie. I forgive you, but you are no longer part of my life.
                    —*An anonymous 7th-grade PeaceWorks Student*

\*   \*   \*

How can you describe the gift of a student giving you a letter like this one to read? The ultimate trust was created between this young girl and me that she could reach into her heart after such suffering. This is what teaching is about to me, this kind of moment. I don't care what any questionnaires say about what we DO or DON'T do in PeaceWorks. I DO care about these YOUNG PEOPLE that many have let me in and to whatever extent they have let me in.

\*   \*   \*

The class lesson on forgiveness was the very last lesson in the 16-week PeaceWorks course. We see clearly in these narratives the collective function of narratives in solidifying TKF's mobilizing narrative of peace through forgiveness. Echoing through each and every narrative are messages that forgiveness is "very hard sometimes," that it is intimately connected with other emotions like anger and pain, that forgiving doesn't guarantee the expression of other emotions such as love or respect, and that it takes time and courage for students to identify with and connect to the mobilizing narrative of forgiveness.

The revisioning of teaching and learning revealed in these narratives beckons all of us to consider who we are as teachers—what we are willing to disclose, what we are capable of comprehending about who students are and what they necessarily bring with them to class, and what it means to be "care-ful" teachers—full of care in our relationships with our students.

*   *   *

I sit in silent spaces wondering about what they wonder about on this evening and what their worlds present to them and how I can help create a world they like to look at and a place where they can come to "voice." I listen to their voices.

- I will forgive my neighbor for killing my uncle.
- I will forgive my history teacher at my old school. She said I was not smart in front of the class.
- When my dad tells me that I'm useless when I do something wrong. That hurted my feelings big time! I was mad at him and I'm still mad because he says it all the time. Dear dad: I would really appreciate if you didn't yell at me.
- Something I will forgive is that I will try to help my brother to stop drinking. He drinks too much because his daughter has a brain tumor.
- I ask for forgiveness for myself because I hate myself and especially my health. Cause when I was small, like 13, I took drugs cause I went with the wrong crowd. I had a problem with my body for that I shaked too much but I stopped and I'm recovering right now.
- I forgive myself because I always hate myself.
- Dear XX: I forgive you for killing my mom, but when I am 18 years of age you are still going to get death row. Forgivingly, XX
- I think I was a 3rd or 4th grader when my mother got a phone call from my aunt saying that her brother has been shot. And so we went to the hospital as fast as we can and saw that my uncle was okay. Everybody was hurt, because my uncle is an innocent man. I heard that two men came up to him and shot him. I was mad, very mad but I forgave them because I knew of course I couldn't do anything and because I don't want anybody else hurting.
- I want to forgive my dad for leaving me and my mom and not having a better relationship with me. And I also want to forgive him for waiting so long to come back in my life.

- I am still trying to forgive God for taking away my mom.

## INTERPRETING REVELATIONS: NARRATING TO CREATE WHOLENESS IN A BREAKING WORLD

In order to create wholeness in a breaking world, we must listen carefully to the stories young people tell us about violence and the peace they are trying to craft. We also must listen to the voice of any one person who offers us revelations about the wake of events that surround and silence the voices of young people as they try desperately to make sense of violence. Public health initiatives such as TKF's PeaceWorks promotes healthy choices and nonviolent behaviors among our most vulnerable youth (e.g., youth who live and go to school in neighborhoods that have a record of violence or whose family situations may not provide healthy role models). We see, too, how the stories that the students tell each other become strategic resources for change. This is especially true when the teachers listen and learn from the stories, revisioning the role they can play in mobilizing each and every story students tell as a resource for moral reflection.

The day-to-day living of PeaceWorks, as students and teachers make their way through the trials and tribulations of teaching and learning about peace, illustrates the power of mobilizing narratives (Jacobs, 2002) and emergent webs of storytelling in organizing for social change. In the final section of this chapter, we offer interpretations of the functions of these narratives for students, facilitators, and those who care to listen and learn from the stories told.

The PeaceWorks' narratives embody a pedagogy of peace and hope, re-envisioning teaching and learning through the mobilizing narrative of TKF. The voices of these young people offer us valuable insights about seeking space, reciprocal trust, being noticed, and healing. We see, too, how the narratives function in some of the same ways described by Sharf and Vanderford (2003). But, we also see how their voices mobilize these functions in the context of teaching peace in a broken world.

PeaceWorks creates the gift of space, an emotional space for voices to be heard. Young people come to classes where they are respected by people who are role models for respect and trust. They are encouraged to open up pieces of themselves in different ways and means—emotions they often suppress or deny. And still we hear adults asking, "What's wrong with these f'in' kids today?" Few spaces exist in a breaking world for youth simply to be, and to be heard. We see in Maggie's narratives a web of storytelling that serves the collective function of mobilizing community and the individual function of students finding their place in this community. Maggie shares:

PeaceWorks has helped me touch the part of kids that is within, that part of them that may feel lonely, unloved, or unheard. I have seen this process happen week after week, I have written about just small pieces and snippets of this process. I have been witness to the beginning of release of pain, sorrow, and neglect. I have been part of the nurturing and strength. In fact, I have been ALL these things and on BOTH sides. They have nourished me and allowed me to release in this SPACE created for all of us. I know my willingness to learn from them opened up paths for trust in both directions. And you know what, there were many difficult moments, and this program isn't perfect, but it DID something, it created a space to let them BE WHO THEY ARE.

The narratives reveal the reciprocal process of learning and teaching peace. As a staff member teaching PeaceWorks, it is clear that Maggie enacts similar emplotments in her own life—that her experience leads her to live life differently—to story her world in new ways.

We see four distinct morals in Maggie's narratives and what she recounts about her communication with adolescents: (a) quest for validation (b) search for independence (c) engage respect, and (d) claim dreams. In their quest for validation, students seem to feel as if they have lost control of their identity. They exert power and dominance in the form of physical and verbal violence against one another, and at times, their teachers. Students, as well as Maggie, voice frustration as time after time, the adult figures at school and in the community let them down. "You don't care about me" echoes in the stories about what a "teacher" should be like. In this way, the students' voices become a mobilizing narrative for adults to embrace—to communicate in ways that validate students.

Students search for independence when control is lost. Stereotypes and labels abound; students voice a need for independence and a place to just be. We see young people seeking space for sensemaking in their lives within the difficult formative life passages they encounter in a problematic world (Geist-Martin, Ray, & Sharf, 2003). The young people in PeaceWorks look for an opportunity to share their experiences about the world they live in, a place where they can ruminate on both their hope and loss. Students identify with TKF's mobilizing narrative by embodying forgiveness and hope amidst the violence and loss in their own lives.

Respect emerges as a pattern in the narratives where students reveal feelings about loss of respect, and ultimately control, in their very own systems of learning. Within this system, at home and at school, the youth feel broken and disenchanted, seeking agency and voice. We understand how important reciprocal respect becomes for students as they voice the need to experience respect in their relationships with others. The voices remind us about the significance of role-modeling values as a narrative resource for creating and practicing peace. Maggie's narratives express her attempts to have students see her as genuine and full of love, love reserved for them. Time and again we hear her saying, "I'm different from the rest." In return, her students' narratives reveal their collective respect for her compassion and patience. They've found common ground as they've bonded. Their revelations lead to trust.

Together, students and teacher work to construct and claim collective dreams for themselves within a broken world. The narratives, particularly the letters of forgiveness, represent avenues and resources for students to voice the lessons they have learned. Above all, they begin envisioning a future—a deserved future for themselves. Visions of hope replace a once bleak space, empty of goals and dreams. It is within this space that young people realize that change can occur, first within themselves and then to be transferred into their communities. These narratives function to accomplish validation, independence, respect, and dreams for the students and teacher.

## Healing the Broken World: Designing a Reclamation

We challenge health communication scholars to expand the way they define and approach illness (i.e., individual and/or familial experiences) toward a standpoint that recognizes how societies can be broken through senseless violence. We see clearly in the narratives offered by Maggie and the PeaceWorks' students how narrative activity evinces healing potential for systemic as well as individual ills. These narratives offer an important resource for health communication scholars–practitioners. We offer these stories as a call to action for scholars-practitioners in the communities in which we live and work.

The nature of students learning peace and the teacher teaching/role-modeling peace is a cyclical process in so many respects. The process is a mirror of reciprocity. The energy exchange–the learning and teaching and teaching and learning–serves as a commodity for healing. Because violence affects the fabric of the world, this reciprocity acts as a currency of exchange that serves to heal the composition of narratives on personal, cultural, and societal levels. This process provides opportunities for shared illumination, reflecting new understandings and newly shared sustenance for one another.

The classroom scenes, poems, and reflections of PeaceWorks are composed of narratives that function in very specific ways for students and the teacher. At the same time, how these narratives function together in interaction is revealed in the three processes:

*Deliberation.* Teacher and students together deliberate dilemmas and in the process, liberate themselves from the ways that narratives have functioned in the past—in their lives as "at risk" students and in teacher's lives, describing what these at risk students are exposed to and become on a daily basis. This liberation often comes with struggle in the process of inventing new ways of de-liberating the self or being at odds with self in opposition to "categories" that young people have been put in previously.

*Recognition.* Teacher and students together appreciate one another's narratives as valid and worthy. In the process, these narratives function to communicate a sense of the value and worth of each other's voices.

*Reclamation.* Teacher and students together bring back, recover, and cultivate narratives that sustain peace and sense of self in this space of sustenance and forgiveness. Narratives function to allow a student to cry out against violence in order to regain and restore peaceful, respectful, and forgiving communication.

In witnessing these narratives, it becomes clear that the narratives of students and the teacher function generally as sustenance that either fuels emotions or nourishes newly "tried on" emotions. PeaceWorks offers young people the space and opportunity to think, feel, and communicate in ways that clearly differ from the dominant narrative scripts they, too often, automatically speak and live. In the PeaceWorks classroom, teacher and students together create counternarratives and undermine the stories of domination in their lives. In some cases, students seem anxious to live out these counternarratives outside of this safe space. Teacher and students alike learn that narratives can function in ways that lead them to feel important, noticed, empathetic, cared for, and hopeful about living life more peacefully.

# IV

## Narrative Sense-Making About Self and Other

∽

### INTRODUCTION

### Christina S. Beck
*Ohio University*

*I shivered as I stood by the phone booth in the dark gas station parking lot. My husband, Roger, answered, and I asked quickly, "Have you heard from Mom?" "Yeah," he responded, "they really don't want you to come."*

*Tears welled up in my eyes as I listened to Roger's account of his conversation with my mother in Indiana. "Apparently, your grandma thinks that Grandpa will think he's going to die if you come so they want you to turn around," he explained.*

*I looked at the lonely stretch of highway to my right and paused. My 90-year-old grandfather had been rushed to the hospital earlier in the day, and I wanted to be by his side. I had cursed the 6-hour drive between us as I pushed the speed limit to get to him, but now, after 3 hours on the road, I hesitated. If I kept driving, what would that communicate to Grandpa? Would I kill him by just showing up at the door? But if I go home and he dies anyway, could I live with my choice not to say good-bye?*

*I decided to press on. I hated driving on Friday nights, especially on snow-covered country roads. Yet, I knew that I needed to get to my grandpa. He had always been like a father to me, and I adored his patience, his kindness, and his quiet resolve to battle through the horrible toll that age had taken on his once-strong body. He loved to work with wood, yet arthritis froze his hands, preventing him from carving and hammering. He valued his independence, yet arthritis crippled his knees, confining him to his scooter except when he tried to use his walker in the house. I smiled, though, as I thought about Grandpa's insistence upon driving to his job as a Walmart greeter and his refusal to cut back on his hours or to give up his task of calling Bingo for elderly Walmart customers every Tuesday morning. He's a fighter, my Grandpa. He's a fighter.*

*Three more hours passed. The clock ticked 10:30 p.m. as I pulled into the hospital parking lot in Warsaw, Indiana. I parked by the emergency department because I knew that the front door would be locked. As I left the car and walked to the entrance, I flashed back to the preceding Monday—the day that Grandpa fell and broke his arm. At first, he had refused to allow us to bring him to the hospital. Finally, he had agreed. Tears filled my eyes as I remembered Grandpa on the stretcher, waiting for a room to open up in the emergency department. I had attempted to reassure him as he spoke about the pain. "Well, it won't be long now," he had said, "I won't have to put up with it for much longer."*

*I pressed the elevator button to get to the Intensive Care Unit (ICU), praying that Grandpa didn't know what he was talking about, hoping that he didn't instinctively realize that the end was near. My heart pounded as I turned the corner to the nurse's station in the ICU. How would Grandpa react to my visit? What would Grandma say when she found me there in the morning? Would the nurses even let me see him at this hour of the night?*

*"Hi," I said to a woman at the station. "I'm George Groscost's granddaughter, and I just drove from Ohio to see him."*

*"That's great," said the woman who I would come to know as Ruth. I paused, adding that "My grandma is worried that he'll die if he sees me. He might think he's dying."*

*"Honey, he'll be glad to see you," Ruth promised me. "He's rather out of it anyway, but you can stay right here and talk to him."*

*I stood at the threshold of the dorm-size room, noting the tubes, wires, and monitors. Grandpa's lips were parched, and a mask covered his nose. He opened his eyes, widening them in surprise as he caught sight of me.*

*"Hi Grandpa," I greeted him as I moved quietly to his bedside. "Mom said that you needed some tender, loving care, and no one can take care of you better than I can." I touched his arm and smiled my most reassuring smile.*

Throughout this volume, we emphasize the essential nature of narrative for health care experiences and interactions. Earlier chapters explore the implications of personal narratives in public dialogues about health issues as well as the consequentiality of narrative for organizing health care events and resources. In this section, we take a more microanalytic approach to narratives and health communication, focusing on personal and relational narratives as co-constructed, emergent, and dynamic mirrors of (and, reflexively, contributors to) health care experiences. Within that context, the chapters in this section continue to highlight core themes regarding narrative theorizing and health communication—the conundrum of enacting conflicting and/or multiple identities during complicated health interactions, the inherent temporality of narratives, and the confusion stemming from our postmodern turn away from absolutism.

*I watched as my mom and grandma left for lunch, sipping my Diet Coke and reflecting on the events of the preceding evening. I had spent the night with Grandpa, comforting him when his pain medication didn't seem to work and when he begged to go home. "Come on, come on," he had urged. "Let's go home now. Let's go now." My chest ached as I said "No." What right did I have to tell him that he couldn't leave the hospital? Who made me the boss of him? Yet, he repeated his requests for freedom, and I recurrently refused.*

*He had seemed so thirsty, and I tended to his requests for drinks of water by holding a straw in his mouth. Who would have done this if I hadn't come, I thought? How could Mom and Grandma just leave him here alone?*

*When he drifted off to restless sleep, I tried to get information. Apparently, he had collapsed in his recliner at home. At 90, he still lived with Grandma in their ranch-style home on a quiet street. He was severely dehydrated, and he had suffered a heart attack, likely because he had not been taking his heart medication. After he had broken his arm earlier in the week, he had been very groggy, thus he depended on my mom and Grandma for his medication and for insisting that he eat and drink. Grandpa could be very stubborn, and my mom and Grandma could be, well, less than assertive. Roger and I had worried about meeting his basic needs when we left only a few days earlier. We should have stayed ... we should have just found a way to stay longer ...*

*Hours passed ... my mom and Grandma came back to Grandpa's room in the ICU and then departed again for the night. My sister arrived. I never really get along with my sister or my mom—very different personalities, very different people. However, on that evening, we aligned with the goal of helping Grandpa ... Unfortunately, we didn't know how.*

*"I WANT TO GO HOME!" Grandpa begged.*

*We had learned that he had an infection. "Grandpa, you have a bug, and we need to zap the bug and then you can go home," I responded, trying to lighten the mood.*

*His eyes grew large. "Zap the bug?" he asked.*

*"Yeah, as soon as we get rid of the infection—"*

*"Zap the bug?" he interrupted.*

*"Yeah, Grandpa, we're going to zap the bug," I repeated.*

*"Zap that bug," he ordered.*

*"Okay, Grandpa, that's what the medicine is doing," I replied.*

*"Let's go home now," he barked.*

*I sighed and slumped in my chair. Grandpa started to lift his leg to get out of the bed. "Grandpa, what are you doing?" I asked.*

*Teresa and I held Grandpa in bed, pushed the call button to implore the nurses to help, and reflected on strategy for nearly 3 hours. He drifted between delusion—reliving long-ago days on his old family farm and fearing the need to chase his beloved dog, Mickey, when he couldn't move out of his scooter—and demands to escape the hospital. "If you ever loved me, Christie, you will get me out of here now," he commanded, adding "Why are you doing this to me?"*

*Finally, we started to wonder why we were being so insistent. What was the prognosis? If this is it, if he's going to die, do we have the right to insist that he die in the hospital? Can't he just go home and be in his favorite recliner? What were we doing here, anyway? We looked up at Ruth, the night nurse, yearning for inspiration and assistance. With compassion in her eyes, she said, "So many people love your grandpa from Walmart. I'm not going to let him die on my watch."*

*At 4 a.m., Ruth entered and commanded us to leave the room. We needed rest, and she had an idea for Grandpa. I fell asleep on the waiting room couch. Around 5:30 a.m., I awoke and darted back to the room, mad at myself for succumbing to slumber. Grandpa was sitting up in a recliner, calm and ready for breakfast. Teresa smiled. "He just needed his recliner," she said.*

Through a strange twist of fate, I was working on this book when my grandfather's health took a turn for the worst. As I wrestled with my feelings, responses, and contributions to the emergent narrative, I wondered what was going through his mind, how he grappled with the frustration of fear, losing control, and pain. This health situation stemmed from Grandpa's arm, Grandpa's heart, and Grandpa's infection. Yet, the rest of us—my mom, grandmother, and sister, the health care staff, myself—implicitly contributed to how events would unfold. This health narrative became our own as well as his, personal as well as relational.

Notably, health narratives constitute messy, fluctuating, temporally and relationally bound enactments that ebb and flow, extending from the past and reshaping what can be in the future. Through my individual and interactional choices, I co-authored the emergent narrative.

During that weekend with my grandfather, I thought about what might have ensued if I had decided to go back to Athens after that conversation with Roger on the gas station pay phone. Even that decision would have contributed to Grandpa's emergent health narrative. ... Perhaps he would not have had someone to offer water to him, given that his crippled hands could not squeeze the call button. Perhaps he would have been strapped to his bed if he tried to leave with others there instead of us ... perhaps ... perhaps ...

For much of that weekend, my previously coherent grandfather ranted, making little sense to me. As his health deteriorated during the following week, an oxygen mask covered his mouth and nose, preventing verbal interaction. He employed hand signals and followed conversations between family members and health care providers with his eyes, but I was struck by his loss of control. Staff members performed procedures on him, administering drugs, changing bandages, moving his limbs, poking and prodding him. At one point, I tried to commiserate with him by saying that he must feel like a bad science project.

Although he could still think and feel, increasingly, family and ICU staff members co-defined how his narrative would ensue, and through those inherently defining moments, we co-crafted ongoing narrative experiences that enveloped all of us. Roger kept reassuring me that I didn't really possess agency for removing Grandpa from the hospital—after all, I was only the granddaughter. However, I knew that I possessed the power to impact Grandpa's experience—I pressed nurses about pain medication and his oxygen flow, and I convinced a night nurse to permit my grandfather's dog, Mickey, to make an early morning visit to the ICU. In so many ways, through actions large and small, we collectively co-constructed what this experience would be ... for Grandpa and for each of us, even for the health care providers who fought to "help" Grandpa for 10 days.

Ultimately, we clashed about what constituted "social support" for Grandpa and each other and what roles we should respectively assume in enacting it. In this medical drama, who should assume the role of director? Grandpa had directed his own life just fine until now, but we implicitly usurped that control by insisting that he stay in the hospital. Did we really get to decide what's "best," just because we happened to be in the room and able to talk without an oppressive mask over our mouths? Should an unfamiliar nurse or doctor or respiratory therapist get to dictate treatment simply because that person happened to be on duty at a particular time and place? As the chapters in this section illustrate, the enactment of health narratives inherently extends from the accomplishment of overlapping individual and relational identities that can (and often do) clash with how people might prefer to present themselves or relate to others.

The situating of Grandpa's illness in terms of the available (and non-available) participants also fits within the broader temporal context of this health saga. Grandpa fell ill in an era of managed care, hospital cutbacks, and medical bureaucracy. He broke his arm in the week between Christmas and New Year's, and we couldn't obtain adequate home health care to assist my ailing, 87-year-old grandmother who had broken her own shoulder during Christmas shopping, or my mom, who had to juggle her own life and work commitments to assist them. Although we called every agency in town, staff members were committed to other clients or on holiday break. The timing compounded an already bad situation, isolating my grandparents from much-needed help.

Just prior to Grandpa's accident and hospitalization, Grandma's hearing aid gave out, and she struggled to hear. Without her replacement hearing aid, Grandpa's own wife couldn't understand his muffled cries for help nor doctors' explanations as Grandpa's kidneys started to fail. As the chapters in this section highlight, the temporal nature of narratives flavors the ways in which we co-construct our personal and relational health stories.

I will remain forever grateful to Ruth, the ICU nurse, for dragging that recliner into my grandfather's room in the wee hours of a Sunday morning. By permitting Grandpa to sit up in a chair, despite his frail condition, she offered him a precious gift—a gift of familiarity, a gift of dignity. Nearly a week later, another ICU nurse, Beth, became my co-conspirator when she allowed me to bring Mickey, my grandfather's dog, right up into Grandpa's ICU room. Grandma and my mom nearly had a fit. "You can't take that dog up there," my mom admonished me, "It's just not done."

In the spirit of postmodernism, health care participants (including health care providers) increasingly herald a blurring of "right" and "wrong," "acceptable" or "inconceivable," regarding treatments, roles, and even behaviors in a hospital setting. As the chapters in this section powerfully attest, narrative sense making encompasses individual, dyadic, and family efforts to sort through considerations and constraints in order to co-determine what can (and should) count as right or acceptable in a particular circumstance at a specific time.

In chapter 15, Barbara Sharf shares her personal struggle with a surgeon who failed to work with her as a co-participant in the emergent health narrative. From her unique vista as a health communication scholar as well as a health care participant, Sharf details the consequential and rhetorical nature of co-constructing workable relational identities between health care providers and health care seekers, especially in light of clashes between perspectives on health care roles, relationships, and medical decision-making. This chapter serves as an excellent exemplar of the ways in which such divergent perspectives become powerfully evident through interaction and emerge as barriers to the accomplishment of medical goals for both participants.

Beach and Mandelbaum (chap. 16) underscore issues of relational and personal identity and temporality in their microanalytic exploration of conversations between a health care provider and a patient. Through their analysis, Beach and Mandelbaum expose the critical importance of interaction for emergent health narratives. In a series of conversations, a patient repeatedly hints at an underlying reason for a developing health situation—his mom had a stroke, and he's struggling to manage the stress. By not pursuing this strand, the health care provider neglects valuable opportunities to affirm and explore important aspects of the patient's broader life and health situation as well as to play a more far-reaching (and integral) role in the patient's ongoing health narrative. This chapter provides an outstanding addition to the literature on health and narrative through its illustration of how co-constructed interactions between health care participants implicitly contribute to (and reflexively exhibit) core dimensions of health narratives.

Keeley and Koenig Kellas (chap. 17) echo the significance of interaction between health care participants in their chapter on final conversations. Highlighting the voices of survivors, this contribution to our volume emphasizes family members and friends as co-participants of the dying process—individuals who shaped the experiences of their loved ones as they also reframed and redefined their respective sense of self and relationship with others. Especially given the literature's tendency to characterize narrative as an individual construction, this chapter offers intriguing insights into health care experiences as shared, relational co-constructions that may result in multiple (and potentially divergent) narratives.

In chapter 18, Bosticco and Thompson detail the role of narratives in the bereavement process, artfully demonstrating the temporality of narratives as well as the plurality of acceptable ones in contemporary society. Given that their research participants had lost offspring, the crafting of stories represented a reshaping of individual and relational identities—whom could each be without that particular child? What would their lives be like now, compared to before the loss? What could be the "right" way for each to tell the story of the child's loss and to position the loss within the broader context of life now? Notably, this chapter constitutes a compelling contribution to our volume in light of its description of the reconfiguring and function of emergent, temporally and relationally bound narratives.

Finally, O'Hair, Scannell, and Thompson (chap. 19), feature the ways in which cancer patients achieve agency through narrative. Given the plethora of current treatment options, cancer patients confront the challenge of sorting through choices while also considering concurrent identity issues and relational constraints—What kind of person am I if I choose Option A instead of Option B? Risk Taker? Survivor? What will my doctor think? How can I tell my family and friends that I'm not going to do Treatment X? Do I really have a choice? This chapter showcases the ways in which answers to such questions frame (and get framed through) emergent health narratives, providing an important companion to literature on medical decision making and health care identities.

As I learn and "re-realize" through my own health care experiences, the co-construction of health narratives is poignant, powerful, and personal. Fraught with the complexities of modern medicine and choices of alternative health care, complicated by economics, politics, and institutional rules and regulations, and mangled with conflicting relational commitments and personal priorities, health narratives implicitly emerge as messy, conflicting, and multifaceted. They fluctuate and change, driven by new developments, new perspectives, altering values, physical limitations, and perhaps even fear.

We cannot escape participation in health narratives, especially those that directly involve us and our loved ones. Even our absence from a bedside marks a contribution to a loved one's emergent story. However, as the chapters in this section attest, despite the conglomeration of mixed emotions and physical frustrations, our co-constructed narratives about health care experiences can afford us the opportunity to reflect, to interpret, and to strive to make sense from situations that seemingly defy sense-making, if we embrace such a contemplative process as part of our own ongoing life story.

# 15

## How I Fired My Surgeon and Embraced an Alternate Narrative

∾

**Barbara F. Sharf**
*Texas A & M*

Here's the thing. Like many other academics in this country, I enjoy a comfortable middle-class lifestyle that includes having adequate health insurance, permitting access to practitioners, facilities, and medications when needed. Unlike most of my colleagues, I've spent the greater part of an academic career studying communication between patients and physicians. I applied the narrative paradigm, emphasizing health citizenry and patient empowerment. Having worked with clinicians for many years, on several occasions I have benefitted from privileged networks and specialized sources of information (as the following tale illustrates). So, even as I found myself in *this* situation—5 days before the most extensive surgery I had ever faced and totally at odds with the surgeon I had selected—I appreciated the irony of my predicament. Irony, however, definitely took a backseat to emotional upset, anxiety, and, yes, panic, as I tried to find the best way to address this problem, one that threatened my current and long-term well-being. This story illustrates how the communicative road toward patient autonomy and clinical partnership became detoured by the pain, fatigue, and stress of illness, then was blockaded by significant differences in expectations and styles between me and my doctor. It portrays how the ideal of active patient participation becomes complicated and encumbered in the actual context of serious illness and the still very powerful traditional medical model.

## PRELUDE

*Narrative rationality ... offers an account, an understanding, of any in-
stance of human choice and action, including science. At the same
time, narrative rationality ... provides a basis for critique.... [implying]
that "the people" judge the stories that are told for and about them and
that they have a rational capacity to make such judgments.*

—Fisher, 1987, pp. 66–67

Though I knew for some time that I had degenerative arthritis in my
right hip, I lived with a version of what sociologist Arthur Frank (1995)
called the *restitution narrative.* In his typology of illness stories, the
restitution plot posits that health problems can be remedied and the
body can be restored to "normal." Because I knew that damaged bone
and cartilage cannot be restored to its former state, that definition did-
n't quite apply, but for the first four years following diagnosis, medicine
and exercise helped me lead a very functional, if not quite normal, existence. However, within a year after a stressful move from Chicago to
College Station, Texas, my health took a distinctly downward turn.

When an orthopedic surgeon first told me that I was destined to have
a total hip replacement (hereafter, THR), I did not want to believe his
prediction. Later, when a second orthopedist offered the same treatment recommendation, I accepted that this surgery loomed in my distant future. Both doctors explained that the implant lasts for about 10
to 15 years, and given my relatively young age, it was in my best interest
to wait as long as possible. The second surgeon said I would know
when the time was right—the pain would be intolerable. Like thousands of other arthritis sufferers, I decided to stall, doing all I could to
manage my pain. I tried a variety of medications, which at best took the
edge off, allowing me to work—not as effectively as I would have liked,
but I managed. I became deeply immersed in patienthood, with both
conventional and complementary approaches—rheumatology, chiro-
practic, podiatry, physical therapy, smelly topical salves, cold and hot
compresses, water aerobics and swimming, hot tubs, Pilates class,
guided imagery, herbs, massage, and acupuncture. Searching for relief
took a great deal of time, effort, and money, crowding out work, social,
and leisure activities. Still, with the encouragement and skill of my
doctors, therapists, and instructors, I got through another 4 years. It
was obvious, however, to me and everyone around me that my condition was getting much worse. I walked with a pronounced limp, climb-
ing stairs was increasingly difficult, and there was hell to pay for
gardening, my favorite pastime. I was tired and stiff much of the time,
able to sleep only 3 to 4 hours a night because I'd wake up in pain, then
be unable to fall asleep again. Eventually, I suffered from constant

pain, radiating from my hip down to my knee. And chronic pain does great damage to mind, spirit, and psyche. Frequently, I was depressed and distracted, difficult to live with. In Frank's (1995) terminology, I had transitioned into a *chaos narrative*, a plotline in which all seems to go wrong and out-of-control, with no promise of getting better. It was time to have my hip replaced.

## A Double Whammy

> *The body is not a territory to be controlled by either the physician's treatments or the patient's will.*
>
> —Frank, 1991, p. 62

THR is considered to be elective surgery because it does not constitute a lifesaving procedure; thus, I was able to plan for it in advance. In late fall, I decided to finish the academic year and to schedule the surgery at the end of the spring semester. Making a commitment to get through the coming semester meant fulfilling several tasks on a grant project, completing recruitment and admissions for our departmental graduate program, teaching a seminar, and completing promised writing projects. Completing these obligations would take considerable effort, but I felt it was do-able.

During November and December, I fell ill with a flu that I wasn't able to shake, a sign of being physically and mentally overextended. Still, I made three long-distance trips to attend an academic convention and family events, and I went through the usual crush of pre-Christmas preparations that often kept me up very late in order to complete. I felt exhausted, but continued the habit developed over many years of making demands on my body in order to do what I determined needed to get done.

However, the second day of the new year, my body quit of its own accord. I woke up feeling completely stiff and achy from head to toe, barely able to move. This was not just pain from my hip; something new and even more ominous was happening. Searching the Internet, I read descriptions of fibromyalgia; alarmingly, this condition, characterized by rigidified muscles, sometimes exacerbated by a bout of flu, seemed to fit very well with what I was experiencing. My rheumatologist confirmed my self-diagnosis a few days later. Fibromyalgia is one of those mysterious pain syndromes experienced by many but that cannot be verified by lab tests and for which neither causes nor consistently reliable remedies are known. I knew about people with fibromyalgia who had to stop working for a year or more, or even permanently. Fortunately, I also talked with a few who found ways of continuing with life activities, so at least a degree of recovery seemed possible. For the next 3 months, my life was marked not only by pain, but also debilitating fatigue and disability. My world quickly became much smaller in scope. I became too tired to talk with people on the phone or to return nonessential e-mails. Any travel, other than car trips, was out of the question. I could no longer even walk across campus or carry my work in a shoulder bag. The rheumatologist's mandate to get a decent night's sleep became a major objective. Completing the responsibilities of spring semester now was a challenge that demanded all my remaining strength.

In this context, I began the process of making arrangements for hip surgery. I wanted it done in a large, urban center where many such operations are performed, informed by the most current research versus having the procedure in the rural community where I live. For the previous 3 years, I had served as a consultant to a health services research center in nearby Houston. One of my colleagues there is a nonpracticing rheumatologist who does research on osteoarthritis. Earlier in the fall, I had asked her for recommendations about the top orthopedic surgeons in the city. I confirmed her recommendation with my rheumatologist, who had recently moved to College Station from Houston. Thus, I felt fortunate to have obtained an appointment with the surgeon who had been recommended as "A+" technically and "A++" for communications skills.

Uncharacteristically, I had not done extensive reading about THR before going to my initial appointment. Earlier I had done preliminary research; by January, however, I was simply too ill and too tired to do more. Dr. Rigor was a taciturn man, the senior physician in a large group practice devoted to bone and joint ailments, situated in an opulent clinic affiliated with a large private hospital. He greeted me courteously, taking a scant history. When I mentioned our mutual colleague who had referred me, he briefly acknowledged his working relationship with her, as well as with Kathy, a second colleague at the research center whose mother had her hip replaced by him. He never asked about my relationship with these individuals or what kind of work I do. Following X rays and a physical examination, Dr. Rigor proclaimed, "Well, you don't need knee replacement," a remark that I found disconcerting as I had never even considered that possibility. He then confirmed my need for hip replacement, providing a simple description of the surgery, extensive preparatory steps, and lengthy recovery process. When I asked about what kind of physical therapy I would need, he assured me that I would receive sufficient therapy in the hospital following surgery. The doctor's declaration that I would not be permitted to put any weight on the right leg for at least 6 weeks after the surgery led me to ponder over the next few months how I could possibly hop on my left foot for that stretch of time. Our meeting concluded with instructions for setting a surgery date by contacting his surgical nurse, Ginny, a personable, knowledgeable young woman. I had the impression that the doctor repeated this canned, 15-minute presentation for new patients several times a day. For my part, I had not distinguished myself as a patient. I asked few questions because I frankly did not know enough to ask much. Instead, I tried to listen and absorb the information he had offered. As I left his office, I wondered, if Dr. Rigor represents an A++ in communicating with his patients, what would a B– or a C+ be like? I met Marlynn, my husband, who was waiting for me in the outer reception area. "Well," I shrugged, "I wasn't bowled over, but he's a surgeon, after all," referring to the generalization that surgeons as a specialist group tend not to excel in interactional skills.

In the 2½ months that followed, I gave little thought to Dr. Rigor and the major surgery that lay ahead. Instead, I was focused on the immediate challenge of surviving the exacerbation of fibromyalgia. A medication prescribed by my rheumatologist intended to relieve pain and facilitate sleep did neither, but instead resulted in the adverse side effect of severe chills. Nearly every evening, I experienced a cold sensation from deep within, resulting in uncontrollable shivering that I could not relieve by putting on several layers of clothes and a comforter. A good friend in Chicago, alarmed by what she heard, tried to convince me to get a consultation at the Mayo Clinic. With her assistance, I corresponded with a kind physician from Mayo who was willing to set up appointments for me with appropriate specialists, but the mere thought of having to travel on three flights to arrive in icy Minnesota in February (not to mention the associated expenses) was inconceivable to me.

For years, I have used Frank's work, which champions the importance of voicing patient narratives, in my teaching and research. But only in this period of acute illness did I come to fully appreciate the meaning of the title of his first book, *At the Will of the Body*. In this volume, Frank (1991) describes important lessons learned after first undergoing a heart attack, followed by prostate cancer a year later. These life-threatening interruptions resulted in a redirection of Frank's identity, work, and life history. For a long while, arthritis had gradually and surreptitiously altered many aspects of my existence, a process I tried to resist in every way I could. Now I understood that no matter what my intentions, the demands and limitations of my physicality dictated my plans and actions, in effect becoming the plotline of my life's story, supplanting other possibilities. As an unexpected complication, the immediate intensity of fibromyalgia displaced my attention, not only from personal and professional agendas, but also away from the anticipation of surgery, diverting valuable time and energy from educating myself about the next major challenge that I would soon be facing.

## What Story Am I In?

> ... stories concern action and experience. To put the matter simply, sto-
> ries are about someone trying to do something, and what happens to
> her and to others as a result.
>
> —Mattingly, 1998, p. 7

My deep immersion in what Virginia Woolf (2002) referred to as the "daily drama of the body" (p. 5) continued until mid-March. By that time, I stopped taking the troublesome medication, halting the nocturnal chills. The weather in Texas had begun to warm up, and my garden beckoned. I started swimming in a heated indoor pool once a week with a friend. I did physical exercises to bolster upper body strength in preparation for walking with crutches after surgery. Simultaneously, I practiced guided imagery on a nearly nightly basis, visualizing relaxation of my taut muscles and mind. The stressful graduate student recruitment process was winding down. Perhaps the confluence of all these events worked to move me to another plane. Though pain, fatigue, and stiffness continued, along with a sharp, persistent neckache, my condition leveled off, rather than escalated. With 2 months to go until the surgery now scheduled for mid-May, I emerged from under the mantle of unmanageable misery with a moderate increase in energy and assumed a take-charge stance.

I communicated at length with two individuals who had had THR operations within the past year. One had experienced several complications and was not recovering quickly or particularly well. The other person was very upbeat in reflecting back on the surgery and recovery. Despite these differences, I learned that both had extensive, long-term physical therapy following their operations, and also relied on a good deal of help at home following their hospital stays. The second person talked at length about the excellent decision-making process that he and his surgeon had used in choosing which type of hip implant would be optimal for him. I was becoming acutely aware of the many aspects of this experience that I had not discussed with Dr. Rigor, and the several tasks that I needed to accomplish before checking myself into the hospital.

This kind of perceptual shift involves the phenomenon that medical anthropologist Cheryl Mattingly (1998) referred to as *emplotment*, the process of an individual becoming aware of what life plot or story she is enacting at a particular point in time. The structure of lived experience stimulates the creation of narratives in two ways: a present recounting of past events and the development of new, unanticipated stories that bridge the present with the future. According to Mattingly, "Narratives, one could say, are about the unintended consequences of action....

[they] do not merely refer to past experience but create experiences" (p. 8). She further develops this concept with the notion of *therapeutic* emplotment as a means of constructively redefining an illness experience in order to find a new way to retell an old story, "a way of framing a practical decision about what to do" (p. 72). In my own case, I transitioned from a dominant plot of severe, debilitating illness that, in effect, paralyzed my ability to take action to one of a proactive patient determined to prepare for surgery.

My revised emplotment impelled new courses of action. In retrospect, it's clear that the dominant theme characterizing nearly all my actions was my attempt to gain a degree of control in a life that had slipped into disarray. I began cooking meals on weekends to freeze in readiness for when I might not be able to prepare food. I made arrangements for a physical therapist to visit my house in order to suggest what alterations would be needed during my recuperation. Gradually, I began to accumulate postsurgical equipment—crutches, a comfortable armchair, a potty seat, an extender tool for when I would not be able to bend or reach.

Other concerns were more difficult to resolve. For the first time in my adult life, I faced a period of enforced dependence (e.g., I was prohibited from driving a car for 8 weeks after surgery), and I worried about how I would manage during what I jokingly called "my confinement." Though Marlynn planned to accompany me to Houston for my hospital stay, he would soon need to resume extensive travel for his job. To my everlasting relief and gratitude, loyal friends and family from faraway places volunteered to give up pieces of their own lives to help me. I felt overwhelmed by such generosity. By mid-April, the first few visitors made their plans. My sister and two close friends would fly to Texas in succession, respectively from North Carolina, Virginia, and Minnesota, each having rearranged her own commitments at home.

Concurrently, I researched details related to the surgery. I searched the Internet, reading Web sites established by both physicians and knowledgeable patients. I poured through descriptions of hip anomalies, surgical techniques, varieties of replacement implants, and potential complications. I now gave a great deal of thought to the device that was going to become part of my body. In January, Dr. Rigor told me that he would be using minimally invasive surgery that decreased the incision by half the usual size of 8 to 12 inches. My reading on the Internet indicated that this procedure had only been practiced for about a year; the overall objective, despite differing techniques, is to reduce scarring, pain, and recovery time. I became familiar with the various materials used in the replacement implants. The devices are composed of an artificial femur bone, the femur head, and a shank fitted within a ball-like cap now predicted to last about 20 years. Contemporary femurs are commonly made of titanium, but the heads may be plastic, metal, or ceramic. The implants may be cemented to existing bone structures or "press fit" so that the natural bones eventually grow around the replacement parts, holding them in place. I had already committed to the press fit option, which requires a longer recovery but is ultimately more durable. I now looked for indications of what materials would offer me the best chance of longevity. The more I learned, the more questions I had for Dr. Rigor.

Peter, another physician, and the closest of my colleagues at the research center in Houston, talked with me about my ongoing concern about the lack of a clear plan for physical therapy. "Why didn't I think about this before?" he said. "My sister is a physical medicine/rehab doc in Pittsburgh. Let's arrange a conference call with her." I gratefully accepted that favor, and a few days later, we spoke with his sister who routinely cares for THR patients transferred to her service within 2 to 3 days following their operations. She described the range of functions with which she works with patients for an average of 3 to 5 days. Of primary importance to me was hearing her perspective of what would be involved in regaining strength and a normal gait.

Following the directions I had been given by Dr. Rigor, I e-mailed Ginny, the surgical nurse, to ask my questions. She was generous with her time and effort in providing informative answers to several concerns, and helped me to set up presurgical appointments in Houston. According to her, I would be in the hospital for 3 days and be able to make the 90-mile drive home after discharge. Opportunity for physical therapy outside the hospital was uncertain, depending on insurance coverage. Although I now leaned toward the metal-on-metal combination implant, Ginny informed me that Dr. Rigor had already determined he would use a metal and plastic combination—without input from me. I found the absence of discussion about the various options disturbing, prompting me to ask Ginny if I could have a conference with Dr. Rigor. Two weeks prior to surgery, I was due to come to Houston to make a self blood donation, a precaution taken in case I should need extra blood during the surgery, as well as to attend a patient education session with the nurses who would care for me after the operation. Ginny e-mailed that Dr. Rigor would fit me into his appointment schedule for that day. This appointment contrasted with the usual protocol. Typically, after the initial consultation, Dr. Rigor did not meet with patients again until the day before surgery. Thus, I welcomed this unexpected opportunity and looked forward to a discussion with him about issues that remained unresolved for me.

## My Plot Boils Over

> *... the fabula of story—its timeless underlying theme—seems to be a unity that incorporates at least three constituents. It contains a plight into which characters have fallen as a result of intentions that have gone awry either because of circumstances, of the "character of characters," or most likely of the interaction between the two. And it requires an uneven distribution of underlying consciousness among the characters with respect to the plight.*
>
> —Bruner, 1986, p. 21

When I arrived at the orthopedic clinic and was ushered to an exam room, Ginny greeted me cordially. I thanked her for all she had done on my behalf and gave her a small purple glass prism as a token of my appreciation. The atmosphere in the room immediately chilled as Dr. Rigor entered with a dour expression and arms crossed over his chest. "So you're the patient who has been taking up all of Ginny's time," he greeted me irritably. That remark set the tone for the visit. He began to give the same presentation I had heard in January. "You've described the operation to me before. I've been talking with other patients and doing reading, and I now have more specific questions." I had been forewarned by my rheumatologist that the surgeon might not give credence to the fibromyalgia diagnosis. I had this possibility in mind when I explained that I had experienced severe symptoms of fibromyalgia since January. I expressed concern that this condition might complicate my recovery. He answered, "It shouldn't have an effect." The tone of his response conveyed an additional message. I said, "You don't believe in fibromyalgia, do you?" "No, I don't," he confirmed. I moved on to the topic of the implant and mentioned, as a result of my reading, that I was interested in the all-metal device; I also said that I valued his expertise and wanted to hear the reasons for his selection. I had hoped to hear a convincing explanation, but his reply caught me off guard. Quite simply, he stated, this practice used the metal and plastic implants made by a particular manufacturer with all patients, and he knew them to be good products. "What about differences in age, life style, and patient preference?" I asked, futilely. "Is there clinical evidence that would help me understand why this is the best choice for me?" But there was neither further information nor negotiated decision making offered. Next question?

I moved on to the topic of rehabilitation, expressing my concern that 3 days in the hospital might not provide sufficient physical therapy. He informed me that this was the limit of insurance coverage. Acknowledging awareness of regional variations in insurance policies and surgical philosophy, I told him about my conversation with the physical medicine physician. "That's impossible," he replied. I was dumbstruck; in effect, he was saying that the other doctor was a liar. I tried another tack. "Look, once I leave here and go home, I'm on my own. I'd like to know that there is a plan in place." Again, he surprised me with his response:

> You're such a good arguer. Why don't *you* call Blue Cross and see if you can get them to approve more time in the hospital? In any event, I don't approve of your going home in 3 days. Traveling that distance in the car so soon after surgery increases your risk of a blood clot. I'd like you to remain in Houston for at least 5 days postsurgically. Seven days would be even better. You and your husband can stay in a hotel.

Ginny, who was observing, interjected her apology for giving me erroneous information. Was this prudence or punishment, I wondered? Why was I just hearing about a hotel stay now, when I had been asking these questions for 6 weeks? And still, there was no discussion of a long-term therapy plan for when I did return home.

As an afterthought, Dr. Rigor said amicably, "It's too bad that we can't offer you the better medication for preventing blood clots." I asked what that would be. "Oral medicine," he said. So what would I be receiving? "Well, you'll be injecting the medicine in your abdomen for 10 days," he stated matter-of-factly, as though I should have known. I had not heard about this part of recovery from anyone I had talked to or anything I had read. Admittedly needle-phobic, I felt myself becoming very upset at the thought of sticking myself in the stomach. "Surely you knew about this, given all your reading on the Internet," he commented dryly. Anger got the best of me. "Are there any other unpleasant surprises I should hear about?" I asked on my way out of the office. Never had I felt so disempowered in communicating with a physician.

In the days following this encounter, my discomfort with my predicament continued to increase. Could I suppress these feelings and just get through the procedure? What other options could I pursue at this late date? If I changed my plans for surgery now, what about the people who had made complicated arrangements to help me recuperate? If I delayed the surgery to find a new surgeon, who would be around later to help me and would I be forced to take a leave from work in the fall? These questions swirled about in my head over the next few days. I felt extremely unsettled by Dr. Rigor's imperious behavior and equally unhappy with myself that I had made these discoveries so late in the game. I talked through my misgivings with family and close friends. They listened sympathetically, although it was difficult for them to know how to comfort or support me. In the end, of course, *I* would have to decide what to do.

After speaking with the head nurse in the hospital unit I would be going to after surgery (a lovely, experienced woman who gave me hope that I would be in good hands despite the surgeon); a spokesperson from Blue Cross (who confirmed the 3-day limit, but also told me that if the doctor wanted me to stay longer in the hospital, the insurance would uphold his judgment); my local physicians (who reminded me that I did not have to go through with this surgery); and even a representative from a competing hospital (who said that I would be receiving comparable treatment at both institutions), I was still trying to make this situation work, but additional questions had arisen. At the risk of further evoking Dr. Rigor's ill-will, I felt I had to speak up—it was now or never. Again, I e-mailed Ginny, but she wrote back saying Dr. Rigor would be contacting me, himself, by phone. And call he did, but without information about our respective schedules, there ensued 4 days of frustrating telephone tag. Finally, on a Thursday morning, 5 days before the scheduled surgery, I reached him. Apparently with my e-mail in hand, he proceeded to give terse replies to my questions, again, with no hint of give and take, only an attitude of "This is how it will be." In the course of answering queries, he now revised the time that Marlynn and I would be staying in Houston postsurgery to 10 days ("I'm looking out my window at the medical center Radisson. You could stay there.") When he finished going through my questions, he asked, perfunctorily, "Anything else?" "Yes," I responded. "I'm very afraid of going into surgery with someone who is so pissed off at me." If Dr. Rigor was surprised in any way, he did not show it. "It's true," he agreed.

> I did not like your behavior in my office last week—that remark about "unpleasant surprises" was out of line. You have a bad attitude, you're high maintenance, and if we weren't so close to the date of surgery, I'd advise you to find another surgeon. Nonetheless, I'm a professional. I can separate my feelings from my work. I'll be able to perform your surgery just fine. You know, you really ought to talk with your colleague Kathy about the hip replacement I did for her mom. I'll see you on Monday.

End of conversation.

I was livid. There was no way I wanted to see Dr. Rigor again, let alone for him to perform my surgery. Even if he could pretend to separate his personal feelings from his work, as a patient, I had no such obligations or pretensions. Psychiatrist Arthur Kleinman (1988) is one of the foremost progenitors of the idea that physicians, as well as patients, create stories as a way of representing their respective explanatory models of illness. Dr. Rigor and I were far beyond Kleinman's distinction between doctors' narratives of disease, characterized by verifiable signs of organic disorder, and patients' narratives of illness, characterized by the fears, concerns, and experiences of living with a disordered body, in effect, "dis-ease." In addition to all of that, we did not like each other. He thought I was uppity and time consuming; I thought he was authoritarian and insulting. In no way did we see eye to eye about how patients and physicians should relate to one another or how medical decisions should be made. Yet, interestingly, both our stories were constrained by an encroaching deadline, the day of surgery. Dr. Rigor felt bound to honor his commitment to do the operation. I felt bound both by the arrangements that had been made by others to help me and also the knowledge that, if the surgery were to be delayed and rescheduled at some unknown time, I might be left with no one available to help. Time had run out, and I had to reach a final decision.

## Intersecting Narratives

> *To think with a story is to experience its affecting one's own life and to find in that effect a certain truth of one's life.*
> —Frank, 1995, p. 23

A vignette that I had read in a book a few years earlier came to mind almost immediately after my phone call with Dr. Rigor. In her autobiographical memoir, *The Scalpel and the Silver Bear*, Lori Arviso Alvord, self-described as the first Navajo woman surgeon, shares how she has attempted to integrate the Native American healing traditions with which she was raised with her education in Western biomedical practices (Alvord & Van Pelt, 1999). She recalls a gall-bladder surgery she did on a Navajo reservation that went very wrong when the patient unexpectedly suffered a stroke that resulted in severe disabilities. In retrospect, Dr. Alvord tries to understand why some procedures go badly, despite the skillfulness of the surgeon. Pondering this problem from a Navajo perspective, she comes to a realization that all matters related to the surgical situation must be harmonious and in balance. In her terms, if the healer fails to set an example for the patient to "walk in beauty," there are likely to be poor medical outcomes. In reviewing the circumstances in which this particular surgery had taken place, Dr. Alvord recognized that she had substituted for a sick colleague without first establishing a trusting relationship with the patient. During the operation, a new nurse made several errors, was inattentive, then defensive when corrected, and she [Dr. Alvord] herself had been angry and stressed. From that point on, she resolved to find ways to maximize harmony in the surgical suite. In recalling this memoir, I became acutely aware that I was not only angry with Dr. Rigor (and he with me);

I also fearful of his doing this procedure. With so much disharmony in this situation, I did not believe the surgery could or would go well. Dr. Alvord's story strongly resonated with my own and helped me to be in touch with the full range of emotions that I had been resisting, in the hopes that things would work out.

A few hours later that day, I decided to act on Dr. Rigor's recommendation and speak with my colleague, Kathy, in Houston about her mother's experience. I had not done so earlier, assuming that Kathy would underscore Dr. Rigor's surgical prowess (after all, he would not have wanted me to talk with her unless he was sure she would tell me a success story). In retrospect, I admit that assumption was a huge mistake. In fact, Kathy corroborated that her mother's surgery had gone very well and that her mother and Dr. Rigor had a good relationship. "But, Barbara, I wish you had come to me before. Dr. Rigor was great for my mom, because she asks no questions. I never would have recommended him for *you*." Hearing Kathy's rendition of her mother's interactions with the surgeon helped me understand in a deeper way why things had gone so poorly between him and me. At the same time, I was aggravated at myself for not having had this conversation with Kathy much sooner.

Coincidentally, my friend, Peter, e-mailed from Houston that afternoon, asking how things were going. I wrote back a short summary of the disasterous conversation with Dr. Rigor. Peter asked me to call him at home that evening. By the time I finished the workday, I was emotionally distraught. Marlynn was in Minnesota, tending to another problematic family situation. To further complicate matters, our telephone lines at home were out of order, so I spent most of that evening with friends who provided the comfort of their presence, allowing me both to verbalize my thoughts with them and to make and receive calls from their phone.

After several attempts, I finally reached Peter at his home. Both he and his wife Maria are physicians. They have also been patients through four high-risk pregnancies that followed the problematic birth of their first child. Of the four high-risk babies, each fervently desired and named soon after conception, one died 4 days after birth, and the next two were lost in miscarriage; the fourth child survived a harrowing pregnancy that had threatened the lives of both mother and baby. Peter had previously shared with me a very personal essay he had written that focused not only on the circumstances of the four pregnancies, but more emphatically about the doctor–patient relationships, both bad and good, that influenced the management and outcomes of these life events. Their first obstetrician had been inattentive to the physical signs of fetal distress and remained oblivious to Maria's and Peter's fragile emotional states. The second obstetrician, who managed the last three pregnancies, grew more sensitive over time to their suffering. She came to be an integral part, even a co-author, of their story. At the same time, both Maria and Peter found better ways to voice their needs and fears. Through his own emotionally stressful experiences, Peter became a firm believer in active patient involvement as an essential component of patient–physician partnership and clinical decision making.

The story of Peter, Maria, and their babies was unspoken but definitely present that Thursday night when he and I spoke. "Maria and I have talked about your situation. Do you want my advice?" Yes, I indicated. Peter minced no words. "Fire this guy. What he said to you was inexcusable." I agreed, but I expressed my worries about the consequences of canceling the surgery. Peter's next words put my concerns into a reordered perspective.

> If you delay having the surgery now, your friends will make adjustments; things will work out. If I need to come stay with you at a later time, I will. But if you go to surgery with this doctor, and for whatever reasons, it doesn't go well, you will forever regret having done so. And even if the surgery does go well, this guy doesn't like you, he will be trying to avoid you afterward, and will not be looking for what he needs to be seeing. You will not get the care you need and deserve.

Then he added, "Remember the story I shared with you about our obstetricians?" This conversation, informed both by Peter's experiences as a physician and as a patient, was the last story I needed to hear that night. All three narratives that had intersected with my own during the course of this pivotal day settled the doubts that had so greatly been troubling me.

The next day, I found an e-mail message from Ginny written late the night before. She wrote, "I know I would try to learn all I could, if I were having surgery, just as you are. I believe you are going to do very well, and will be happy with the outcome of your surgery. I'll see you Monday!" That afternoon, I called to cancel my Monday appointment and my surgery on Tuesday. Dr. Rigor had left for the day, as had Ginny. Since he has no voice- or e-mail, I wrote a letter, detailing my reasons for canceling. I wasn't yet sure what my next step would be, but a huge weight had been lifted—of that I was certain.

## POSTSCRIPT

*What we are finding is that after writing about traumatic experiences, unlike writing about superficial topics, individuals begin talking more*

*to their friends, laughing more, and using more positive emotions in their daily language.*
                                              —Pennebaker, 2000, p. 14

I was unbelievably fortunate. I spoke with the director of the research center in Houston, who agreed that neither Dr. Rigor nor I would be at our respective best for the surgery. She offered to make some phone calls on my behalf. The next Thursday, Marlynn and I had an appointment with the orthopedic surgeon from the competing hospital. Although it was late in the afternoon, he spent over an hour examining me, explaining his surgical philosophy, and answering my questions. He agreed with my preference for the implant, and he was able to cite the most recent research comparing the efficacy of various devices. His rule was that I could put 50% of my weight on the operated leg after the surgery, which meant more mobility and no hopping on one foot. Barring complications, he said I would go home on the third day after surgery. He promised that I would be given a physical therapy plan to practice at home. As we left his office, I felt the pain in my neck that had bothered me for months perceptibly ease. My sister and friends managed to change airline reservations and places with one another so that all were able to travel to Texas without penalty. I underwent a successful THR one week after the original operation had been scheduled. My chaos narrative had finally ended.

It wasn't a perfect experience. I still had to have blood thinners injected into my stomach (adeptly administered by my sister). Two days after the drive home, the operated leg swelled to twice the size of the other one and turned amazing shades of red, purple and chartreuse from thigh to toe, necessitating a scary trip to the local emergency room to test for a blood clot (luckily, it was not). I still fatigue easily and experience severe pain from time to time when I overexert physically. Progress is not continuous, but rather a jagged back and forth. On the flip side, although I am not moving as well or as gracefully as I might like, I am making constant strides and doing so much better compared to how I was a year ago. In retrospect, although I remain angry with Dr. Rigor on several counts, I have an appreciation for his candor, which ultimately contributed to reshaping the conclusion to my story.

## REFLECTIONS

*... there is nothing as theoretical as a good story.*
                                              —Bochner, 1998, p. 349

Throughout my recovery and in thinking through how I would approach writing this chapter, my story of illness and healing transitioned into the third genre identified by Frank, the *quest narrative*. According to Frank (1995), "Quest stories meet suffering head on; they accept illness and seek to *use* it" (p. 115). This autoethnographic essay (Ellis, 1997) pays homage to some of the many scholars who have significantly contributed to my own understanding of the concept of illness narrative while simultaneously seeking to unpack the several layers of meaning that comprise my own. My final task is to identify how my particular saga relates to narrative theory more generally, as well as to an enhanced concept of *patienthood*.

I consider, first, the ways in which narrative makes meaning(s). My illness narrative fulfills five previously identified, socially constructive functions (Arntson & Droge, 1987; Sharf & Vanderford, 2003). In telling this story, I attempt to *make sense* of my experiences, using collected memories, journal entries, and archived e-mails. It is chronologically structured, but a chronicle is not the endpoint; the plot focuses on figuring out how and why I dealt with a problematic physician–patient relationship in the ways that I did. In so doing, the story also *warrants* (and occasionally critiques) the decisions that I made. Not surprisingly, by having the last word in retrospect, I succeed in *re-gaining a sense of control* that was often lost to me while many of these events actually occurred. Perhaps less predictable, my story reflects *changes in self-identity* that morphed with the stages of sickness I experienced, illustrating that it can be extremely difficult to be a coherent, resonant storyteller in the midst of an ordeal. The construction of an illness narrative (or any story of suffering) requires some form of perspective, whether through the passage of time, feedback from a listener, or some other structure that invites reflection on the story told, even as the story is being lived (Allison, 1994). Finally, this account works to *build community*, though not in ways I have thought about before. I do not seek to entice readers to unite against authoritarian physicians or identify with me, a character who is not a heroine, but a highly flawed, often confused participant in this drama. In the end (for I did not have this intention going into this project), I judge it to be a cautionary tale, a story with a moral imperative of sorts, that invites audiences to consider what not to do, how to look for danger signs of an unworkable relationship earlier on, and how to get out of the mire.

A second implication of this work is the relationship between narrative resolution and patient participation. Two concepts that constitute active patient participation are *engagement with one's illness experience* and *negotiation of decision-making* between providers and patients (Sharf, Haidet, & Kroll, 2005). Dr. Rigor and I were at ideological odds about our clinical relationship; he declined any attempts I initiated to negotiate with him. To remain as his patient would have meant conceding all control of decision making to him, the scenario that ostensibly provoked my dilemma.

The less obvious aspect in the plot centers on *engagement*, a sense that one can influence the course of one's own experience of illness and health-seeking versus *fatalism*, a sense that one's illness course is predetermined and unchangeable. Envisioning engagement as a continuum, I place myself closer to the engaged end, but not all the way there. And why not? I became stuck! Feeling trapped in a chaos narrative, I became so embedded in one version that I was unable to envision alternative sequences. Not perceiving variant endings resulted in a period of emotional upheaval and a temporary inability to take actions in my own behalf. Conversations with a few key *intercessors*, friends who, in effect, got between me and a predetermined bad ending, helped me to interpret the development of my story differently and to see that alternative emplotments were possible, despite time constraints.[1] Once I was able to get unstuck, to perceive options still available to me, I felt empowered, energized, and capable of taking actions instrumental to actualizing a different and improved story. Clearly, the process of moving toward full engagement is a major struggle, even for a person who has relevant expertise, access to information, personal and social voice, ample interpersonal support, privileged connections, and financially feasible alternatives. For individuals lacking many or all of these resources, overcoming a sense of fatalism and overpowering chaos would be extremely onerous at best.

The final consideration I would like to address involves the *exponential power* of narrative, that is, the resulting force of stories that build on one another to deepen and accentuate meaning. Narratives derive from specific circumstances at particular points in time with characters having individual needs, motives, and emotions in context with one another. Through their creation, narratives consciously shape historical understandings of the events to which they refer and may also have immediate impact in terms of actions and choices in the moment. Stories also indefinitely lodge in fluid sociocultural spaces, what Burke (1957) referred to as "the 'unending conversation' going on in history" (p. 97) that allows them to be recollected and recreated in entirely different situations, achieving influence in ways not anticipated by the original storytellers. This aspect was particularly evident in how Lori Alvord's tale of surgery gone awry and Peter's and Maria's rendition of personal struggle in the attempt to have healthy babies somehow became interwoven with my own account. Furthermore, I am convinced that juxtaposing them in the course of one critical day significantly increased their impact on my own story.

In a unique sense, these stories served as a significant source of social support at the time I needed to make a decision about whether or not to stick with my originally planned surgery. Many individuals—my husband, sister, close friends and colleagues—who were there to listen sympathetically as I weepingly talked with them about my dilemma, later confided that they were pleased that I made the decision to part ways with Dr. Rigor. However, they felt constrained in sharing that opinion at the time, anticipating quite sensibly that should I decide to go ahead with the original surgery, they would have further undermined my trust in him, negatively impacting the outcome. They carefully maintained neutrality in offering comfort and support. Of all my confidants, only Peter gave me direct advice, impelled by his story of the difference it had made to have an obstetrician that he and Maria felt was on their side. Stories cannot be neutral; they convey a point of view, a particular perspective. The tales about poor outcomes related to problematic patient–physician relationships clearly and strongly made implicit, persuasive arguments that reflected on my own situation, and ultimately made an important difference in shaping my narrative.

Just a few last thoughts. I realize that Dr. Rigor—if he bothers to think about this episode at all—has a different version of this story to tell, which is his prerogative, but he will need to find his own venue. Writing this chapter has forced me to reconsider and search for lessons from a difficult experience. The process of storytelling has a force all its own.

## NOTES

1. Thanks to Paul Haidet and Tony Kroll for their help in understanding the role of narrative embeddedness, alternatives, and intercessors in the unfolding of this tale.
2. I am most grateful to Dr. Christina Beck for encouraging me to commit to this essay at a time when I felt incapable of taking it on and to Dr. Carolyn Ellis for her insightful, supportive feedback.

# 16

## "My Mom Had a Stroke": Understanding How Patients Raise and Providers Respond to Psychosocial Concerns

∾

**Wayne A. Beach**
*San Diego State University*

**Jenny Mandelbaum**
*Rutgers University*

In the following transcribed excerpts, drawn from a routine medical interview, a patient repeatedly discloses that "My mom had a stroke." On three different occasions, over the course of a single medical encounter, the patient invokes his mom's illness as a significant factor influencing key health behaviors that are eventually discussed: excessive drinking, inadequate exercise and diet, and sleeplessness. However, he does so in the midst of producing other actions: (a) explaining his drinking, (b) offering mild disagreement with the interviewer, a physician's assistant (PA), and (c) explaining why he does not exercise. In response, despite patient's repeatedly invoking the serious impact that his mother's stroke has had on his life and his health, interviewer does not take up these psychosocial matters, nor even minimally acknowledge them. Because the patient presents these serious lifeworld experiences three times, at times quite dramatically, it seems anomalous that the PA does not address them in some way.

This chapter focuses on how patients present and interviewers respond to psychosocial problems during medical encounters. We reveal how it comes about that the interviewer pursues a biomedical agenda in lieu of addressing patient's health-relevant issues (e.g., see Maynard, 1991; Beach, 2001; Beach, Good, Pigeron, & Easter, in press; Heritage & Maynard, in press; Roter & Hall, 1992; Stivers, 2002), actively drawing attention toward bodily symptoms—blood in his stools, a pancreas damaged by alcohol, high cholesterol, high blood pressure, and excess weight—and not taking up concerns that are made available, and could be heard as "root" (Barbour, 1995; Felitti et al, 1998) or psychosocial problems underlying the patient's symptoms: stress caused by being a caregiver for both his mother and father. Although the patient makes it clear that he takes these commitments seriously, he also frames his caregiving efforts as rational explanations contributing to his poor health habits.

More specifically, we examine how, in each instance, the patient raises "Mom's stroke" not as the focal, or main action of his turn, but rather as part of the implementing action, or vehicle for producing the focal or main action (i.e., the psychosocial impacts of caring for family members):

- In Excerpt 1, he introduces the matter of his mother's stroke as part of an account for, or justification of, his drinking;

- In Excerpt 2, he offers "Mom's stroke" in order to note the onset of his drinking, as a way of disagreeing with the PA's claim that his stomach ailments might be related to his pancreas;

- In the third occasion (Excerpt 3), patient invokes "Mom's stroke" to account for his failure to exercise.

In each case, the matter of his mother's stroke and the problematic implications her condition has for his life, are raised in the service of some other action—indirectly, not as something to be addressed in its own right. In the ways these matters are introduced and structured, then, the PA is not sequentially obligated to take up the patient's psychosocial, lifeworld issues. They are not announced as the "main business" of the turns in which they occur. Rather, their introduction is subordinate to, or a vehicle for, other primary and ongoing actions. For instance, they are not introduced as announcements of good or bad news, to which some sort of response to and eventual appreciation of the valence of the news delivery would be relevant (see Beach, 2002; Maynard, 1997, 2003). Nor does the patient initiate story prefaces seeking the interviewer's alignment before producing an extended telling (e.g., see Beach, 2001; Jefferson, 1978; Mandelbaum 1989; Sacks, 199).

For example, over 30 years ago, Terasaki (1976; also in press) observed how talk that may appear to do the work of "announcing" may not be treated by the next speakers as an "announcement." "It appears that features of the design and placement of the item in the overall structure of the conversation contribute as much to its recognition as do content considerations." (p. 3).[1] Kitzinger (2000)[2] also notes that a similar phenomenon can occur in utterances in which speakers "come out" as lesbians or as intersexual. Speakers may "embed" their coming out in a position that it is not presented as "announcing" news for appropriate acknowledgment, uptake, and assessment. Coming out, in these instances, is not the primary activity. Rather, it is embedded in other social actions, and it is these other activities that get taken up by next speaker: "*Not* presenting information about one's sexuality as news has decisive consequences for shaping the course of the talk's development. If it is not announced as news, recipients have to work hard to receive it as such." (Kitzinger, 2000, p. 185).

The interviewer in the case examined faces a similar predicament. Although psychosocial matters are raised, they are in each case embedded by the patient as accomplishing some other actions (i.e., accounting, disagreeing), and produced in such a way that it is these actions that are made relevant to be taken up by the PA. We now consider both how this embedding of psychosocial matters is recurrently achieved as well as the consequences of their embedding for interviewer's responses throughout this medical interview. In lieu of directness, scholars widely recognize the offering of cues or clues as common behaviors produced by patients during medical encounters (e.g., see Beach et al., in press; Gill, 1998; Gill, Halkowski, & Roberts, 2001)—resources for introducing psychosocial matters impacting emotional and physical health and thus, the quality of life. Because interviewers do not actively seek what patients only hint at, one consequence is that no "official" attention is provided for them to be addressed during interaction. However, as will be evident, patients' indirectness is not tantamount to the lack of significance for health and well-being. Thus, the findings of this study provide clear implications for both patients (in terms of how they present issues that have relevance to their health, but which interviewers may not ask about), and for interviewers (in terms of pursuing psychosocial matters that may have health relevance, even if they are raised only tangentially).

While attending to patients' concerns clearly does occur (e.g., see Beach & Dixson, 2001; Beach & LeBaron, 2002), recent research has consistently revealed a host of delicate moments arising from patients' attempts to describe and offer lay diagnoses of their condition (see Beach, 2001; Gill et al., 2001; Jones & Beach, in press; Peräkylä, 2002; J. D. Robinson, 2001; Stivers & Heritage, 2001). One primary set of social activities involves moments where patients voluntarily elaborate about their lifeworld circumstances, raising matters that could be heard to extend beyond what care providers were focusing on in prior questions. Within these elaborations, patients often disclose primary concerns, matters that may or may not be aligned with biomedical diagnoses but are nevertheless put forward as concerns. This chapter shows three environments in which this can occur, and explains how it is that a care provider could come to fail to take up a patient's psychosocial concerns. Our analysis addresses each of three instances involving "Mom's stroke" in the order in which they occurred. The contiguous nature of these social activities is thus preserved and used as a resource for this analysis. Observations can then be offered not only about each set of moments, but also their serial and cumulative organization over the course of a single medical encounter. Implications for communication and patient-centered care is raised and elaborated.

## DATA AND METHOD

Interactional materials are drawn from a corpus of videorecorded and transcribed medical encounters within a large health maintenance organization (HMO) located in the southwest United States. All names and references to individual's identities have been removed to guarantee anonymity of speakers—PA and a 43-year-old male patient undergoing an annual health appraisal. The presenting problem nominated by the patient at the beginning of the interview is severe, persistent diarrhea.

Conversation analytic (CA) methods are employed (see Atkinson & Heritage, 1984; Drew & Heritage, 1992; Heritage & Maynard, in press; Pomerantz & Fehr, 1997; Sacks, 1992). This mode of analytic induction is anchored in repeated examination of recordings, in unison with systematic inspections of carefully produced transcriptions. Priority is given to locating and substantiating participants' methods for organizing and thus accomplishing social actions. It is an explicit and working assumption of this research method that participants continually and intrinsically achieve, through an array of interactional practices, displayed understandings of emergent interactional circumstances. The overriding goal, in examination of both ordinary/casual and institutional (e.g., medical) encounters, is to identify and describe patterns in interaction through which everyday life events are socially constructed.

## DRINKING AS A DELICATE MATTER

Excerpt 1 begins with a series of progressive and increasingly specific questions by the PA about the frequency, quantity, and nature of patient's drinking behaviors (see Appendix with transcription symbols):

1. "Do you drink?": #2:3-4

INT:    <u>Do</u> you <u>drink</u>?

PAT:    Um hm.

INT:    <u>How</u> often do you <u>drink</u>?

PAT:    <u>I</u> usually have something °everyday° before >I <u>go</u> to bed<.

INT:    Okay and about how many drinks per day [do you drink]?

PAT:    [ Maybe three].

INT:    And what <u>is</u> it that you're <u>drink</u>ing?

PAT:    Usually <u>vod</u>ka a:n: (0.2) °some kinda mixer ↑diet (.) seven <u>up</u>°
        [or something.]

INT:    [°O k a y °. .hh] Now. (.) <u>drinks</u> (0.2) in: the <u>con</u>text of
        des<u>crip</u>tion uh <u>usu</u>ally has different <u>mean</u>ings ta different
        peo<u>ple</u>? .hh About <u>what</u> <u>quan</u>tity per <u>drink</u> would you say
        that you're having.

PAT:    In terms of fingers or [$uh heh heh heh heh huh$].

INT:                       [Yeah. Are you- are yo    ]u having a
                       <u>shot</u>? Are you <u>having</u>
    a:=

PAT:    =>Probably about a shot<.=

INT:    =°I see.° .hhh [And you-

PAT:    [>But that isn't- I mean <u>that's</u> just been in the la:st< (.)
        f:<u>our</u> years or <u>five</u> years that I've been  [°doing that °  ].

INT:                               [>But you've b]een
                  doing that everyday<
    (.) for the past four or five ye[ars?

PAT:                             [↑Pretty mu:ch. (.)

INT:    °Okay.° (.)

PAT: →   **My mom had a <u>stroke</u> (.) five years ago and u:h I <u>have</u> to
        go every night after work and help (.) my dad out with
        her <u>so:</u> = .hh when I come <u>home</u> just ta un<u>wind</u> $I have
        a few drinks$ and then >go to bed<.**

INT: →   Have you ever noticed any **<u>blo:od</u> in your stools or <u>bla:ck</u> stools?**

Notice that once interviewer establishes patient's drinking, he next
queries "<u>How</u> often do you <u>drink</u>?" Patient's response, "<u>I</u> usually have
something (everyday) before >I <u>go</u> to bed<." leaves unspecified both
an exact *frequency* and what he drinks. Yet, his drinking most "°every-
day°" makes available a potential drinking problem for the interviewer
to subsequently address, although it is not offered here *as* a problem.
Note that the patient volunteers that he drinks prior to going to bed.
Later in this excerpt, he makes clear that he seeks to unwind following
a day of work and caring for his mom and dad.

PA next continues to gather information by addressing the quantity
of patient's drinking. His "Okay" responds to patient's prior contribution by minimally acknowledging it before moving into a next question,

"and about how many drinks per day do you drink?" (see Beach, 1993, 1995). This "Okay" action provides a brief glimpse into one resource employed for keeping the discussion focused and on track to accomplish an agenda an interviewer is pursuing at any given point in time.

It is of some interest across the excerpts analyzed herein, then, that the initial attempt by the patient to volunteer even minimal information is met with some enforcement: Subtly but decidedly away from topics and issues indirectly raised by the patient, and thus not raised by the interviewer as he relies on "Okay" to move the medical encounter forward on his own terms.

It could be argued that, in providing the information regarding <u>when</u> he drinks ("before I go to bed"), the patient might be making available to the PA something that could be heard to be related to why he drinks. It is clearly not germane to how much he drinks, but locates it in the patient's day, and could be heard to be the beginnings of an account (explanation) for why he drinks (Buttny, 1993; Heritage, 1983; Scott & Lyman, 1968). Mentioning the timing of the drinking when it has not been actively solicited could be heard to be a way of making available to the physician that there could be more to report regarding the drinking, such as the reason for it, that may be tied to when it occurs. This is not made actively relevant in any way, but the provision of a piece of unsolicited information could make available to the PA the opportunity to probe further in order seek a reason for its provision. The PA merely acknowledges the information and moves on to the next question regarding how much the patient drinks.

In overlap ( [ ] ) and response, patient's "Maybe three." suggests that an exact "metric" for assessing "how many" drinks is an ambiguous task (see Halkowski, 2000). So too is providing an exact answer to interviewer's next "And what <u>is</u> it that you're <u>drink</u>ing?," as patient again qualifies that it is usually vodka and some kind of mixer. It is this interplay, between the interviewer's seeking specific answers and the patient's repeated offerings of hedging and inexact assessments, that his next question is designed to elicit a more specific quantification of how much the patient actually drinks:

> 2. "In terms of fingers": #2:3
> PAT:      Usually <u>vod</u>ka a:n: (0.2) °some kinda mixer ┼<u>diet</u> (.) seven <u>up</u> °
>              [or something.]
> INT:      [°O k a y °. .hh ] Now. (.) <u>drinks</u> (0.2) in: the <u>con</u>text of
>              <u>descrip</u>tion uh <u>usually</u> has different <u>mean</u>ings ta different
>              peo<u>ple</u>? .hh About <u>what</u> <u>quan</u>tity per <u>drink</u> would you say
>              that you're having?
> PAT: **1→** In terms of fingers or [$uh heh heh heh heh huh$].

```
INT:                          [Yeah. Are you- are yo ]u having a
           shot? Are you having a:=
PAT:       =>Probably about a shot<.=
INT:       =°I see.° .hhh [And you-
PAT: 2→                    [>But that isn't- I mean that's just been in the
           la:st< (.) f:our years or five years that I've been [°doing that ° ].
INT: 3→         [>But you've b]een doing that everyday<
           (.) for the past four or five ye [ars?
PAT:                                        [↑Pretty mu:ch. (.)
INT:       °Okay.°
```

First, PA's "°Okay.°" acknowledges the patient's response of "-diet
(.) seven up °[or something.]", closing this sequence. "Now" shows
that he is moving on to something else that could be heard to have its
basis in what precedes it. Because descriptions of quantity mean
different things to different persons, the interviewer seeks a more
specific "objective" measure from the patient. Patient offers a candidate metric: "In terms of fingers or [$uh heh heh heh heh huh$]."
As patient raises his left hand for interviewer's inspection, he
forms different finger combinations (one to three) to symbolically
portray possible measures for the amount of liquor in a glass. The
fact that patient's verbal and visual depiction are followed by laughter ($uh heh heh heh heh huh$) may mark the somewhat awkward
yet humorous and even delicate nature of his gesture and topic.
Although the activity "at hand" (literally, in this instance) could
simply be constructed by the patient as funny, the patient also exhibits awareness that the problem he addresses—quantity of alcohol consumed—is ultimately a serious matter requiring resolution.
Discussing excessive drinking is delicate in almost any environment, particularly a medical one (see Haakana, 2001). Discussing
such personal matters with a stranger also contributes to the delicacy of these moments.
    In overlap, the interviewer translates the patient's "fingers" analogy
and gesture into a more common metric—"a shot?"—which patient's
"Probably about a shot." essentially confirms as a reasonable estimate
and the interviewer quietly responds with °I see.°. It is here (2 →), before the interviewer can complete what appears to be a next question
("And you-"), that the patient qualifies the amount of his drinking by
stating that he's only been drinking like that "in the la:st < (.) four years
or five years." This oblique reference to "the last four or five years"
could make available to the PA that there is some circumstance that began 4 or 5 years ago that prompted the drinking. Similar to "before I go
to bed," this information is not directly sought by the PA, and although

it is hearably relevant to the current project (providing an objective measure of how much the patient drinks) it offers another kind of objective measure of how long the drinking has been going on, and raises an unexplained question: Why 4 or 5 years? While this issue constitutes something the PA could take up, it is packaged in the service of minimizing the longevity of the drinking, and thus is not officially proffered as that on which talk should now be focused: It is produced officially in the service of quantifying the drinking, rather than raising psychosocial matters that might have prompted the drinking.

The prior sequence is possibly complete at this point. Indeed, the PA has acknowledged the patient's response that he has "probably about a shot" with "I see," showing that this question has received its answer and that the sequence is closed. Thus, patient's attempt to minimize the extent of the drinking by limiting it to the past 4 or 5 years reopens it, providing for the possibility of further talk regarding this matter. Again, the PA is not put in the position where actively pursuing a psychosocial matter is made directly relevant, because it is raised officially in the service of quantifying the drinking. That he provides this attempt to delimit the extent of his drinking at this moment may also evidence his recognition that he could be found at fault for excessive drinking—and seeks to minimize possible blame associated with his actions (e.g., see Beach, 1996; Heritage, 1983). Thus, patient may be seeking to situate his drinking within significant (as yet unarticulated) lifeworld events.

In response (3→), interviewer checks his understanding of patient's quantification of his drinking. The words the patient provided for characterizing the extent of the drinking are used by interviewer as a counter assertion (see Beach, 1996; M. H. Goodwin, 1990) for characterizing the extent of the drinking. The patient then confirms this hearing, and PA's "Okay" shows that he takes it that this sequence is closed.

This action is, curiously, akin to how cross-examining attorneys do not simply query opposing/unfriendly witnesses but construct accusations shaped to attribute wrongdoing and even challenge the believability of witnesses' stories/testimony (see Atkinson & Drew, 1979; Drew, 1978, 1985, 1992; Metzger & Beach, 1996). Here, interviewer's not taking up the patient's reference to "f:our or five years" bears resemblance to some modes of interrogation designed to restrict contributions from question recipient. On such occasions, it is not uncommon for those whose narratives (or potential narratives) have somehow been constrained or challenged— as with courtroom witnesses and even during news interviews (see Clayman & Heritage, 2002)—to continue by offering a fuller explanation substantiating their position, defending their argument, or even pleading for their innocence. The patient orients here to the problematic character of drinking to this extent, and seeks to provide some psychosocial information that explains and justifies this extensive drinking. Such an explanation is not actively sought by the PA—he has shown with his sequence closing turn, "Okay," that he takes this sequence to be officially closed. However, it may be generated by a possible hearing of the PA's understanding check, "But you've been doing that everyday (.) for the past four or five years?" as also embodying an accusation or critique of the patient.

The patient then uses this opportunity to provide an account of what happened 5 years ago that could be heard to at least explain what could have prompted this drinking:

3. "My mom had a stroke": #2:4
PAT:  →   My mom had a <u>stroke</u> (.) five years ago and u:h I h<u>ave</u> to <u>go</u>
          every night after work and he<u>lp</u> (.) my dad out with her <u>so:</u>
          = .hh when I come <u>home</u> just ta un<u>wind</u> $I have a few
          drinks$ and then >go to bed<.
INT:  →   Have you ever noticed any <u>blo:od</u> in your stools or <u>bla:ck</u>
          stools?

This excerpt begins with a report of his mother's stroke. As Kitzinger (2000) noted with regard to "coming out," his mother's illness is presented at a point in the utterance (here, in the beginning), such that it is not presented as an announcement to be responded to. Rather, it is followed by a report of his obligation: "I have to go every night after work and help (.) my dad out with her." This volunteered information further legitimates the extremity of his situation (see Pomerantz, 1986)—a caregiving obligation from which there is little "time out"—efforts aiding both his ill mother and dad (presumably, mom's primary caregiver).

Importantly, however, he next formulates ("so:") that his drinking is a consequence of his caregiving efforts. In this way, he clearly accounts for having a few drinks. The report is produced quite overtly in the service of explaining how (and why) he comes to be drinking so much.

As patient volunteers "when I come <u>home</u> just ta un<u>wind</u> $I have a few drinks$," additional and key information is disclosed: (a) A need to "un<u>wind</u>," which implies ongoing stress; (b) A delicate orientation to drinking, marked by laughter ($$) demonstrating patient's awareness that a discrepancy exists between his drinking and what good, appropriate patients might do to preserve their health (Haakana, 2001). As noted, such actions are routine during medical interviews, particularly when patients portray their behaviors as knowingly unfavorable and thus potentially unhealthy. Through these efforts, it is clear that the patient works to account for his drinking as a resource for coping with difficult family responsibilities. He also designs his account to better inform interviewer of the difficult life circumstances he is facing. Such an account could make relevant an offering of reassurance and compassion about his troubling situation (actions discussed in the conclusion of this chapter). However, because it is produced specifically as a postexpansion of a series of exchanges regarding the quantity of his drinking, the PA could possibly hear it merely as accounting for these actions. Further, the mention of his mother's stroke is positioned at the beginning of this unit of talk, removing it as far as possible from the part of the turn designed to be responded to. That is, although the life circumstances the patient produces could be taken up here, they are produced at the beginning of the turn, not as an announcement for immediate response, but rather in service of another action: accounting for excessive drinking. They are not produced as an announcement in their own right. Their position in this part of the interaction—as the reopening of sequence (question by PA, answer by patient, acknowledgment by PA), providing a report of circumstances that can be heard to be accounting for the facts established in the immediately prior sequence—mean that the interviewer is not put in the position of "having" to respond to the psychosocial concerns that are the vehicle for the action of accounting for the quantity of drinking. Yet the patient raises serious life concerns, framing them as directly relevant to (that is to say, generative of) the health-related matter currently under discussion.

In the next turn, interviewer continues with, "Have you ever noticed any <u>blo:od</u> in your stools or <u>bla:ck</u> stools?" While bloody or black stools may be symptomatic of damage caused by excessive drinking, and thus are biomedically relevant, the interviewer can be seen here to be missing a prime opportunity to support and talk further about the serious, and clearly closely associated issue that the patient has depicted. As interviewer chooses not to deviate from "the biomedical agenda," a "window of opportunity" for being empathic and connecting with the patient has thus been passed by (see Bellet & Maloney, 1991; Branch & Malick, 1993; Lang, Floyd, & Beline, 2000; Spiegel, 1999; Suchman, Markakis, Beckman, & Frankel, 1997). His lack of uptake overlooks the patient's disclosure of directly relevant, personally private, and delicate information. Moreover, the significance of the patient's "lay diagnosis" (Beach, 2001) for treatment and possible referral is (at this moment) left hanging. Essentially, the interviewer chooses to sustain a focus on physiological matters in lieu of a practical description of his directly relevant daily lifeworld experiences.

## Summary

To briefly summarize Excerpts 1 through 3, patient's initial and tangential raising of the family context influencing his drinking were not pursued by the PA. The patient's subsequent and fuller depiction about "my mom had a stroke," produced to account for his heavy drinking, is not taken up. Instead, interviewer pursues his questions about physiological matters. Although the patient has progressively introduced details of his psychosocial situation, often as subordinate rather than focal matters, interviewer has chosen to focus exclusively on biomedical concerns. This option is in no small part made available by the way the patient raises these concerns (i.e., as an account rather than an announcement, and located in a part of the turn that removes it from that which is directly response relevant).

## A DISMAYED RESPONSE

The patient's second reference to mom's stroke occurs approximately 9 minutes following Excerpts 1 through 3, soon after the completion of a physical examination, and thus during a phase of diagnosis and treatment (Byrne & Long, 1976). Interviewer begins with a projection of what he will do next (go over a list of items "quite uh germane to your health") that could be heard to indicate that the upcoming matter is delicate (Schegloff, 1980). He then proceeds to offer a recommendation, that he shows he is making with the support of his supervising physician, that relies on a possible diagnosis of pancreas trouble provoked by excessive drinking as the cause for the persistent diarrhea that the patient has come in with. The first issue addressed is drinking, an elaboration raising concerns about possible damage and "ill effects born by the uh alcohol":

4. "mom's had her stroke": #2:22-23
INT:    Now um .h I want to go over some things which I uh (1.0) found and they're quite uh germane to your health. And one of those is the uh (0.3) drinking that you mentioned?
PAT:   Um hmm.
INT:    You said that you're having (.) five <drinks a day> and there are con- some concerns. (.) Uh those concerns are number one, .hh uh alcohol does effect your pancreas, .hh an:d uh that may have some effect upon .hh what's going on with your diarrhea.=I've >had the opportunity to speak< with my mentoring physician, .hh and uh he's recommended that we do some additional tests on ya (.) pt .hh one of which is called a serum amylase.=That- that'll give us an idea .hh of

how your <u>pan</u>creas is functioning.=What your <u>pan</u>creas does
in your <u>body</u> is it produces various en<u>zymes</u> that <u>aid</u> in
di<u>ge</u>stion as well as producing <u>insu</u>lin and <u>glucogons</u>, which
is used in the regulation of your (.) blood sugars so we're
going to <u>test</u> that. The other thing [we're].

PAT:                                                  [Blood] sugars were pretty
low [ normal ].

INT:           [Yeah yeah y]ou're not a <u>dia</u>betic.=<u>So</u> (.) when we're
checking your amylase .hh we're not <u>check</u>ing for diabetes,
we're <u>check</u>ing to see if your <u>pan</u>creas .hh is being <u>damaged</u>
from the alcohol. .hh <u>The</u> <u>other</u> thing we want to look at is
<u>how</u> your <u>liver</u> (.) is <u>func</u>tioning .hh and to <u>see</u> if there is
any <u>ill</u> ef<u>fects</u> born by the uh <u>al</u>cohol so we're going to do
some liver function test (.) as well.

PAT: **1→ Oh but the daily you know the °drinking° everyday at
night has been just since my mom's had her stroke the
last four- four or five years. (.) >The diarrhea's been<
since I really think nineteen years at least [( probably)].**

INT:                                              **[ Okay but ]
sometimes these things-.**

PAT: **1→ >But I'll check it.< I don't know I $hmph$.**

INT: **2→ NOW (.) we're also going uh to send a referral to Doctor
Dorsey who is your designated primary care physician.**

PAT:      He is?

INT:      And [uh:::-].

PAT:           [°I've ] never been there.°

The PA attributes to patient his reporting that he has "five <drinks a
day>"—emphasized by being spoken slower (< >) than surrounding
talk. (Patient actually reported having "Maybe three, " but does not correct PA's summary.) Informed that his pancreas may have been adversely
affected by alcohol, which may explain patient's ongoing problems with
diarrhea, interviewer's discussion with his mentoring physician (a common practice for PAs) has given rise to the prescription of additional tests
(e.g., serum amylase). Next, interviewer explains this test and moves to
describe for patient how the pancreas functions in the body. A query by
patient seeks confirmation of low blood sugars, which interviewer apparently understands the patient as implying that this indicates that he may
be diabetic. The PA rejects this concern by stating he [the patient] is not
diabetic. He also again emphasizes the need to determine if the patient's
pancreas has been damaged, and that the liver will also be tested.

The PA's lengthy overview is met with surprise by patient (1→), indicated by a turn-initial "Oh." As Heritage (1984, 2001) has noted, "oh
prefaces" routinely treat prior speaker's positions as "questioning the

unquestionable" (2001, p. 4), actions which are misconstrued if not altogether inaccurate, inappropriate, or even inapposite (see also Beach, 1996). Such "oh prefaces" also project nonalignment as speakers move next to reassert contrary positions, as the patient's "but" indicates. He reemphasizes that his daily drinking, at night, "has been just since my mom's had her stroke the last four- four or five years." This declaration is followed by a reporting designed to clarify his problems and reveal an inconsistency in the interviewer's reasoning: Because he has experienced diarrhea for at least 19 years, how could this ailment be caused by drinking the last 4 to 5 years?

Essentially, the patient has challenged a portion of PA's diagnosis. We have shown that, when patients proffer their own and/or question an interviewer's diagnosis, such contributions are treated with hesitation and indirectness—as though patients are resisting adherence to a biomedical model in which physicians address diagnosis, and only subsequent to data gathering and physical examination. By displaying interactional resistance to distinct and mandated phases of clinical interviews, traditional and biomedical procedures are repeatedly challenged. In turn, physicians routinely resist opportunities to expand on actions soliciting early requests for diagnostic information (Jones & Beach, in press).

Here the patient reports facts—the duration of his drinking, and the duration of the diarrhea—leaving the PA to formulate the upshot of the report (Drew, 1984). This technique of a "novice" reporting circumstances and leaving the "expert" to formulate its (disagreeing) "professional" implications has been noted in the library setting also (Mandelbaum, 1996). In the library, as is perhaps also the case here, such a technique may be used as a "delicate" method for disagreeing with a professional, because it provides resources for the professional to revise his professional opinion. Although, the patient is not soliciting an early request in the present case, he clearly offers an alternative analysis of relationships between his drinking and diarrhea, and in this way, makes available a possible disagreement with what the PA proposes doing. In response, with "Okay but sometimes these things-.", The PA begins what could be heard to be a contesting of the patient's action. Patient then builds a contrast to his prior turn (indicated by "But") and offers uncertainty: $(1\rightarrow)$—">(probably). But I'll check it.< I don't know I \$hmph\$," thus altering his position. "But I'll check it" registers his concern, and the decision to comply regardless. Here, the patient displays recognition that, although his counter to the interviewer's position is potentially unfavorable, so too is he aware that his speculation about how long his diarrhea has occurred—initially marked with more fervor—is tenuous. Three specific actions are relevant here: (a) Patient states a need to "check" the claim he has advanced; (b) claims insufficient knowledge (Beach & Metzger, 1997) with "I don't <u>know</u>"; and (c) laughs with $hmph$. Taken together, patient qualifies and backs off of the accuracy of his position, expressing some doubt and deference in the presence of a medical expert. Such actions are exceedingly common during medical interviews: "since patients are overwhelmingly tentative in their various solicitations, they reveal distinct orientations to their actions as delicate maneuvers while also legitimating physicians' authority and expert knowledge" (Jones & Beach, in press, p. 31; see also Gill, 1998; Gill et al., 2001). This delicacy may be further indexed when the patient completes his utterance with laughter ($hmph$).

In response, (2→) PA's "NOW" is a way of moving on to the next activity and is followed by the PA moving on to the next recommendation that he has for diagnostic testing. However, the patient's mentioning his mother's stroke serves as the method he uses to implement the primary action of this turn, questioning the PA's assumptions about the patient's pancreas. Further, it functions as an enforced attempt to draw attention away from patient's reported history and toward a referral to "<u>your</u> designated primary care physician." Doing so essentially curtails further elaboration of the patient's attempt to clarify interviewer's diagnosis. It also makes clear that although patient treats such matters as relevant to his medical history and thus diagnosis, they are best addressed (if at all) by another medical expert he will "<u>send</u> a referral to"—a relationship patient reports being unaware of because he has "never been there.°"

## Summary

In this instance also, the patient's mother's stroke is raised as part of the method for implementing another action. Here, he delicately lays grounds for disagreeing with PA's diagnosis. When he mentions that "the daily you know the drinking everyday at night has been just since my mom's had her stroke the last four- four or five years," this is done as part of contesting the physician's claim that the diarrhea has been caused by heavy drinking. The case is completed by building the contrast that the diarrhea has "been since I really think nineteen years at least probably." He is building a contrast between the duration of the drinking (4 to 5 years, prompted by the Mom's stroke) and the duration of the diarrhea (roughly 19 years). The focal action here calls into question the diagnosis the PA has offered. Patient reports circumstances that put him in the position to infer that a pancreas damaged by heavy drinking is unlikely to be the cause of the diarrhea, because the diarrhea is of much longer duration than the drinking.

Again, it would be possible for PA to take up the psychosocial matter of the mother's stroke and its impact on the patient, but this would involve beginning a quite different line of action than the one under way. Clearly, an important issue for care providers to consider is when and how to take up such matters, especially those that may underlie a set of potentially serious health problems (as appears to be the case here).

## A SERIES OF OPPOSITIONAL COUNTERS

The third and final reference to mom's stroke occurs nearly 3 minutes following (Excerpt 4). Interviewer offers specific advice for patient's drinking, namely, to "cut down" to no more than two ounces (shots) a day and if that continues to be a problem, contact the chemical dependency program. Attention is then drawn to "the need to exercise," as interviewer queries "... are you exercising at all?"

Again, the matter of his mother's illness is subordinated to another principal activity—accounting for a failure to exercise:

> 5. "Not since my mom got sick": #2:25-26:
> INT: Okay. pt .hh Now in terms of um (.) your drinking, .hh need
> I say (.) you certainly need to cut down. (.) Ideally no more
> than (.) two ounces a day. pt .hh Um: If that might become a
> problem area for ya .hh we do have a chemical dependency
> program.= I've circled the name and the phone number
> and you may call them at your leisure.
> PAT: °Okay.°
> INT: And I'd like to um (.) talk about some other things which
> are certainly important. One of tho:se is u::h (.) the need to
> exercise and I didn't ask ya are you exercising at all?
> PAT: 1→ °Not since my **mom** got sick.° >I **used** to **bike ride**< three
> **miles but I- I hadn't had time.**
> INT: 2→ **Well exercises (.) even if it's no more than just walking**
> **for thirty minutes non stop three to five days a week .hh**
> **is a valuable tool. pt And uh it's certainly-**
> PAT: 3→ I- I don't have thirty minutes <either. $heh$ But what I **do**
> **is like> when I came here (.) is I took the stairs instead**
> **of the elevator.**
> INT: [Uh hmm ].
> PAT: 3→ [ I **always** t]ry to take the stairs at work (.) **rather than**
> **call somebody in the next office.**
> INT: Uh hmm.

PAT: **3→** >I'll **walk** over there so I **try** to get as much exercise as I
can **that**< way but setting time aside $ I **just** don't$ **have**
it.

INT: **4→** **Well-** what **I'd** like to **do** though is just **uh**: (.) **tell** you
that that (.) is something that you should consider **doing**
in the future. And the **reason why** is it does help to **raise**
your good cholesterol.

PAT:        [ Um hm].

INT: **4→** [ It produ]ces chemicals in your **brain** which helps to **deal**
with anxiety and stress. .hh It uh [helps].

PAT:                                                  [ I lo ]ve to exercise.=

INT: **4→** =Good. (.) Helps to **lower** your **blood pressure, and it**
**certainly** helps you with **weight**. And >**there's** a little
guide< to sort of help you with that. .hh And > here's a
little handout< I'd like to share with you.

Without hesitation, in response to PA's question about exercise, patient provides his mother's illness as an account for not exercising: "Not
since my <u>mom</u> got sick." (1 →). The occurrence of mom's stroke is again
invoked as an event of considerable magnitude in the patient's life: It is
invoked as an account for his drinking and now for not exercising (e.g.,
not riding his bike 3 miles). The immediacy of patient's response also
reveals mom's stroke as a benchmark date for assessing the time he has
available to invest in health-promoting activity. This utterance marks
the third time that this particular psychosocial matter has been raised
in direct connection with the patient's serious health problems (excessive drinking and failure to exercise). As we have observed, in each case,
it has been raised as part of the implementation of some other action
such as accounting for his unhealthy conduct, or making available evidence that could counter the PA's attempted diagnosis. Yet, it is nonetheless surprising that, given the clearly pressing and recurrent nature of
the patient's concern, the PA continues to *not* take up his concerns.

Because "mom's stroke" is not presented as the patient's direct and
only problem at any point in the interview, the PA does not exhibit being
compelled to acknowledge or pursue these psychosocial matters. In
the ensuing series of turns, as the interviewer continues to promote the
value of exercise, patient continues to indicate his positive attitude toward exercise but his inability to make time for it. In (2→), by reassert-
ing the importance of exercising, the PA treats the patient's prior turn
(1→) as his accounting for not exercising. Similarly in (3→), patient
again accounts for his lack of exercise by reporting his lack of even 30
minutes and offering what he does instead (taking the stairs). In response, the interviewer minimally acknowledges, and the patient continues to give examples indicating his willingness to exercise. Yet, the

patient does not state making exercise a priority over his other daily activities. Finally in (4→), the PA prefaces his report of another advantage of exercise with encouragement to the patient to "consider doing" it "in the future." This recommendation indicates that the PA still considers the patient to be in need of persuasion in the face of the patient being resistant to exercise regularly. The patient's "I love exercise" continues to positively assess the value of being physically active, yet leaves hanging an inability and/or unwillingness to enact an exercise plan because of the time constraints his mother's illness imposes.

This orientation by the interviewer is consequential for the unfolding of this interview, which resembles a series of reciprocal counters not unlike those noted earlier (see Excerpt 2). For example, just as the interviewer's (2→) fails to pursue patient's problems, so too does patient (3→) immediately dismiss the interviewer's suggestion: "I- I don't have thirty minutes <either. $heh$". Here, the patient treats as delicate his discounting and thus challenging of interviewer's proposed "walking" solution. Similarly, just as the patient produced an extended utterance establishing the relevance of his efforts to exercise (3→), the interviewer also provides a series of reasons for compliance: Raising good cholesterol, reducing anxiety and stress, lowering blood pressure and weight. His reference to "anxiety and stress" is the closest he gets to addressing the concerns the patient has nominated throughout this entire medical interview. It is noteworthy, however, that "anxiety and stress" are raised here as part of a generic and itemized list (see Jefferson, 1990) for advancing health through exercise, not as tailored to the patient's unique circumstances. In the end, a compromise does not emerge where the patient might somehow increase his exercise in the midst of work and caregiving responsibilities.

### Summary

For the third time, the patient uses his mother's health as an account for medical-related noncompliance. In turn, the PA does not utilize opportunities to address how the patient's mother's illness, and the caregiving responsibilities he takes on, reveal key health implications. However, it is once again clear that the particular ways the patient raises his mother's health situation remain embedded, that is, in a position in the ongoing turn where they are not made available as that which "should" or even "must" be responded to.

## DISCUSSION

Close analysis of the social actions comprising this medical interview reveal that the patient's references to his mother's illness are not straightforwardly produced, such as an announcement requiring response and assessment by the PA. In sequential terms, the patient's accounting, disagreeing, and explaining of his daily circumstances provide resources for interviewer to not directly address and pursue mom's stroke—as consequential for the caregiving the patient provides, as impacting how the patient lives an unhealthy lifestyle, or as an ongoing and serious health matter requiring medical attention. These issues are not addressed in this interview, and we have advanced sequential, "structural" reasons for their not be taken up by PA: Local, embedded, and systematic explanations for why and how the patient's troubling life circumstances—not presented to be taken up, but in the service of explaining his drinking and life circumstances—do not get discussed. Technically, then, interviewer does not disattend concerns that patient did not make directly available as topics in their own right.

No claim is being made that the PA lacks concern for the patient's health condition. It is possible that the patient benefited, perhaps in significant ways, from participating in this medical interview. It is also possible, as with Excerpt 2, that the patient is anxious to connect his drinking firmly to his mother's illness, not just as an account for his behavior, but also to show that it is short-term conduct—at least in contrast with his long-term diarrhea—and may in fact not be as relevant as the PA is intimating. However, clearly, the interviewer did not seek elaboration on the patient's family dilemma, and thus further talk about the relevance of mom's stroke to the patient's health and lifestyle was constrained. Left unexplored, then, are potential "root issues" (see Barbour, 1995; Felitti et al., 1998) contributing to ongoing health problems and how such knowledge might shape not only diagnosis, treatment, and referral but, ultimately, mortality and morbidity. Thus, our findings should not be taken to imply that, by not further discussing patient's mom's stroke, better medical care was necessarily provided.

In writing this chapter we have had the opportunity to discuss these and a host of related and complex issues, which may be summarized as follows:

- What relationships exist between (a) a technical, sequential basis for interviewers not addressing concerns raised (but not raised to be directly addressed) by patient; and (b) acknowledging, reassuring, and offering support for patients' troubles even though they are not presented as primary topics for discussion?

- What windows of opportunity are passed by when not addressing "cues or clues" offered by patients about their condition, and what implications arise for the ongoing quality of care?

- What interactional evidence can be provided about "compassionate" care in the midst of indirectly provided concerns by patients?

Indeed, the materials examined herein exemplify recurrent problems in not only providing medical care but also establishing sufficient interactional explanations for the organization of medical interviews. As noted, a long-standing and primary concern with understanding patient-centered care involves the diverse ways patients offer "cues or clues" about their concerns, how (or if) these behaviors are addressed by providers, and overall impacts on healing outcomes (e.g., see Balint, 1957; Barbour, 1995; Beach & Dixson, 2001; Beach & LeBaron, 2002; Cassell, 1985; Engel, 1977; Frankel & Beckman, 1988; Gill, 1998; Gill et al., 2001; Heath, 1986, 1988, 2002; Jones & Beach, in press; Lang et al., 2000; Levinson, Gorawara-Bhat, & Lamb, 2000; Marvel, Epstein, Flowers, & Beckman, 1999; Mishler, 1984; Stivers & Heritage, 2001; Suchman et al., 1997; Waitzkin, 1991). However, how are "cues or clues" to be evidenced as interactional achievements, and in response, how do medical experts address (or not) patients' concerns (whether indirectly or directly raised)? The interactional moments examined in this chapter make clear that, over the course of a single medical interview, a distinction needs to be made between how a patient repeatedly verbalizes concerns about his mom's stroke, and how he does not actively invite pursuit of an obvious and important set of health-related topics (see Beach, 1996; Pomerantz, 1984). Similarly, other work is moving forward, such as ongoing examinations of how cancer patients' subtle and directly produced verbal and nonverbal expressions of "fear" get responded to by oncologists (Beach et al., in press).

It is important to emphasize that speakers' reportings about their worlds "are in fact extraordinarily complex speech events" (M. H. Goodwin, 1990, p. 230), progressively and collaboratively built in and through conjoint, moment-by-moment actions (see Beach, 2000; Mandelbaum 1989). Across a wide array of both ordinary conversations and institutional encounters (see Drew & Heritage, 1992), conceptions of "narratives" as uninterrupted monologues, produced by single speakers, are inadequate if and when the achieved character of human interactions remain the grist for the analytic mill. From the materials examined herein, it is possible to extract key moments of the patient's "narrative" and integrate his concerns into a coherent framework. The result would appear something like the following:

I usually have something ° everyday ° before >I go to bed< → >But that isn't- I mean that's just been in the la:st< (.) f:our years or five years that

I've been ° doing that ° → My mom had a <u>stroke</u> (.) five years ago and u:h I
h<u>ave</u> to <u>go</u> every night after work and h<u>elp</u> (.) my dad out with her <u>so:</u> =
.hh when I come <u>home</u> just ta un<u>wind</u> $I have a few drinks$ and then
>go to bed< → Oh but the <u>daily</u> you know the ° drinking ° everyday at
<u>night</u> has been just <u>since</u> my <u>mom's</u> had her stroke the last <u>four-</u> four or
five years. (.) >The diarrh<u>ea's</u> been< since I really think <u>nine</u>teen years
at least (probably) >But I'll check it.< I don't <u>know</u> I $hmph$.   °→ Not
since my <u>mom</u> got sick.° >I <u>used</u> to <u>bike</u> <u>ride</u>< three miles but <u>I-</u> I hadn't
had time. → I- I don't have thirty minutes <either. $heh$ But what I <u>do</u>
is like> when I came here (.) is I took the stairs instead of the elevator →
I <u>always</u> try to take the stairs at work (.) rather than call somebody in
the next office → >I'll <u>walk</u> over there so I <u>try</u> to get as much exercise as I
can <u>that</u>< way but setting time aside $ I <u>just</u> don't$ <u>have</u> it.

From this extracted "narrative," a claim could be advanced that the
patient repeatedly attempts to raise that and how his mom's stroke
continues to influence his life. Yet to whom does he raise the fact and
with what interactional consequences? Viewing the patient's "narrative" as solely produced does provide a user-friendly opportunity to
comprehend the basic gist, or plotline, of the drama he is portraying.
What is inevitably lost, of course, are the interactional contingencies
co-produced by the interviewer and the patient animating this encounter: As we have shown, each utterance is designed as responsive to not
just any but specific social actions, and in turn, makes available to the
next speaker particular and relevant understandings of evolving
courses of meaningful conduct—behaviors that, by definition, could
not and would not be produced by individuals apart from this embedded context (Goodwin, 2003). Inherently, social phenomena—such as
extended answers to prior questions, delicately produced laughter,
raising concerns indirectly, or not addressing topics related to mom's
stroke—would therefore not be available for examination. The lack of
embedded contexts would be a great loss if what we seek to understand
is how communication shapes, and is shaped by, illness and wellness.
Nor would a much wider range of social activities be available as a resource for better understanding the interactional organization of medical interviews—for their own sake as interesting forms of institutional
involvements, and/or to improve communication between providers
and patients.

These are critical issues as medical care systems seek innovative
ways to preserve wellness, medically and morally (Bergmann, 1992).
The consequences of artificially separating body, mind, and spirit are
nontrivial for the human condition. When patients' basic needs and
concerns are unmet—even as a result of their inability to raise them directly—patients seek return visitations, including ERs, because their

stated problems were not heard and attended to in prior encounters. Satisfaction, loyalty, and compliance is compromised in ways severely impacting healing outcomes. Despite increasing technological sophistication, malpractice suits escalate as basic communication problems between patients and providers drive the machinery of litigation (see Levinson et al., 2000). Resolving these disjunctures begins with giving priority to basic social actions: How the patients construct and the providers respond to lifeworld experiences throughout history taking, physical examination, and diagnostic and treatment discussions. Any prescriptions we offer about how to improve these critical moments must remain sensitive to actual practices employed by lay and medical experts (Heath, 1986), accessible only through close examination of recorded and transcribed encounters. The alternative is to propose vague solutions for nonexistent interactional problems, or perhaps worse yet, specific but misdirected remedies further restricting patients' disclosures.

## NOTES

1. For example, consider the following excerpt and discussion by Terasaka (1976):

        (3)   [NB:—2]
        1   B:   So, Elizabeth'n Will were s'poze tuh come down las'night
        2        but [there was death 'n the fam'ly] so they couldn'
        3        come so Guy's asked Dan tuh play with the comp'ny deal,
        4        so I guess he c'n play with'im. So,
        5   A:   Oh good.

    In this example, the news of the death (indicated by brackets) is not remarked on, whereas the news that the golf game will take place is received as assessable news. Our suggestion is that a major factor in the recognition of announcements by speakers is to some degree independent of the content of the events they report and resides, instead, in the organization of their presentation in the talk.

    Thus, announcements should be differentiated from talk about occurrences that might otherwise appear to be announceable but can be shown to have been "buried" in their presentation. There are additionally instances of talk in which a recipient treats some talk as news to them, which were not marked by the deliverer as announcements.

2. We are grateful to Gene Lerner for pointing out the relevance of this article.

## APPENDIX: TRANSCRIPTION SYMBOLS

In data headings,"SDCL" stands for "San Diego Conversation Library," a collection of recordings and transcriptions of naturally occurring interactions; "OC" represents "Oncology," followed by vernacular extracts drawn from the video-excerpts being analyzed (e.g., "feeling (.) lately").The transcription notation system employed for data segments is an adaptation of Gail Jefferson's work (see Atkinson & Heritage, 1984, pp. ix–xvi). The symbols may be described as follows:

: Colon(s): Extended or stretched sound, syllable, or word.

_ Underlining: Vocalic emphasis.

(.) Micropause: Brief pause of less than (0.2).

(1.2) Timed Pause: Intervals occurring within and between same or different speaker's utterance.

(( )) Double Parentheses: Scenic details.

( ) Single Parentheses: Transcriptionist doubt.

. Period: Falling vocal pitch.

? Question Marks: Rising vocal pitch.

↑↓(( Arrows: Pitch resets; marked rising and falling shifts in intonation.

° ° Degree Signs: A passage of talk noticeably softer than surrounding talk.

= Equal Signs: Latching of contiguous utterances, with no interval or overlap.

[ ] Brackets: Speech overlap.

[[ Double Brackets: Simultaneous speech orientations to prior turn.

! Exclamation Points: Animated speech tone.

- Hyphens: Halting, abrupt cut off of sound or word.

> < Less Than/Greater Than Signs: Portions of an utterance delivered at a pace noticeably quicker than surrounding talk.

OKAY CAPS: Extreme loudness compared with surrounding talk.

hhh .hhh H's: Audible outbreaths, possibly laughter. The more h's, the longer the aspiration. Aspirations with periods indicate audible inbreaths (e.g., .hhh). H's within (e.g., ye(hh)s) parentheses mark within-speech aspirations, possible laughter.

pt Lip Smack: Often preceding an inbreath.

hah Laugh Syllable: Relative closed or open position of laughter

heh

hoh

$ Smile Voice: Words marked by chuckles and/or phrases hearable as laughed-through

# 17

## Constructing Life and Death Through Final Conversation Narratives

ᢙ

**Maureen P. Keeley**
*Texas State University-San Marcos*

**Jody Koenig Kellas**
*University of Nebraska-Lincoln*

*Authentic conversation has the power not only to enhance how people cope practically with dying, but to illuminate and enrich the very meaning of life for [people] and [their loved ones] alike, as they enter the sacred moment of mortal time together.*
—McQuellon & Cowan, 2000, p. 312

Five years ago, I (Maureen) had the opportunity and privilege to spend about 9 weeks with my mother during the last 4 months of her life. When my mother and I faced the terminal time that we would have together, I remember being thankful for the opportunity to talk with her and to hug her often. I also know that it was one of the most difficult but meaningful experiences of my life. My experience with my mother at the end of her life also prompted my scholarly interest in this important and unique interactional context, so I began my journey to understand more about final conversations (FC). I started asking others to share their experiences with me, and over the past 18 months, I have been privileged to hear many wonderful stories about FC.

I have also shared my FC story with numerous people, and in that sharing, I have gained insight into myself, about my relationship with my mother, about dying, and about communication as a whole. In one

365

of those many conversations, my friend and colleague, Jody, and I discussed the narrative nature of FC. We talked about how FC have the potential for helping survivors to heal, not only because of the value gained by having the conversation with the loved one in the first place, but also because telling the story of the FC after the loved one has passed often serves as a way of making sense and coming to terms with the death. Narratives about the loss of a loved one have been shown to have positive benefits for the tellers (e.g., Sedney, Baker, & Gross, 1994; Weber, Harvey, & Stanley, 1989); however, research has not yet examined how stories about FC have specific health benefits for tellers.

Combining the personal insight and experiences of a participant interviewer with the insights of a scholar who has yet to experience a FC with a loved one, we bring our combined strengths to this chapter. Together, in what follows, we explore FC stories in an effort to shed light on the role that narratives play in constructing our health and lives in the light of death. After a brief discussion of the relevant literature, we present a study of 40 FC narratives and the themes that emerged as central to the teller's experience in coming to terms with the death of a loved one.

## THE DEATH CULTURE

We live in a culture and a society that has removed death from our view (D. Heinz, 1999), thereby complicating and obscuring the meaning of death. For most of us, "death has become remote, no longer an integral part of life, but a fearsome and unwelcome visitor" (Callanan & Kelley, 1992, p. 31). Most people consider death to be depressing and morbid (Kubler-Ross, 1969, 1997). When a loved one is diagnosed with a terminal illness, most people in the United States are at a loss for what to do and do not even know what to say (Moller, 1996). D. Heinz (1999) refers to the death experience as "the crisis of our age" (p. xix).

One consequence of our society's attitudes toward death includes neglecting those most affected by the loss of a loved one. Medical professionals and other "outsiders" often overlook and forget family members, friends, neighbors, and co-workers during the death process (Callanan & Kelley, 1992). According to Callanan and Kelley, "An impending death sends ripples through all the relationships in the life of the dying. Each person involved has his or her own set of issues, fears, and questions" (1992, p. 2). If we are to make sense of death and the process that we all go through when we are faced with death (our own or a loved one), we must gain a better understanding of the survivors' perspectives and their stories.

Previous research exploring survivors' experience of the dying process has looked mainly at bereavement, focusing "… our attention on what has been lost or on the pain of missing" (Hedtke, 2002, p. 286). Taking a primarily bereavement perspective suggests that all survivors postpone grieving and healing until death occurs. However, individuals who experience a terminal amount of time left with loved ones attest that the anguish begins almost immediately because the "diagnosis of a ... terminal illness abruptly and intensely brings the reality of human mortality home" (McQuellon & Cowan, 2000, p. 313). Potentially, communicating and spending time with dying loved ones may sow the seeds that lead to healing, and thus, an exploration of communication at the end of life from the survivors' perspective is warranted.

## Communication at the End of Life

Talk provides a way to create meaning out of senselessness that often accompanies death. Communication enables us to advance connections with those who are dying. These conversations and connections may help us to begin to look at death as it really is, as a normal part of life, and not as a rigid trajectory of grief (Hedtke, 2002). As Hedtke asserts, contemporary society requires a reconstructing of the language of death and grief.

If we can reframe how we talk about and experience death in society, people may begin to understand and accept that the time constraints that accompany an impending death create a clear opportunity for people to engage in an "authentic conversation" (McQuellon & Cowan, 2000, p. 312) with their dying loved ones. For everyone involved, the examination of "one's life in the face of death can lead to richer meaning and more life-giving forms of thinking, feeling, and acting" (McQuellon & Cowan, 2000, p. 315). Facing a terminal amount of time potentially frees us (as well as the dying) from past constraints, from busy schedules, and from the myth that we have limitless time to communicate with our loved ones. Past research confirms that communication at the end of life has benefits for the terminally ill and implies a significant impact for those who continue living (Aiken, 2001; Kubler Ross, 1969, 1997). Despite this preliminary research, scholars have not yet examined the implications of communication at the end of life for survivors. Further, we also lack scholarly reflection about the benefits that survivors experience as they make sense of such conversations after the loved one has passed. The following section reviews literature on narrative and explores storytelling as a vehicle for making sense of death and communication at the end of life.

## Narratives of Loss

Little research has focused on survivors' experience of death, or on how FC impact that experience. Literature on narratives, on the other hand, has examined how people narratively make sense of the world and the events of their lives (e.g., Bochner, 2002; Bochner, Ellis, & Tillman-Healy, 1997; Bruner, 1990; Fisher, 1989) and how people who have experienced a traumatic event cope with trauma through the process of telling stories (e.g., Pennebaker & O'Heeron, 1984; Weber, Harvey, & Stanley, 1989; Wigren, 1994). Taking a narrative approach to FC can illuminate the survivors' experiences in many ways. In particular, three features/approaches central to narrative theory may be useful in understanding FC experiences. First, all human behavior is narrative in nature; second, meaning-making through narrative is contextual, temporal, and complex; and third, stories serve the function of helping us to make sense and meaning out of our lives.

Perspectives that view all human communication as narrative in nature have opened the door for interpreting conversations as narratives. Fisher (1989) asserts "viewing human communication narratively stresses that people are full participants in the making of messages, whether they are agents (authors) or audience members (co-authors)" (p. 18). Bruner (1990) also saw stories as individual constructions and as genres in our minds, against which we evaluate the world around us. Conceiving of narrative ontologically (e.g., Bruner, 1990; Fisher, 1989) suggests that people make sense of important life events by organizing them and assessing them against a storied form. This body of literature offers justification for taking an interpretive narrative methodology to understanding FC because it privileges narrative as the means by which we assess our conversations, relationships, and our place in the world.

In addition to viewing narrative as central to our communication and our cognition, narrative theory also depicts stories as complex, dynamic, temporal, and contextual. Narratives are inextricably linked to social and historical time (Fisher, 1989; Somers, 1994). For example, we can at least in part understand the nature of FC narratives by recognizing their situatedness in the modern "death culture," which attempts to minimize talk and stories about death (D. Heinz, 1999; Kubler-Ross, 1969, 1997). In addition, narrative context is important to understanding FC because FC narratives not only concern the cultural setting in which the events are being told (e.g., death culture; the "lived context of the events being retold"), but they also reflect the context of the events themselves (e.g., final conversations; the "living context of the telling itself"; see Babrow, Kline, & Rawlins, chap. 2, this volume). In other words, FC narratives are rich and complex because they reflect the context in which the FC events occurred as well as the context in which the story is being recounted. According to Ochs (1997), narratives allow us to fuse these aspects by uniting our pasts, presents, and futures. She explains:

It is our cares about the present and especially about the future that organize our narrative recollections of past events. Narrative serves the important function of bringing the past into the present time consciousness. That is, narrative provides a sense of continuity of self and society. But perhaps even more importantly, narrative accounts of past events help us to manage our uncertain future. (p. 191)

A narrative understanding of context and time may help to illuminate the functions of FC and the ability of FC narrative to both reflect and affect our experiences.

Finally, a third body of research on narrative illuminates the sense-making function of narratives. More specifically, research highlights important links between the telling of difficult or traumatic stories and the psychological and health benefits for the teller of the story. This research has clear implications for those interested in health communication because it suggests—and we are further convinced by our own data—that the telling of stories is therapeutic in many ways.

Pennebaker and his colleagues (e.g., Pennebaker & Beall, 1986; Pennebaker & O'Heeron, 1984), for example, discovered that talking about trauma relates positively to both mental and physical health. The growing field of narrative therapy also offers testament to the psychological and physical benefits of telling stories of loss. Mishara (1995) argued that, by putting trauma in narrative form, storytellers transform themselves from self (victim of trauma) to other (character in story), and this self-transcendence provides the essential key to making the trauma a past experience. Reflection on the meaning of the experience is also essential to this process. According to Mishara (1995), "When ... narration is not used to bring about reflective insight, it loses its healing power" (p. 192).

Indeed, one of the central tenets of narrative therapy rests on people's ability to "restory" their lives. According to Monk, Winslade, Crochet, and Epston (1997), stories help to shape our lives, but ignored lived experiences go unstoried or unnoticed. Sedney et al. (1994) argued that the absence of stories about death can stifle a person's ability to make sense of the experience, explain his or her role in the event, and experience emotional relief. Forgoing stories may also contribute to family secrets, limit family communication (Sedney et al., 1994), and people who do not hear stories of death in their families may have trouble communicating about death later in life (Book, 1996).

On the other hand, stories about the death of a loved one help people experience emotional relief, assign meaning to the experience, bring family members together, and open up lines and facilitate communication (Sedney et al., 1994). In addition, these narratives teach lessons about family communication rules surrounding the topic of death (Book, 1996).

Our data suggests that FC constitute an important final stage in peoples' relationships; and provide survivors with an invaluable opportunity for personal growth and healing. Further, our data suggests that survivors may miss the opportunity to learn valuable lessons and potentially restory the experience in meaningful and beneficial ways if they leave FC untold. A narrative approach to understanding FC experiences illuminates identity, sense-making, and communication as contextually situated, important characteristics of FC stories that both affect and reflect our experiences.

## METHOD

### Participants and Procedures

We conducted 42 retrospective interviews in a private office; two were not used in the data analysis because of differences in the data-collection process (e.g., interview protocol and online interview). The sample consisted primarily of White, female participants with 33 female and 7 male participants: 33 White, 4 Hispanic, 1 Black, and 1 Asian. Participants ranged in age from 21 to 85, with the average age of the participants being 40.6 years. We employed a snowball sampling technique to recruit participants (Lindlof, 1995). To participate in the study, participants had to meet two criteria. First, they had a FC or experience (nonverbal interaction) with a loved one, with both participants' knowledge and understanding that one of them was dying. Second, they had to possess a clear recollection of the FC interaction, which took place any time between the diagnosis of "terminal amount of time to live" and the actual death.

The amount of time between the loved one's death and the interview regarding the FC averaged 6.9 years (range from 3 months to 27 years). Given the exploratory nature of the study, we used a semistructured focused format with open-ended questions for the interview protocol (Kvale, 1996; McCracken, 1988; C. J. Stewart & Cash, 2000).

*Procedure.* After the participants were comfortable and signed the informed consent form, they completed a questionnaire concerning demographic information and the nature of the relationship with the FC partner. Following 10 minutes of free-writing about their FC, we interviewed participants orally about their FC, relying on a 23-question interview schedule (see Appendix). A certified grief counselor assessed all questions for relevance and utility.

Additional questions emerged during individual interviews. Interviews averaged 90 minutes (ranging from 60 to 120 minutes). All of the interviews were audiotaped and transcribed verbatim. The interviews resulted in 526 single-spaced pages of data.

## Data Analysis

We wanted to reveal people's experiences and to make sense of this phenomenon that we call final conversation narratives by explaining the recurring patterns of meaning that were revealed during the interviews (Creswell, 1998; Miles & Huberman, 1994). Employing grounded theory (Strauss & Corbin, 1990), we identified emergent themes through both open and axial coding. In order to identify the themes, we used the constant comparative method by reading, rereading, and reflecting on the participants' statements in order to identify the important messages in each category (Straus & Corbin, 1990).

After the data set was coded, we used the negative-case analysis technique to ensure that categories were not forced on the data (Erlandson, Harris, Skipper, & Allen, 1993). Once the data was identified, categorized, and coded, we conducted a reliability check between us and had a reliability of 84%. Participant checking utilizing 8 participants (20%) also confirmed the findings that the themes and structures were consistent with their FC experiences.

## RESULTS

Four primary themes emerged in the analysis of the FC narratives: (a) (re)constructing individual identity, (b) (re)constructing relational identity, (c) sense-making and healing, and (d) lessons about communication. The following section discusses the findings.

### (Re)Constructing Individual Identity Through Final Conversations

The first major theme that emerged in our analysis of the FC interviews illustrates the importance of final conversations for helping the survivors grapple with, learn about, and come to terms with their own identity. According to Fletcher (2002) death often brings about an identity crisis for the surviving individuals. Research on narrative identity suggests that one of the primary purposes of narrative activity is the evaluation or construction of self (e.g., Brockmeier & Carbaugh, 2001; Bruner, 1997; Bruner & Kalmar, 1998; Cohler, 1991; Linde, 1993; Somers, 1994). In particular, Somers (1994) reminded us that "narrative identities are constituted and reconstituted *in* time and *over* time" (p. 624, italics in original). The participants in our study confirmed that FC experiences forced them to reevaluate their identities, but they asserted that FC also significantly helped them to redefine themselves in a productive light. The process of defining and redefining self emerged in the context of both the remembered events (i.e., part of the plot of the FC story included the assessment of identity) and in the context of the telling (i.e., identity was reassessed during the FC interview). Three primary categories emerged that explain the ways in which tellers learned something about their own identity in the process of having FC. Categories include: myself and others, others telling me about myself, and seeing myself in a different light.

*Statements about myself and others* refer to any statements about the teller's own identity that he or she noticed during the process of having a FC. Although FC involve collaborative constructions, people spent a fair amount of time in their narratives discussing and analyzing their own individual identities and their roles in the FC and death process. For the most part, these statements characterized the tellers as either tentative and doubtful about their roles in the experience or as significant and important.

Participants in this study who lost parents at a young age expressed doubts about the manner in which they approached the FC. Karen,[1] now an adult, recognizes that:

> I was 15 and ... I didn't, I didn't really have the maturity and sureness of myself. And you know ... it's completely uncharted territory. And at 15, I, uh, I can remember one time when he was in the hospital ... that I was in the room with him alone. And I just kinda sat there in the chair and I didn't know what to do and he was sleeping. And, you know, thinking back ..., I wish I had hugged him or done something. But ... I was 15. So, you know, it's not a terrible regret I have, but had I been a little older, you know, I would have. (LL 114–124).[2]

The remainder of Karen's story suggests that the narrative helped her to make sense of her identity in relation to the FC experience. Sedney et al. (1994) supported the importance of narrating death in that children "... are apt to assign a meaning to the death that involves a negative, painful perception of themselves. A story about what happened can provide another way to impose meaning on their experience that is open to clarification in discussion with others ..." (p. 4).

Constructing FC narratives also contributes to adult survivors' identity construction. People who have lost loved ones as adults communicated similar doubts. Grace expresses such internal second guessing:

> You question whether or not you did enough. You question your own ... actions. You question your own conversations. You question whether you

told them enough that they were loved and whether you, uh, listened enough to their ... feelings and so forth. And whether you were projecting your feelings more than you should have ... I think that, that gave me some self doubt ... I had to sit down and examine what I had done and what I should have done. (LL 278–284)

Although death can cause a crisis of identity (Fletcher, 2002), FC also helped people to recognize positive aspects of their own identities. For instance, Roxanne realized that she helped to facilitate a peaceful and rewarding final conversation with her father:

But, I think because I was nonjudgmental and respected, you know, and just listened openly, I think it gave him a sense of belonging and being respected ... And loved. And ... by the same token, I was honored that he opened up and shared that with me. (LL 453–455)

FC narratives reflected tellers' doubts about themselves. However, FC also gives survivors the opportunity to recognize their own individuality in reaffirming ways. The ability to evaluate oneself in a positive light in the face of FC experiences may have important implications for understanding psychological well-being in relation to death. Although we discuss sense-making as another emergent theme at length, the process of narratively evaluating identity in the FC context clearly links with the healing process. Life story research, for example, suggests that the ability to create a coherent sense of self in response to adversity is essential to a sense of solace and well-being (Baerger & McAdams, 1999; Cohler, 1991). In addition, narrative therapy offers the concept of *reauthoring one's stories* (Monk, Winslade, Crocket, & Epstein, 1997), which may be important for tellers of FC narratives in the process of questioning the coherence of their identities. Telling FC stories may be an important step in evaluating and affirming identity.

In addition to examining their individual identities, people telling FC narratives also reflected upon themselves in relation to others and the roles they assumed in response to the situation. Sedney et al. (1994) warned that the absence of stories about death may handicap a person's ability to make sense of what happened, and that one important aspect of that process involves explaining their own role in the events.

In relation to the dying person, participants at times described themselves as "the caretaker." Sam's recognition of his role as caretaker helped him to reconcile this role in other aspects of his life. When asked how his perceptions were impacted by these final conversations, he explains:

I made peace with my role in life as a caretaker of others. Up until then, I found myself always in caretaker positions, but it also ... had a lot to do with being an adult child of an alcoholic. You know ... I always saw that as pathological. That somehow I'm always allowing myself to be pulled into situations where you know there's kind of a co-dependent thing going on here ... And then, I guess ... when all of a sudden you're dealing with real, real dependency for good reason ... it kinda makes all that stuff look kinda silly. I kinda ... got over that. (LL 393–401)

Although Sam took pride in his role as caretaker of his mother, Cathy avoided that role with her husband. She recounts that "I was not the caretaker ... I had to make sure I wasn't the caretaker. I had to make sure he didn't get the sense, too much of a sense that I was getting stronger than he" (LL 548–550).

Cathy's struggle to balance her identity with her husband similarly reflects a common theme that emerged in statements about myself in relation to others—*role reversal* between the dying and the surviving. Children of dying parents often described the FC experience as punctuated by the role reversal between child and parent. Lori (#25) struggled with becoming the parent and dealing with FC in which she had to take on the difficult role of "gatekeeper." She recalls:

... When he got sick, part of the painful [FC] were when I would have to be the gatekeeper. And he would come and try to convince me that he was fine and that he could drive and he could do this and he could do that. And I felt awful. I really felt awful about that. That was very painful... the roles were reversed. You know, I was the parent and he was the child, which was really awful. But it was the way it was. (LL 726–734)

Although statements about myself in relation to others often reflected the difficulty of managing FC, people also recognized the precious nature of *recognizing self* in the final moments of the loved one's life. Claire* celebrates herself in relation to her FC with her uncle, asserting that "I know whenever I was with him I felt like I could do anything. I felt really strong ... when I was with him; I became the person I wanted to be. I was just real confident" (LL 567–569).

*Others telling me about myself statements* refer to any instance in which the dying person or anyone present for the FC makes a statement that confirms or redefines the storyteller's identity for him or her. The most prominent instances of this category emerged from the stories of daughters' FC with their fathers and wives' FC with their husbands. Daughters consistently discussed the invaluable nature of having their fathers confirm their identities for them and how these FC contributed significantly to their current *self-esteem*. Weber et al. (1989) argued that stories of loss help tellers achieve better self-esteem. Examination of the FC narratives in this study suggest that self-esteem may, in part, depend on the confirmation and encouragement from the dying parent, particularly when fathers affirmed the self-esteem of daughters. Ruth describes this encouragement poignantly in the description of her final conversation with her father: "... He did a lot of like ego reassurance. 'You're wonderful, you're wonderful, you're wonderful.' And now, hmmm, I guess there's still a little 5-year-old part of me that still thinks that way. Like I know my daddy loves me and is so proud of me" (LL 139–142). Similarly, Claire* recognizes that her uncle spent the majority of their time during FC building her self-esteem. She noted, "The message was, I am, you know, I am somebody ... I think that on his ... side, he felt like that was the most important thing to leave with me" (LL 224–227). The narratives reflect a sense that fathers (and uncles) knew how important their final words to their daughters would be.

For wives, the messages from their dying husbands included themes of *strength and encouragement*. Victoria's husband passionately reassured her that she had the strength to survive him. She explains:

I just got really scared he was gonna die and I screamed at him, "You, you can't die. I can't live without you!" And I remember that he was still strong enough, he grabbed me by the shoulders and flung me around and just right in my face, were these really gleaming ice blue eyes and said "Yes you can. Yes you can if you have to. And you will do it well." (LL 15–19)

FC narratives often reflect the selfless nature of the dying person and the impact that their words have on the identity of the teller. This finding may not be surprising, given Gergen's (1994) contention that individual identity is relational in nature. Tellers report gaining strength and a clearer sense of self through their FC experiences. For example Brenda* (#27) was surprised by her own strength; Ellen (#28) realized she could handle things as a "grown up" in a way she had not anticipated before; and Victoria (#2) took her husband' belief in her and "grew up at that moment" (LL 75–76).

This aspect of FC also highlights the importance of context and time associated with these stories. During the FC experiences, the loved ones helped to bolster the esteem of the survivors. In the present and future tellings of the FC story, the survivors use these experiences to reaffirm and continue to construct their current identities as important. Linde (1993) referred to stories whose primary point involves an evaluation about the speaker as life stories and acknowledges their significance because of their extended reportability and their ability to help people understand self-identity. Unlike "statements about myself," in which tellers were able to question the coherence of their own identity in relation to the FC, "others telling me about myself" serve as important episodes in the FC for affirming identity in the past, present, and future. Life stories, or self-narrations, emerge as products of discourse (Bruner & Kalmar, 1998), implicitly social in that their coherence must be negotiated with others (Linde, 1993). Our data suggest that tellers negotiate their identity with the dying loved one and reaffirm that identity in the present telling by citing the other as an important source for their present identity affirmation.

*Seeing myself in a different light* included statements in which the storyteller explicitly explained how this experience changed the way she saw herself or the way she acted. These statements, reflect a culmination of the lessons learned from the other two types of identity statements just reported. For example, loved ones encouraged survivors to realize their strength, and, in turn, survivors acknowledged a *new sense of strength and openness* that resulted from the FC experience. Brenda* voices surprise by her own strength; Ellen realizes that she can handle things as a "grown up" in a way she had not anticipated before, and Roxanne explains that FC made her "A whole lot less judgmental. My actions, a whole lot more compassionate. I'm much more open because I've experienced something that was really not rational. I think it's made me much more spiritual, and ... open" (LL 255–257).

Perhaps the greatest impact on identity during FC emerged not only in retrospect, but when the dying person changed the tellers' sense of themselves because of something they said during the FC. Tory gained a tremendous sense of peace and satisfaction during one of her many conversations with her brother about what they would miss about each other when he passed. She describes the most meaningful part of their FC:

> He goes, "I'm going to miss the fact that you always have a band aid for my wounds." ... I kinda stopped, I was like "I didn't realize that I did anything like that for you." ... I gave him another way of looking at things or just listening ... it was such a good feeling for him to say that ... because all this time, I thought I was more needy of him than he was of me. (LL 155–178)

Somers (1994) referred to the stories people tell about their lives as "ontological narratives" and asserts that "ontological narratives make identity and the self something that one *becomes*. Thus, narrative embeds identities in time and spatial relationships. Ontological narratives affect activities, consciousness, and beliefs and are, in turn affected by them" (p. 618). The participants in our study who saw themselves in a different light were clearly affected by the FC experience, and they use the FC narratives as ways of both reflecting and affecting, or enacting, their new sense of selves.

## (Re)constructing Relational Identity Through Final Conversations

The second major theme that emerged during the FC narratives focused on statements that reflected what the storyteller learned about his or her relationship with the dying person. Stories both affect and reflect relational identities (e.g., Koenig Kellas, 2003). Our data indicates that FC impacted emergent relational identities in three key ways: (a) uniqueness/importance of the relationship, (b) strengthening the relationship, and (c) confirming the relationship.

*Uniqueness/importance of the relationship* refers to instances in which the tellers portray themselves as having a unique relationship with the dying persons and/or describe themselves as important in the situation because of the unique relationship. Tellers of FC narratives realized the uniqueness and special nature of their relationships either because of final words of confirmation from their loved ones or because of their ability to communicate with the dying person when no one else could. Josie's FC with her father reinforced for her the importance of their relationship to him:

> You could see it in his eyes that ... we are the apple of his eye; for some reason that ... sentence just sticks out ... I always knew ... that we were important to him and everything, but I never knew how much until right then. Because he was just, "You know, y'all are my life. Y'all are ... what I've lived for and done all this for ... I'd be a totally different person if you all weren't here." (LL 121–127)

As this example illustrates, the dying person can communicate relational uniqueness explicitly. The storyteller also evidenced the importance of the relationship when he or she clearly assumed a particularly pivotal place in the dying person's FC experience. Roxanne describes the distinctiveness of her relationship with her father as evidenced during her FC:

> ... that communication didn't happen with anybody but me. But I think that's because I was the most attuned to him, listening to his stories and trying to, I dealt with him on a different level than the others ... I think it was on a more spiritual, soulful type level that we were attuned like that. (LL 92–95)

Tellers also described relational uniqueness in terms of *unexpected relational roles*. Brenda* recalls her FC experience by acknowledging that she and her grandmother were more like "significant others" than grandmother and granddaughter. Claire*'s uncle made sure to tell her that he thought of her as a daughter and his favorite in the family.

Finally, Victoria's husband illustrated the uniqueness and importance of their relationship in their final conversation on the night he passed away. Victoria recounts, "And then he ... said 'I want the luxury of being held to earth only by your love. Not to be connected to anything else.' ... he'd let everything else go" (LL 57–58). Tellers of FC narratives consistently celebrated the relational uniqueness that emerged in their FC experiences.

*Strengthening the relationship* statements included those in which the tellers describe how the process in some way improved or strengthened the relationship. For people who had experienced difficult relationships with the dying loved one, FC appeared to be particularly instrumental in building relational cohesion. Katherine* used the FC to tell her mother for the first time that she loved her. Victoria recognizes the FC experience as part of an ongoing process of healing and repairing the relationship with her mother. She recalls:

> It's more complicated with her. It wasn't just the final conversation. There were a lot of things that happened in the last years, years that changed the way I felt about the relationship. But, I think having the final conversation, being able to be the one who was there at the end, put a cap on my forgiveness and acceptance of her. (LL 145–148)

People who experienced positive relationships with loved ones prior to the FC experience, on the other hand, often reported a sense of *transcending the current relationship* through FC. Claire* describes her relationship during her FC as "... Intense. Really ... powerful ... closer than close ... I thought we were close before, and it was like we just opened up this new door and ... just more emotion. More ... love I think" (LL 468–473).

FC also offered tellers a sense of *closure and completeness* to the relationship. Weber et al. (1989) cited establishing a sense of closure as an important benefit of stories of loss, and the storytellers in this study confirmed its importance in their FC narratives. Ellen appreciated her FC with her husband because: "I completed my relationship with him. I didn't walk away thinking 'Uggh, I should have said. I didn't say. I coulda said. I wanted to say.' There wasn't anything ... that we didn't really say. And in the final analysis ... the most important things were all said" (LL 609–611).

Finally, FC reflected tellers' ability to *confirm the reality of the relationship*. These statements describe the overall characteristic of the relationship between the teller and the dying person, whether the statement reflects a negative or positive relationship. Tellers explained that they understood things about the relationship they had not realized and also learned how much the dying person loved them. For example, Roy's mother told him a powerful story about what he considered to be "the most important thing that ever happened to her," yet she had never shared the story with anyone else (LL 256–257). Because of their FC, he maintains, "Well, that's part of the reason that I knew she loved me best" (L 470). He, in turn, thanked her for being the most powerful influence in his life.

FC narratives allow people to *reaffirm and celebrate* their relationships with the dying person, and they also gave people the opportunity to *recapture parts of the relationship that had been lost*. Participants described a sense of knowing they were loved, even if that feeling had not been present prior to the final conversation. FC offered people a needed clarity about their relationships, illustrated by Katherine's* conclusions about the FC with her mother. Katherine* explains that "It changed my kinda definition of what [love] is. Of course she loved me. And of course I loved her. How silly to spend half my life thinking that there wasn't love between us just because we didn't say the words" (LL 166–169). Ultimately, FC narratives reflect the paramount importance of celebrating, making sense of, and/or remembering relational uniqueness between the teller and the dying loved one. In so doing, they support Bochner et al.'s (1997) assertion that "storytelling is not only the way we understand our relationships, but also the means by which our relationships are fashioned" (p. 310).

## Making Sense of and Coming to Terms With Death: The Healing Process

The third major theme that emerged from the FC interviews highlights the power of conversation for sense-making about death and healing. Nadeau (1998) stressed that the process of sharing experiences enables individuals to interactionally construct personal meanings of death. Clearly, as we have already demonstrated, one important aspect of storytelling includes reconciling *identity* in the face of adversity or traumatic events (Cohler, 1991). In addition, our analysis of the interviews clearly indicated three categories that reveal how FC help people come to terms with *death*: (a) making sense of death, (b) mapping out how to heal or take advice from the dying person, and (c) taking away positive lessons for life.

*Sense making statements* reflect the tellers' understanding of the final conversation, of death, or of the loss, in a way that helps them come to terms with the process. These statements reflect a cognitive process that occurs in the storytelling, indicating the teller has processed the meaning associated with the FC experience. These statements are not surprising, given that a number of scholars cite meaning-making as the central function of narratives (e.g., Babrow et al., chap. 2, this volume; Bochner et al., 1997; Bruner, 1990; Weber et al., 1989). At the end of life, family members often take the time to share stories with one another prior to the actual death of the loved one, resulting in a shift in the meaning of death for the individual members and/or the whole family (Nadeau, 1998). Participants shared with us the fact that their perspectives on death changed drastically because of their FC. Betty Lynn's new understanding of death following her FC and final interaction with a close family friend exemplifies such a shift:

> It's okay to die ... its okay to die. There is, there is a God, or whatever you want to call the higher power. For me it's God ... there is a hereafter. There is a place for us to go. We aren't just living here as a dead end thing, [and] when we die it's over with ... you know it [the FC experience] took away a lot of that fear of dying. And it just made ... dying a part of living, a part of that process. (LL 192–198)

This *shift in perspective* resulted directly from the interaction with the dying loved one. The sense-making emerged from reaffirmations about their beliefs or achievements of a new understanding regarding their loved one's belief regarding their meaning of death and/or an afterlife (i.e., it is a natural progression and the next stage of my life).

In addition to making sense of death because of FC, survivors talked in their FC narratives about experiences following the death of their loved ones that impacted their sense-making about death. Specifically, the tellers came to terms with their loved ones' death because they feel comforted by the *continued presence of the deceased*. Ellen reiterated numerous stories about her husband, Michael, giving her the sense that he was still connected to her. She felt his presence through dreams (LL 222–229) and a touch of Michael's hand on her right shoulder while she was driving (L 264). These experiences and other events allowed her to let go and to come to terms with her young husband's death. She observes that "my life changed after that. I mean, I didn't ... miss Michael any less, but my ability to be here and do my job here, going on in my life and raising my kids had been shifted" (LL 393–395).

Much of the meaning-making which emerged in the FC narratives revolved around survivors' beliefs concerning an afterlife. This strong belief in an afterlife coincides with Nadeau's (1998) findings that belief in an afterlife is a very important categorization of meaning-making in the midst of death experiences. The FC and/or experiences after the death of their loved ones' created a tremendous amount of comfort and peace for the participants.

*Mapping out how to heal together or get advice from the dying person* include statements that describe how the teller has reflected on the lessons given by the dying person for how to come to terms with death and go on living. Individuals talked about the profound importance of their FC on their future decisions. For instance, Sondra notes that her husband explicitly stated:

> "I don't want you to fear death. I don't want you to mourn me if I pass away ... death is a part of life ... don't mourn me, rejoice, because I'm in a better place" ... I'd always thought ... you show devotion to that person for a long time, even past their death. And he said "no, you will love ... your real love for someone is to want the best for them." (LL 19–34) ... [This] conversation made a big impact in why [I] don't have that bitterness. (LL 398–399)

People with the benefit of receiving permission to move on following the death of their loved one expressed the importance of this selfless act of love for their healing process. Victoria talked about other women that she knew that didn't receive permission to marry again from their spouses, how they were burdened with guilt (LL 251–255). Further, she stressed the fact that it does matter what is said during FC because it is often "the person who's dying [that] can lead the others [back to living]" (LL 229–230).

FC clearly helped every person that we talked with to feel better, to adjust to their personal loss, and was a critical part of their healing process. For instance, Victoria (#2) revealed that her FC with her husband ultimately helped to create a beautiful death resulting in tremendous comfort for her during his final days and immediately following his death. Specifically, she states:

> ... it was so beautiful and there was so much peace that ... it took me a lot of years to get how devastating his death had been to the girls [their 2 children]. Because for me it was devastating and I had to rebuild, but he convinced me that it was part of the picture, the way that his story needed to be. (LL264–268)

Clearly, loved ones can participate in the healing process by explicitly talking with the survivor about how to go on living. This finding supports Nadeau's (1998) conclusion that stories shared by individual family members when death is expected impacts (as well as reveals) how well people will cope with their grief following the death.

*Positive lessons for life* is the last category in the sense-making theme, and these statements focus on the lessons that participants learned from FC that they incorporated into their current realities. Sam shared how his FC with his mother taught him that how one faces death can result directly from how an individual leads his or her life. Specifically, he explains:

... the things that are important in the last years or months of your life are
the things that are important ... if you keep that in mind, if you think in
terms of ... is this something today that's gonna make me ... better prepared to face this transition in life that I'm going to be facing? ... And if
you ... face your death with regrets, or with bitterness, or with fear, or
with loneliness ... its because of all the choices that you made in life ... I'll
tell you how this has impacted [my life] ... my wife and I ... [will] sit down
and make 1-year goals, 5-year goals, 10-year goals, and then we [ask]
how do we want to end our lives kind of goals. ( LL 69–87)

These stories often revolved around living a good life by overcoming
fear, from living life from a place of love and not ego, and from learning
the lessons needed from all of our experiences—especially the death of
a loved one. The lessons learned during FC and communicated in FC
narratives seem consistent with Freeman and Brockmeier's (2001)
concept of *narrative integrity*, which suggests that autobiographical
identity depends on our conception of the good life as it "emerges in
line with specific social, historical, and discursive conditions regarding the importance of accounting for the life one has led in line with an
overarching cultural system of ethical and moral values" (p. 83). In our
data, FC narratives reflect an awareness of *morals and values* as central to the sense-making process.

## Communication Practices Resulting From Final Conversation Experiences

Finally, our data indicate that, in addition to (re)constructing identity
and making meaning both during the FC experience and in the retelling, participants also managed the dynamic nature of narrative time
(Ochs, 1997; Ricoeur, 1981b) by translating lessons from FC into current and future communicative practices. The interplay between the
categories in our findings reflects Somers (1994) assertion that "ontological narratives are used to define who we *are*; this in turn can be a
precondition for knowing what to *do*" (p. 618). The fourth major theme
that emerged from the FC interviews focuses on two areas of communicative behavior that participants learned from the actual process of interacting and talking with their loved one prior their death. In
particular, our participants articulated clear lessons about communication that occurs at the end of life as well as their communication with
loved ones in the present.

*Lessons learned about communication during final conversation*
include statements that describe the teller's awareness of the importance of communication at the end of life. Communication at the end of
life ran the gamut from casual everyday talk to very intimate statements of love.

*Everyday talk* conversations, mundane, routine, and, at times, utilitarian, remain an important and valuable part of FC for two reasons. First, everyday talk can reflect the reality of people's relationships (e.g., whether they were testy, silly, etc.) as they had been prior to the terminal illness. Duck (1994) and Duck and his associates (Duck, Rutt, Hurst, & Strejc, 1991) proposed that everyday talk comprises an integral part of maintaining relationships. Thus, everyday talk can be one way that people continue to promote and perpetuate the relationship during the final months and days of the loved ones' lives (Hedtke, 2002). Sam succinctly pinpoints the importance of the everyday talk:

> ... we think we realized at the time, that the interactions that were going on were really important. And it wasn't ... like some kind of major event ... the mundane, you know the unimportant things on the surface, but that were some real valuable things happening during that, that sharing ... you can see little microcosms of my family ... my sisters and me, kind of over talking to my mom. (LL 49–54)

Everyday talk during FC may also return a bit of normalcy to a situation that is very extraordinary. Dana clearly highlights this point when she talks about her conversations with her dying father. She was 11 when he died; he had been fighting a brain tumor for 3 years and was in a hospital for months at the end of his life. Dana remembers how her father often would bring the conversation back to the everyday things: "... he was always so, remember study for the math test ... because what it was ... not only a final conversation, but I was also leaving for the day. So, it was, don't forget ... work on your diorama, and do your projects" (LL 154–157).

Additionally, when a terminal illness extends over a long period of time, participants describe the exhaustion and difficulty of creating new and meaningful ways to say "goodbye" or "I love you," day after day. Thus, the talk about the ordinary (such as Dana's story about a grade earned on a test or Ellen's story about humorous discussions with her husband regarding the extra long hair on his chin) help to make the time a little less strange and possibly relieve the pressure to be profound all the time.

Alternatively, other conversations "complete the relationship ... that leaves nothing left unsaid" (Ellen, L 609–611). To that end, participants talked about the need to participate in honest and as authentic a conversation as possible, with their loved one. For instance, Brenda* recalls:

> I was relieved because I could finally now communicate with her. She knew how upset I was about her dying. And I could finally, I could finally

get our relationship back ... Because, not being able to express that to her, um, kinda put a gap there that had never been there. I wasn't allowed ... so I hid my feelings from her. Tried to anyway ... I didn't have to do that anymore. So it allowed us to be closer again. (LL 452–458) ... I learned that I could cry in front of people and not feel ashamed to cry about someone I love, for sure. (#27, LL 489–490)

These statements also reflect a desire for survivors to utilize their new-found awareness and appreciation concerning the importance of communication at the end of life in future interactions with dying loved ones. Betty Lynn summarizes beautifully what others had stated during their FC interviews. She advises:

Talk about death. Talk about what is happening. Don't let it become this monster that is going to invade you and then take you away from here ... tell the people that you want to tell them that you love them ... don't let things go unsaid ... feel all the feelings ... don't just stuff them away and not have 'em ... (LL 433–437)

Betty Lynn exemplifies the stories of other participants who helped others at the end of their lives by simply being open to and taking the time to really talk with the dying person.

On the other hand, others referred to fear or discomfort as reasons for avoiding a direct conversation about the impending death. Specifically, Cara reports:

I regret not talking ... I wish I wouldn't have tried to block it out that he was dying. I wish that I would've sat there and actually had a conversation with him ... I've never dealt with death before. So, seeing him there was hard enough, but I, I totally regret not talking to him ... I think I'll be able to deal with death differently because I'll ... be able to talk to them a lot differently. (LL 225–247)

Still others talked about being disappointed because they waited for a profound conversation, yet that conversation never came. When the dying person could not engage in an authentic conversation, the survivors found that they could not force the other person to say what they desired to hear or to even participate in a deep conversation. However, Katherine*, like others, came to the conclusion that she could be the one to say what needed to be said for her own closure. She notes:

... it took me days to get myself ready to tell her that I love her ... but I knew that it was my assignment ... but it took me weeks of processing and going and not saying it and going home and thinking ... I didn't do it ... it just had so much emotional baggage with it ... because she had never told me [that she loved me] ... I knew intellectually that I would be so angry if I didn't get this done and she died ... how wasteful. (#30, LL 240–249)

In the end, Katherine* successfully told her mother that she loved her and that she appreciated all that she had done for her, and Katherine* felt a tremendous sense of relief and peace. Others acknowledge that they participated in a meaningful nonverbal interaction to fulfill their need for a deep and authentic interaction. These nonverbal interactions usually involved the powerful and intimate code of touch. In Maureen's case, a hug fulfilled that need. For Roxanne, a squeeze of her hand facilitated closure. A vocalic response (e.g., Jules* received a grunt when no one else could get any kind of response) or a final look at the moment of death (Victoria) also became extremely powerful and meaningful.

*Tools for communicating more effectively in present, everyday, interactions* are statements that illustrate how the lessons learned during FC apply to their current communicative behaviors on a daily basis. Almost everyone talked about the fact that their FC made them realize that they don't want to leave anything unsaid because this experience made them realize that, in reality, anyone could die tomorrow. For instance, Cathy eloquently highlights the fact that we are accountable for what is said or left unsaid in our relationships. She observes that "the responsibility of every sentence ... pretend like it might be the last day with somebody you love and say those wonderful things you want to say" (LL 709–711). A common thread in these stories stresses the value of "seizing every opportunity to communicate" (Tory, L 591). Perhaps, Dana summarizes most clearly what others learned about communicating more effectively in their everyday interactions:

... one of the things I learned is I never know when somebody's last day is going to be. I try to always appreciate them in the present, and tell them ... I love them and how much they mean to me ... [I] don't treat them with disrespect ... If there is something going on, I feel that you have to clear the air because you don't know. Which ties back to what I learned from my dad ... you don't know when it is going to be the last time ... I never leave for work without the goodbye, I love, kiss, kiss, which takes forever. (LL 599–621)

Clearly, these interviews indicate communication within one specific context (i.e., at the end of a loved one's life) has a lasting impact on individuals' current interactions within close relationships. To be able to transcend painful periods in our life and apply lessons learned about communication to our everyday life is a hidden gift of FC.

## IMPLICATIONS AND CONCLUSIONS

Examining FC permits understanding of communication at the end of life and illustrates how narratives help survivors make sense of that process. First, FC narratives offers a unique opportunity for us to learn about ourselves and to confirm our identities by looking at ourselves in a new light or by seeing ourselves through a loved one's eyes. Second, FC narratives enables us to promote ongoing connections between us as survivors and the deceased (Hedtke, 2002), thereby confirming our relationships with our loved ones. Third, FC narratives empower people to utilize communication with their loved ones as a way to begin to make sense of death, their loss, and thereby begin the healing process. Fourth, we were struck by the lessons learned by individuals concerning communication with their loved ones at the end of their lives and how it also impacted their everyday communication practices.

These findings offer important new understanding to the process and functions associated with a subject understudied in the narrative and health communication literature: final conversations. In the process, the findings contribute to, as well as support, existing narrative theory. The stories, most often told years after the death of a loved one, reflect the complexity of narrative time (Ochs, 1997; Ricoeur, 1981b). Participants were able to take the scattered and past events surrounding the death of a loved one and create narratives with thematic meaning about individual and relational identity, as well as lessons about death and communication that affect the present telling and future lived events. FC narratives also clearly reflect social, historical, and relational contexts (Fisher, 1989; Somers, 1994). Situated in a time when the current "death culture" (Heinz, 1999; Kubler-Ross 1969, 1997) encourages minimal talk about death, these stories seem to help people shed the shroud of the death and make sense of difficult events. Our findings confirm previous research on the importance of the extended reportability and coherence of identity narratives (Linde, 1993), as well as the meaning-making and healing power in stories of death (Sedney et al., 1994) and, in so doing, help to position FC narratives, specifically, as an important part of coming to terms with the death of a loved one.

Because of this finding, not surprisingly, most of the FC stories in our study were overwhelmingly positive. At first reflection, it is easy to surmise that there is a simple methodological explanation. Specifically, because participants were self-selecting, people with negative FC may simply have chosen not to participate in the study, thus resulting in a skewed sample. Interestingly, however, the few participants that did have difficult relationships with their dying loved ones also chose to share their stories. Yet, despite the fact that these narratives were often more difficult to share and even negative in part, the tellers ultimately provided a positive spin to the conclusion of the story. Beyond methodology, it may be that participants recall and shape the FC experience in such a way that can help the storytellers minimize their pain or self-doubt, thereby empowering them in a way that helps them to overcome their loss. Further, narrative theory suggests that people are biased by a social norm to focus on the positive aspects of stories. Freeman and Brockmeier (2001) suggested, for example, that people's autobiographical narratives adhere to the cultural, historical, and ethical standards of "the good life." In addition, a societal bias toward positive narratives is reflected in life story research, which focuses on how people can create a sense of coherence in their narrated identities (e.g., Baerger & McAdams, 1999; Cohler, 1991; Linde, 1993) and strands of narrative therapy that promote ways for people to "restory" their negative experiences (Monk et al., 1997).

It may also be important that most of the participants had a lot of time to mourn, heal, and to reflect on their FC before sharing their stories with the interviewer (i.e., the average amount of time from FC to the interview was 6.9 years). Thus, time may have also been an issue regarding the positive nature of the stories. The participants that recalled FC shortly after the death (e.g., 6 months or less), focused more on the actual death rather than on the FC and were more negative in nature (due to the talk about the actual death process). Clearly, having the time to recall and reflect on the actual conversations served an important function in the sense-making process for the participants and likely contributed to the nature of the stories told. Future research might assess how repeated tellings evolve and contribute to the sense-making and healing process.

An alternative conclusion, and an important implication for our understanding of FC narratives, is that the lack of any stories regarding regret[3] constitutes a testament to the importance of communication at the end of life for the survivor. One of the final questions that participants were specifically asked focused on possible regrets and/or drawbacks regarding FC. Every participant in our study stated that the potential for positive outcomes resulting from the FC far outweighed any potential negative risks (e.g., strong emotions, unmet expectations, or negative messages). The finality of death may help people overcome petty grievances and focus their attention on the positive aspects of relationships and communication. This finding may also suggest that people are biased from the outset to look for and focus on the positive stories as a way to have a good ending with their loved one.

Finally, participants stated that telling the story of their FC was very important. All of the participants talked about the value and significance of sharing their FC with the interviewer and thanked her for asking them to tell their story. Sharing their FC story, in the midst of living in a society in which the norm is to not to talk about death and the events that surround it, was perceived to be uplifting, freeing, and healing. Participants cherished the opportunity to tell an important story with someone who was willing to listen, further strengthening the argument that people need to share stories with others. Overwhelmingly, our data suggest that participating in FC and sharing stories about our FC are two important ways that we can "turn toward death together" (McQuellon & Cowan, 2000, p. 318).

## NOTES

1. Most of the participants chose to have their real name used in all publications, however, an * indicates the use of a pseudonym at the participant's request.
2. Participant's interviews were transcribed verbatim. Use of L and LL signifies the line number (L) or line numbers (LL) that correspond with the line numbers from each corresponding transcript.
3. With the one exception of Cara, #20, who attributed her avoidance of genuine conversation with her grandfather to her fear of and lack of experience with death.

## APPENDIX: FINAL CONVERSATIONS INTERVIEW QUESTIONS GUIDELINE

1. Would you share with me your recollection (your story) of your final conversation or conversations with your loved one?

Follow up questions/specific details about one or more of the conversations:

2. What was the most meaningful conversation that you had with this person?

3. Why was it the most meaningful to you? Who initiated this conversation?

4. How did you or he/she initiate the conversation?

5. Were you alone during this particular conversation? If not, who else was present?

6. Who did most of the talking during this conversation?

7. What was the most important thing that you "got out of" (or "took away with you" or "stayed with you") from this "final" conversation? Why?

8. (What do you think the dying person got out of the conversation?)

Nonverbal Experiences:

9. What sorts of nonverbal experiences (anything other than the words themselves—you may need to give some general examples for clarification) stick out in your mind from this time period? AND what did each of the nonverbal experiences mean to you?

10. Which of those experiences were the most meaningful to you and why?

General Questions:

11. How would you characterize your relationship with (name of person) before you knew they were dying?

12. How would you characterize your relationship with (name of person) after you knew they were dying? (If there was a change) What do you attribute the change in your relationship to?

13. How do you think your final conversations made you feel about your relationship to (name the person)? Why?

14. How were your perceptions about YOU (and/or) your actions impacted by this conversation?

15. What were the lessons that you learned from this/these conversation(s)?

16. What aspects of your personal life were changed (if they did) as a result of this experience?

17. What barriers (or obstacles) did you experience in regard to your disclosure (i.e., revealing of yourself, or being able to open up or ask the other person about certain things) during this time period?

18. What were some of the conversations that you initiated and what did they do for you and for your loved one?

19. Any drawbacks to these final conversations?

20. What are the benefits to final conversations?

21. Have you had anything occur that you would consider communication or a sign from this loved one since he/she has passed?

22. Is there anything that the two of you didn't talk about but you wish you had?

23. Is there anything else that you would like to add?

# 18

## An Examination of the Role of Narratives and Storytelling in Bereavement

∾

**Cecilia Bosticco**
**Teresa L. Thompson**
*University of Dayton*

*I had been in my second semester of graduate work when Teresa was diagnosed and began her battle with cancer. When I returned to school about ten months after her death, I found myself still looking for ways to understand what had happened to me. Every class I took, every theory I encountered, every paper I was assigned became a vehicle of explanation. I revised my thesis topic in order to more systematically explore the power of sharing stories in the processing of grief—a power that I had personally experienced among my friends, family and acquaintances.*

—Cecilia Bosticco

Bereaved individuals are "wounded storytellers" in similar fashion to those discussed by Frank (1995). Their bodies, minds and emotions exhibit signs of the "illness" of bereavement, crying out for the opportunity to give voice to their experience. Through the use of storytelling, they begin to make sense of their malaise, to take control of events formerly beyond their power of influence. Cecilia's personal bereavement experience in the aftermath of the death of her 13-year-old daughter provided the impetus for this research. This chapter is based on her experiences and thesis research. She conducted the interviews on which this work is based. Any reference to "I" within this chapter refers to her experiences and perceptions.

In past work, we have overviewed the process of grieving and delineated the importance of family communication in general on the grieving/bereavement process as well as the relevance of narratives/storytelling in bereavement. In the present piece, we report a qualitative study that examines this process more specifically. Although we refer back to research from those earlier reviews, because of the lengthy nature of the present results, we will not begin with a traditional literature review. After reviewing the theoretical perspective that frames the present study, Walter Fisher's Narrative Paradigm, and detailing our methods of analysis, we turn to the compelling stories of grieving parents. Through their voices, we gain insights into the powerful and therapeutic nature of narrative. Although, as Cecilia will attest, narratives prompted by loss cannot erase tragedy, they can bring understanding and resolve for the future.

## THEORETICAL FRAMEWORK

Fisher (1984) viewed narrative as a "master metaphor" (p. 6) rather than as a "particular method of investigation" (p. 2). By proposing that the human species be called "*homo narrans*" (p. 6), he claims a central position for the narrative paradigm such that all other methods of understanding communication flow from this central concept. Fisher argues that storytelling remains intrinsic to the nature of humans and that humans use "good reasons" (p. 7) as criteria for making decisions and communicating in various contexts. Further, according to Fisher, humans create and apply good reasons to fit specific situations according to norms or rules dictated by their history, culture, personal integrity, and experience. As such, Fisher contends that people must choose among all the stories the world has to offer in order to create a good life for themselves.

Each individual participates in his or her life as one who reasons and makes value decisions (Fisher, 1984). Individuals constantly re-create stories. Each story requires an author (a person who tells the story) and co-authors (people who receive the story and the audience that participates in the creation of meaning for the story). The world provides plots and texts that the storytellers creatively retell, making meaning and value judgments as they do so. They rely on narrative rationality to assess these value judgments, gauging both narrative fidelity and narrative probability as essential factors in determining the extent to which they will value a story (Fisher, 1984).

*Narrative fidelity* addresses the "truth" of the story. People make use of learned (but not formal) ways of judging the values expressed in a story. They turn to what Fisher (1985a) called the "logic of good reasons" (p. 349). An individual develops these good reasons based on his or her background, culture, beliefs, self-concept, interactions with others, and past experiences. In other words, a person uses his or her unique blend of personal perceptive tools to measure the veracity of the stories he/she hears or constructs. If a story does not meet these criteria for truthfulness, it fails the test of narrative fidelity (Fisher, 1985a, 1985b).

Narrative probability evaluates story construction. People recognize a specific set of rules or expectations about what makes up a story—a particular sequence of events, sensible causal relationships between important elements, and a distinct framework that includes some things while excluding others. If a narrative does not emerge as a coherent entity that matches what people expect in a story, it fails the test of narrative probability (Fisher, 1985a, 1985b).

Through this framework, then, we investigate the ways in which individuals make sense of loss that defies consistency or coherence, according to preconceived life scripts—the death of a child. The current investigation resembles other works on health and narrative by Frank (1995), Kleinman (1988), and White and Epston (1990), but it extends and further explains some aspects of these scholarly contributions. Much of the work on the therapeutic value of storytelling focuses on what storytelling does to facilitate understanding and meaning-making for the person who is ill. This research looks at a different kind of "illness"—bereavement—and explores the role of storytelling separate from its use by "experts" such as doctors or therapists. As such, this chapter presses the boundaries of current health communication research, contributing theoretical and empirical understanding of healing beyond disease or disability to disruption of life due to premature death.

## Research Question

Fisher's narrative paradigm suggests that people naturally turn to stories in an attempt to understand and find their way through a devastating happening such as the loss of a loved one. Through the use of narratives, they look for "good reasons" for the event and for their emotions in response to it. They create and apply these good reasons according to norms and rules learned from history, culture, and personal experience, fitting with the personal integrity of the individual who measures the rationality of such stories by use of narrative probability and narrative fidelity. From among all of the stories possible to be told, an individual chooses the ones that facilitate a good life for himself or herself and his or her family.

This chapter examines the role of such stories in the grieving and bereavement process. The following research question will be addressed in this study: How do grieving parents use the storytelling process to help them cope with loss and bereavement?

## METHODS

Bereavement constitutes a difficult time for most people, but grief responses vary. One of the critical indicators of a strong grief response to loss is the degree of involvement of the bereaved individual's self image in his or her relationship with the person who dies. The parental role involves an individual in bonds with his or her child, based both on interaction and culturally mandated expectations. These bonds strongly affect the self-concept of the individual. When a child dies, the parent suffers formidable losses to his or her self-concept in addition to the loss of the relationship with the child. These multiple losses usually result in a strong grief response in bereaved parents. Thus, this study engages bereaved parents as respondents in an attempt to assure that the individuals interviewed are reporting from a strong experience of grief.

We employed snowball sampling to recruit participants. Respondents included four White males, one African American female, and five White females. Their children died at ages ranging from 10 days to 40 years. The duration of their bereavement experiences (the time from the death of their child until they were interviewed) varied from 3½ to 30 years. These respondents exhibit wide variance in terms of the age of death of their children, cause of death of their children, and duration of bereavement; however, they hold in common a strong grief experience.

We devised an interview guide to elicit the respondents' personal stories of their bereavement experiences and to guide participants in covering similar topics in their accounts. We sought to provide an opportunity for respondents to talk about their grieving experiences. Our interview sessions lasted for 1 to 1½ hours. We audiotaped all sessions with the permission of the respondents and later transcribed them. We used these transcriptions and the sparse notes taken during the interviews as data for our analysis.

We labeled the narratives and collected similar topics into groups. Narrative analysis of the accounts yielded rich results for the discussion of the research question. Although it is rather unconventional to cite and integrate so much past research in a findings section, the practice brings together various conceptions about stories, including how they work for people, with the accounts of this study's participants to discern how stories were valuable to these bereaved parents. Many examples emerged from the accounts of these respondents that confirmed their use of narrative processes to create meaning, to test action plans, and to make choices that helped them and their families deal successfully with the effects of the loss of their children. In order to protect the privacy of the parents who shared their stories in this study, fictitious names have been used in our description of findings.

## FINDINGS

Fisher's (1984) presentation of his theory of the narrative paradigm provides an excellent organizational pattern for analysis of the data in response to this question. His first premise is that people naturally turn to stories. Brockmeier and Harré (1997) agreed, claiming that people become so practiced in the ability to understand on the basis of narratives, that storytelling becomes "transparent" (p. 272) to them. They tell stories without being aware of doing so.

Schank (1990) asserted that telling a story is necessary to confer reality on an event for the person who has been involved in it. According to Weick (1995), stories "impose a formal coherence" (p. 128) on the disorderly stream of happenings in the world. A story preserves the "connectivity" (Schank, 1990, p. 125) of incidents. Unless a story collects details in a coherent structure, things that happen to people are remembered "cross-contextually"; that is, particular instances are stored along with other instances of similar type and separated from the specific situations in which they occur (Schank, 1990, p. 122). Details that are gathered into a story and given a causal structure are remembered together with the story. Those that are not, are lost to "dynamic disconnection" (Schank, 1990, p. 124). People decide which details to connect to their stories, not realizing that because the story will be remembered as a unit and the other details will dissipate in time, the story will eventually become the reality (Schank, 1990).

An examination of the results reveals common elements in the stories told by the respondents to this survey. Most obviously, they find loss to be very difficult, but those interviewed developed strategies for coping with their losses. All of the respondents came to an acceptance of grief, verbalizing a recognition of the individuality of its process, whether in talking about differences among family members, discussing variations in the sharing of members of support groups, or in wanting others to respect their personal grief journeys. The belief that time and process change the effect of the loss on the individual, but pain, loss, sadness and emptiness remain to some degree, emerged as another common element. Reorganization following loss does occur. The participants voiced a sense of commonality with others who have lost a child, but a feeling that they are "out of kilter" with others who have not had the same experience. Further, each person's story connected deeply to the reality of the loss. Every one of them came to a section of his or her story that brought evidence of strong emotion. One woman cried several times.

## The Therapeutic Value of Emplotment

Four parents in this study narrated experiences that point to their instinctive desire to collect the details related to their children's deaths into a story. For Carl, assembling a plausible story about the night of his son's death was a long but necessary task. He found witnesses to what happened at the party and others confirmed that his son had dropped off some girls at their homes. However, after that, Carl discovered only circumstantial evidence from measurements taken by investigators at the accident scene. Carl had to build his narrative based on his own knowledge of his son's car, of his son's driving ability, and of his son's physical soundness for driving that night as well as on the basis of pure conjecture. Yet, he was able to construct a perfectly believable account that, for him, was a good story of what happened the night of his son's accidental death. The story allows this father to put his son to rest as a responsible young adult who made a slight mistake in judgment and drove a less than dependable car rather than as an irresponsible teenager who deliberately took unacceptable risks with his life. The pain resulting from the loss of his son is immense, and creating the story helps Carl to somewhat ameliorate it by casting his son in the best possible light.

Tess, whose son was killed in a motorcycle accident, admitted that it had been difficult for her to accept the reality of her son's death. During the early part of her bereavement, "If I saw a motorcycle, I had to go check it out. If someone looked like him, I had to go check it out," she said. She felt compelled to collect every report and certificate on which she was able to lay her hands relating to the accident and her son's death. Tess confides, "I had asked my sister to take a picture of [my son] in the coffin so that later on I will know he is really dead." Her desire to find out all the details and to have physical evidence of the death indicated that she needed to build a story from all of the information available so that she could understand and accept what happened to her son.

Beth and Mark, whose son was killed in a military accident, provide the third and fourth examples. Interviewed separately, they both discussed the announcement of their son's death by official military representatives. Beth says, "And they said there's been an accident and your son has been killed. That's all.... So, your initial thing is, 'Well, what happened? Where did this happen? What happened? What's'— you know, no details. They have no details—or if they do, they won't tell you." Mark relates,

They said, "He's dead," and that's exactly the way they said it.... That's all they had.... In fact, we didn't get any details until two days later when his friend brought him home. Then he told us the details.... And we didn't really get the details of everything until the guys came down and we spoke to the guys. And, you know, we got piecemeal details from our sons talking to them and on the side.... They told us the stories ... and it was wonderful for us.

Building the story was essential to them. They naturally sought it. According to Tannen (1988), stories facilitate the development of a relationship between the actual happenings and the people involved. Beth's and Mark's narratives include information about the young military men who came to the funeral and about their abilities to tell stories regarding the son's daily activities at the military station. The stories created connections between the son's military comrades and his family.

As discussed in the preceding paragraphs, stories bind details together at the same time as they create a connection between events and people. Individuals coping with loss desire these qualities of stories. Thus, in cases where individuals lack significant details, such as in a perinatal death situation, survivors may deliberately create memories, a practice often encouraged by therapists (Gough, 1999; Mahan & Calica, 1997; Shapiro, 1993; Worden, 2002). Something as simple as taking photographs of the dead or dying child can be very supportive.

A case of the deliberate creation of details to produce a more positive story occurs in the narrative of the motorcycle victim's mother. She talked about her own sense of helplessness in approaching her son's funeral and about the uncomfortable things that occurred in the funeral her ex-husband had planned at the time of her son's death. She also told about the memorial service that she planned on the first anniversary of his death. By that time, she had time to think about what would have been more comforting and supportive to her in a funeral. She incorporated all of those things in the memorial service—photographs, appropriate music, the people who were present the night her son died. She reported that the first anniversary memorial service "was probably the most healing thing I had done in the whole five years." Due to her deliberate creation of details to remember, she is now able to replace the pain of the original funeral story with the satisfaction of the memorial service.

Fisher (1984) contended that people use "good reasons" (p. 7) to measure how they talk about what happens to them and how they should behave in response. One measure of good reasons results from the establishment of one event as the cause of another. McAdams (1990) talked of the ability of narratives to arrange what happens in orderly patterns that facilitate the discovery of causal relationships. We discussed causal interaction between events as an essential element of a story earlier in this section.

Without exception, our participants indicate in their accounts that the death of a child comprises a good reason for one to experience grief. This acceptance of loss as a good reason for grief represents establishment of causal relationship. Our parents also talk about pain, disorganization, anger, and many other responses as reasonable results of grief. Descriptions of coping strategies and the result of time's passage that lead to a return to a normal or "new normal" exemplify our respondents' recognition of causal patterns.

Another example of the use of good reasons as a measure for behavior occurs when we ask participants to give advice to others who have lost a child. They suggested that any response that occurs as a result of grief is acceptable. They rated the loss of a child as a good reason for a parent to experience a whole range of responses that, according to their experience, should be considered to be normal. Participants recommended that action in response to grief should be accommodated, both by the bereaved and by members of his or her social network. As one father stated, losing a year of volunteerism is reasonable for a person who is taking care of his or her grief needs—finding a way to survive.

## Bereavement Stories as Cultural Artifacts

Fisher (1984) also maintained that people create and apply good reasons for behavior and communication according to basic rules they have absorbed from history, culture, and their own personal experience. Brockmeier and Harré (1997) agreed, asserting that people create stories that define them as members of their social environment. These authors observe that children learn about storytelling in much the same way as they learn language. Children immerse themselves in storytelling from birth, eventually acquiring a repertoire of familiar cultural stories along with a relaxed capability for their use.

Schank (1990) claimed that people use the stories of their culture as lenses through which to view daily events and that they also construct their own stories based on those same common stories. They learn rules or sets of expectations about the kinds of stories that count as acceptable in any culture. Storytellers must match the details and causal patterns of the events they attempt to develop into a story to these accepted rules or expectations. If they cannot, listeners will find it difficult to follow their stories and will object. Schank (1990) called this process "story-fitting" (p. 169). Culturally based stories allow hearers to feel acquainted with what people tell, and they develop a delicate balance between the generality of the cultural story and the individuality of the narrative based on it (J. A. Robinson & Hawpe, 1986).

A good example of the power of a cultural story comes from Ann's narrative. Losing her newly married son to an aneurysm challenged her coping abilities, especially because the kind of support that is currently offered to bereaved individuals was not available when her loss occurred. She found comfort in a religious cultural story—that of resurrection. She believes in a life–death–resurrection cycle that is based in the stories of her Christian religion. Those stories tell Ann that her son is not dead, but experiencing eternal life through resurrection. In the story that she told about him, he was enjoying life with his deceased father, to whom he had been very close, and all of the other relatives she has lost. Her story follows the cultural master story with which she is familiar. Indeed, it is likely that Ann's Christian faith does not just constitute a cultural master story, but is rather an intrinsic part of who she is, what she believes, and how she can heal, spiritually and emotionally. It may well be an integral part of her identity and ability to heal (see Parrott, 2004b).

Another example of a parent connecting to a culturally familiar story comes from Mark. His narrative of the viewing and the funeral was filled with satisfaction and mostly glowing accounts of emotional and spiritual support that he and his family received during that time. Berardo (1988) stated that societies create the rules and rituals surrounding loss to help people cope with it. Such rituals help survivors because they arise from cultural precedents yet possess the power to speak to new situations (Imber-Black, 1991). Although Mark did not directly refer to the cultural stories that were relived in his families' experiences during these days of ritual, he made use of them. The story of his son's funeral and burial re-create familiar cultural stories that are comfortable and comforting because of their familiarity.

Three of our respondents reported that their cultural experience was lacking when it came to providing norms and rules for them in their bereavement experience. The current American culture remains ill at ease with the yearning and searching behaviors that are normal for grievers (Silverman, 1988). This discomfort leads to the subjects of death and bereavement becoming taboos—things not talked about in polite society (Irwin, 1991). This attitude caused these three parents to call for a more open and frank dialogue about bereavement in our society to better prepare people for dealing with it.

Kate, the mother of a 15-year-old girl who died of a chronic disease, spoke at length about her own lack of death and dying experience as she was growing up. She had no good ideas about how to change the general lack of conversation about such topics, but definitely cried out for an end to the taboo status of death and dying in general discussion.

Ann expressed a wish that she had known more about dealing with death before her son died. She had only been to one funeral prior to her own experience with death and that had happened when she was a young wife. May, who had cared for her retarded daughter in her home for 39 years, talked about efforts of others to comfort her, but she complained that those people had not learned how to "walk in the shoes" of the bereaved and, thus, were not very good at it.

Another example relates to the American culture's attitude about God. Three of our participants came across an apparent cultural bias related to trust in God—people seemed very apt to cite "God's will" to explain death and tragedy. Because our participants belong almost exclusively to one particular religion, Catholicism, it may be that the phenomenon of citing God's will at the time of death arises more specifically from their religious culture, rather than from their national culture. Nonetheless, the practice was recognized and rejected by these three respondents. The role of religion and spirituality is just beginning to be recognized in the research on health communication (Parrott, 2004b).

May objects to hearing people try to comfort her by citing God's will. She suggested that it would be more soothing to her to have company or be invited to go out rather than to hear how God felt about her daughter. Beth claimed that God had nothing to do with her son's accident. She blamed it on "horseplay" and the fact that God allows people freedom to do what they will. Things just happen, she believes. God stands ready to sustain and support people through whatever occurs in their lives. Paul, who lost his newborn son, deliberately named the people who taught him about God. He rejected the will of the vengeful God that he was taught to fear. He found comfort in the idea of randomness. These parents experienced and discarded the culturally accepted method of explaining the death of their children because personal experience revealed the cultural story to be lacking.

## (Re)storying and Decision Making

One can explore imaginary and implausible possibilities in stories, according to Weick (1995) and Brockmeier and Harré (1997). Because they can include both known and hypothetical elements, stories can be constructed and reconstructed until they become believable explanations of reality (Robinson & Hawpe, 1986). Hearers can accept that a story may only represent one believable explanation for an event and that other equally convincing accounts might clarify the same situation (Robinson & Hawpe, 1986). Because people view stories in this way, narratives not only have the power to interpret events in a particular way, but also can be used to reexplain the same events when and if the person's meaning and/or experience change (Brockmeier & Harré, 1997, Robinson & Hawpe, 1986). Schank (1990) asserted that insight can be gained through rethinking one's own stories.

May, Beth, and Paul expressed familiarity with the cultural expectation that bereaved individuals should be comforted by assurances about God willing the death of their children. Yet, when they constructed their own stories of bereavement, they rebelled because their experience demanded a different script. These parents could not cope with their loss through belief in a God who wanted them to live the rest of their lives without their children, so they had to find another explanation for why their children died. A new story, unambiguously placing God on their side, allowed continued trust in the higher power in whom they believe and comfort from God's care.

Fisher (1984) asserted that people possess an inbred ability to measure the rationality of stories. They employ *narrative probability* (the way a story fits the rules for a story) and *narrative fidelity* (the veracity or truth of a story) as their criteria. Robinson and Hawpe (1986) supported this premise, stating that when a story is effectively constructed, it is "coherent and plausible" (p. 111). Robinson and Hawpe (1986) concurred that people expect plausibility in the accounts that they hear.

For instance, Kate spoke about all of the people who were present right after her teenage daughter died. She mentioned that her father came into the room and that he was crying. Without further explanation, this fact would not seem out of the ordinary for the situation; however, it held special significance for her at the time, and it was important for the listener to have background about the reason for its significance. To help the listener understand the implication of her father's tears, Kate inserted another short anecdote about her father, saying that he had only cried in the sight of his children three times—at Kennedy's death, at King's death, and at this granddaughter's death. The anecdote clarified an important causal relationship in the first story—the assertion of her father's intense grief at her daughter's death.

In another instance, Paul talked about the feeling of being out of control at the birth of his son. He told a second story that reinforced and enlarged upon the first story. In the second anecdote, Paul talked about how he had always been able to control the actions of his children as they were growing up; however, in the case of his daughter's problem with anorexia, he could find no way to exert that control and to make her eat properly. The "out of control" feeling seems to be a common denominator in both stories, the second anecdote augmenting and explaining the experience in the first story.

Another indication of storytellers' awareness of the need for clear causal relationships regards their attempt to clarify conflicting cause-

and-effect statements that are made in stories. They follow these seemingly inaccurate sequences of events with explanations that appear to have come from their own struggle with the facts and indicate the storytellers' subsequent adjustment of their understanding of the facts so that they make more causal sense.

For example, Kate talked about behaving in an automatic manner for a year after her daughter's death and told of an incident related to paying her water bill. She clearly remembers going downtown with the intention of paying the water bill and thinking that she had done so. However, she received a bill that indicated she had not done so. As she was talking, Kate realized that the facts she remembered and related did not seem to make sense based on the resultant past-due water bill, so she inserted a statement that reflects her own quandary about the situation. She said, "I think what happened is" that she must not have paid the bill because she couldn't find a parking place. She adjusted the story in midtelling to reflect her realization that the first version did not follow the causal relationship story rule.

Kate provided another example of midstory adjustment related to cause-and-effect story rules. She talked about the pain of being physically separated from her daughter for 3 years so far and of the difficulty of thinking about people she knows who have lived 50 years without their deceased children. In the midst of her discussion, she seemed to realize that one solution would be for her to die soon. She immediately moved from storytelling to prayer in a request for a long life. As she returned to the subject of long separation from her child, she acknowledged that others have done it and so will she. She said, "It'll be all right." Kate rejects one logical solution to a difficult situation as quickly as it seems to arise.

The preceding example also illustrates the premises of several other researchers. According to McAdams (1990), stories constitute natural carriers of meaning and motives. They can provide "tools" (Weick, 1995, p. 150) for analysis of events and help solve inherent problems in situations, allowing for discovery of what actions can be taken and what can be learned (Robinson & Hawpe, 1986). Kate allows the listener to hear her realization of the results of her plot dilemma as well as her adjustment of the story so that it fits the effects she wants to occur.

Another example of a storyteller making use of a story as a tool for discerning future actions and beliefs occurs in John's narrative. He talked of efforts that he and his wife made to act on a belief in faith healing on behalf of their daughter, who was born with a chronic disease. They took actions that boldly indicated their faith that she would be healed of her disease. Following the plot of faith healing, they should have been steadfast in believing that God would grant healing in response to their faith-filled actions and that the disease would have left her. However, in the midst of their action, they were unable to follow that storyline. It just did not make sense based on other information they also believed, and they returned their daughter to her familiar medical management routine. During our interview, John was still teased by the promise of faith healing, but he knew that that plot line did not work for him and his family. He told me that he was sad about that because it affected his belief in the power of prayer. He prays in a different way now because he has chosen not to adopt the faith healing storyline as his own. He envies gospel stories because, in them, people receive what he was unable to incorporate into his own story–healing for themselves and/or their children. He has learned that the temptation to retell his story according to a different belief system does not fit with his experience—that its causal relationships are faulty.

Narrative fidelity, according to Fisher (1984) tests the truth of a story. Schank (1990) claimed that the only way new information can be understood is when it connects in some way to one's own stories. In other words, stories "connect the unknown to the known" (Brockmeier & Harré, 1997, p. 279). An integration of these ideas suggests that what people recognize to be true resides in the stories with which they are already acquainted, thus, they judge the narrative fidelity of new stories based on stories they already know and trust.

In Jen's story, we see an example both of the use of story as a "tool" and of a storyteller's ability to make judgments based on narrative fidelity. Jen's newborn son died 10 days after he was born. Her story includes discussion of two conscious decisions that she made during her bereavement. At first, she chose to die, which she attempted to implement via drug and alcohol abuse. Subsequently, she decided not to lose her other child due to her self-destructive behavior, which she executed via treatment and participation in Alcoholics Anonymous. Currently, she is a recovering alcoholic. She has been actively attending AA meetings for 18 years.

Jen now tells the story of her own tragedy and alcoholic response to other women who have become alcoholic in response to tragedy. She hopes to help those other women cope with their problems by telling the story of how she successfully coped with a similar problem. She hopes that the other women can connect their story to hers and find in her recovery a key to their own recoveries. She remains convinced that her story can become the tool to which other women can connect their own experience and from which they can learn to improve their own lives. Her actions demonstrate an inherent belief in narrative fidelity—that her story will ring true for others. At the same time, this constructive retelling of her experience helps allow Jen to build some good out of the painful experiences surrounding her son's birth and death.

Kate's story demonstrates narrative fidelity very clearly. After her daughter died, Kate joined a book club at church that discussed a book that she refused to read. She explained that she knew the book talked about questioning God and that her religious background would not allow her to do so. When she joined a bereavement support group, other parents not only openly questioned God, but they expressed anger at God for what happened to their children. She was shocked because her own story did not allow such behavior; however, she realized that these other parents questioned and expressed anger without being punished (as her story led her to believe would happen). She told me that, although she was not sure how questioning the God on whom one depends can be good for one, she had come to be willing to express her questioning and angry emotions to God, based on the evidence of the other parents in the support group. Up to the point of our interview, her experience had not shown the questioning to be harmful. Kate's measure of the truth of the stories of other parents is her own story. She seems to be timidly testing her ability to adapt her measure of narrative fidelity because of hearing the stories of others.

Carl gives us another example of the use of narrative fidelity. He told about attending a series of support group meetings. He said he had been answering for his wife whenever questions were raised at the group meetings to protect her from dealing with the difficulties of grief. His actions came from a benevolent protector type of male mentality, and he only meant to support her. When challenged by the group facilitator, he became angry, and he could no longer seek support from the group. He actually stopped attending, allowing his wife to go alone. As he talked about this incident, he never admitted that the group facilitator might be right in asserting his wife must do her own grief work. His own story told him that it was good to protect his wife from harm, and it seemed apparent to him that grief was harmful for her. At a different time in our interview, he claimed that he supported her bereavement needs and that his efforts have brought them closer since their son's death. Carl needed to maintain the consistent theme that he supported his wife in her bereavement. That theme reflects the truth of his own story and preserves narrative fidelity for him.

Returning to Jen's story, we see a powerful example of a storyteller revising the plot of a story to reflect changes in both her experience and her insight. During the period immediately following her son's death, when Jen was acting under her self-proclaimed decision to die, she appeared to the rest of society to be doing fine. She went to work. She took care of her daughter. She seemed to move on. This is one story that Jen could tell about that time. Another story about the same time could be that she was not really present for her daughter, that she was only going through the motions of working and taking care of her family, that she was killing herself with drugs and alcohol. When Jen faced the choice of shaping up her life or losing her daughter, she made a second deliberate decision. She decided to work through whatever steps it would take to avoid losing her first child as she had lost her second. Her motives and meaning changed, so she changed her attitude and behavior. Because of those changes, Jen can now tell this second story and allow it to become the basis and reason for the new life that she now leads as a result of alcohol abuse treatment and working the AA twelve-step process. She is conscious of the divergence of the two stories relating to the same time in her life, and she uses them as illustrations to other women of the probability that they can change their own unpleasant stories as well.

Fisher (1984) argued that people pick the stories they want to use from all stories available so that they can make a good life for themselves and their families. A striking example of this premise resides in the story of Paul. He talked about people trying to comfort him with the statement, "It's God's will." He vigorously rejected that explanation along with the story that he associates with it about the nature of God. He recounted coming upon a different explanation (story) that fit his experience more closely—that of randomness. Paul voices satisfaction with the random-event explanation for his son's injury and death, repeating it several times during his narrative.

Paul clearly chooses one story above the other for his own good and that of his family. Accepting "It's God's will" as a cause for his son's death would make him and his family targeted victims of a vengeful God. A story based on that cause would seriously hamper Paul's ability to call on God for support and help. As a father, Paul strives to teach his children about their religious heritage. The "God's will" scenario is impossible for him to reconcile with his own experience, and he refuses to pass it on to his children. On the other hand, if he accepts the randomness of events in the world as the cause of his son's misfortunes, he may call on a God who might allow people to suffer difficulties as part of being human, but who stands with and supports those same people through those difficulties. Paul can then teach his children about God as a caring father rather than a merciless judge.

Mark and Paul gave us other instances of deliberate choice of a story when, without prompting, they both brought up the subject of family definition. Both acknowledged that answering the question, "How many children do you have?" was more difficult for them now that they have lost a child. Now they need to have a prepared reply, unlike before their losses. Paul admitted that he doesn't claim the son that he lost 10 days after birth when asked about his children. In our interview, he gave a practice sentence that might introduce the subject of his lost son, but he found the resulting story long and difficult to tell. He said he was not sure he wanted "to go there" anyway. When the prospect of including his first son (an infant who never left the confines of the hospital) in the conversational story was not satisfying to him, Paul decided to claim only his two living children. His decision seemed to be consistent with the rest of his story. While he cherished the life and death of his first son, he did not usually deal with that memory on a daily basis. Paul's choice of a family definition story reflects his general experience.

In the other case, Mark said that he always claims all four of his sons, even though one died. He expresses satisfaction with the story that he has prepared to support this decision, an account coinciding with his larger bereavement story. He admitted thinking of his son often and keeping reminders of him at home and at the office. His son had been 19 years old at the time of his death, and Mark's choice to continue to include him in the family definition acknowledges the years during which all four sons lived together as a family unit. Brabant, Forsyth and McFarlain (1994) also reported that parents in their study spent effort on developing practiced definitions of their families after a child's death. These authors use Goffman's (1959) *front-stage performance–backstage reality* concept as explanation for this phenomenon; they offer a front-stage story for others that did not include the deceased child in the family definition and a backstage reality within the family that did.

Schank (1990) asserted that people use stories to test the quality of their own decision making. If they can create a plausible and coherent story to support the reason for their decisions and can imagine the same kind of story happening as a logical consequence of them, they then become more confident in the correctness of their decisions (Schank, 1990). People choose the story that provides a good life for themselves and their families (Fisher, 1984).

Two incidents from Kate's narrative exemplify this decision-support function of stories. Shortly after her daughter's death, her son came back from overseas with a boil that needed medical attention. She took him to the Emergency Room at the hospital in which her daughter had died. She reported "losing it" at that time. Her son said that she cried and screamed and behaved as if the doctors were going to kill him as well. She said, "I'm not coming back here ever!" In this story, Kate seems to be a woman totally out of control. However, during our interview, while she definitely remembered the incident, she rejected the story just told and its implications. She corrected her son's version of the story and revised her own statement, "I just said I didn't want to be here—that was all I said. I didn't want to be here at this particular time." The second statement reflects a more reasoned decision—she was upset at the time, but she rejects the idea that she will never go to the hospital again. She told me that she has, in fact, been there since to attend the meetings of a bereavement support group. Kate chooses to support the second version, which reflects clearer thinking on her part.

In the second incident, Kate talked about her decision to get drunk when, at Christmastime, she finally began to feel emotions related to her daughter's death (which had occurred at the end of June of that year). Her decision to drink had unacceptable ramifications. When faced with evidence that drinking to avoid the pain of difficult emotions entailed the physical pain of alcohol withdrawal, Kate quickly changed the story she chose. She realized that alcohol use was not the decision she wanted to make because its story lacks narrative probability for her. Instead of turning to alcohol, Kate started attending support group meetings and the story of her experience there fit more comfortably with the rest of her life. The decision to talk and listen to others in response to her loss resonates better for her than the decision to drink.

Jen's story also exemplifies the way that storytelling allows the testing of decision making. When she came to the second deliberate decision of which she spoke, Jen was able to imagine two separate stories to explain the time between her son's death near the end of October and her entry into alcohol treatment at the beginning of April—one in which she did everything expected and another in which she prioritized alcohol over her daughter. After she was challenged to change in order to keep her daughter, she acknowledged the truth of the second story and changed her initial decision. In light of the second story, Jen realized that her first decision could not work for either her or her daughter. If she wanted to be a good and healthy mother for her first child, she needed to change her response to the death of her second child, and she did.

John's story also serves as another incidence of storytelling helping to test decision making. He and his wife had made a decision to demonstrate their faith in the healing power of prayer by removing their chronically ill daughter from her medications and her accustomed medical regimen. They wanted desperately for God to heal her in response to their faith-filled actions. However, John related being at work one day and having the hair stand up on end on his neck as he imagined the possible results of their actions. As he told opposing stories to himself about the possible outcomes of their actions, he realized that he could not accept the probable ramifications of the plot that took his daughter away from the medicines and routines that had sustained her thus far. John found himself unable to believe that this story of miraculous healing would actually work out to be real. He called his wife, and she confided that the same thought process had been happening with her. They rejected the story of miraculous healing because it did not fit with their experience. They had tested their faith-healing decision by means of narrative, just as Fisher suggests.

John shared another ramification of their decision to return to conventional medical treatment—a crisis of faith for him. He found that their decision no longer allowed him to believe in faith healing. He said he was still intrigued by the idea, but it only made him feel angry and cheated. He talked about having come to the insight that trying to influence God's miraculous action is presumptuous on his part—that he had no right to "decide what is or isn't going to happen." He decided to change the way he prayed in order to safeguard his faith.

Those who listen to stories play an integral role in defining emergent (re)storying of experiences. The "confiding experience" (Harvey, Orbuch, Weber, Merbach, & Alt, 1992, p. 105) brings the comfort and input of other people to the storyteller's process of understanding what has happened. The teller of a story wants it to be understood and accepted by his or her listener(s), so is careful to fashion an account that is well-reasoned and engages the curiosity of the listener (Harvey et al., 1992; Schank, 1990). By listening or refusing to listen to various stories and types of stories, listeners have power to affect what stories are told and, ultimately, remembered by the teller (Schank, 1990).

Parents explained that they want to talk about their lost children, but often others will not allow it. Beth noted that it was especially difficult for her when she mentioned her son's name to someone and that other person turned away, probably because the topic made the other person uncomfortable. Yet, for Beth, talking about her son was comfortable and desirable. When people behaved in such fashion, they refused to hear Beth's story, so she could not keep his memory alive by talking about him.

My own personal experience confirms this hurtful truth. I find myself grateful to people who talk about my daughter's memory, even at the risk of discomfort for themselves. Although my voice may waver, my spirit is always grateful that others keep Teresa alive in their thoughts as I do.

Tess related incidents in which people saw her son's picture and began to challenge her about behavior that might have prevented his death, such as wearing a helmet or taking safety classes. Tess chafed at the memory of such discussions because they portrayed her son in a negative light. She admitted that he had made some mistakes, but he also did many things right. She commented that she disliked having to explain details to people who did not care or had no right to know. These listeners forced her to defend her son and try to justify his behavior when she would much rather tell stories about his dreams and his positive behavior.

Jen talked in very warm terms about the positive influence of a listener—her mother-in-law. She always wanted to encourage others to talk about her lost grandson. Jen wanted to talk about her son and no one (except for her mother-in-law) would allow her to do so. Her mother-in-law's function as a listener encouraged Jen's storytelling, and that process helped her to understand the loss of her son and its consequences.

## SUMMARY

The accounts of the respondents of this study reveal their use of narrative processes in understanding and managing the powerful effects of loss. As predicted by the narrative-paradigm theory, these parents have naturally turned to stories to capture and organize their experiences. They are adept at determining good reasons for events and situations based on the outcomes of their narratives. They make use of narrative processes to test their decision making, to help them decide from among various possible courses what they will do. They choose the most appropriate and helpful narratives to promote a good life for themselves and for those they love from among the stories of their culture, history, and experiences. They engage in storytelling whether or not they have full awareness of its use and helpfulness to them.

Utilizing narrative analysis in this study allowed us to "look inside" the data to discover how storytelling helped people organize the events and emotions of their grief. Our respondents' attempts to construct plausible stories allowed them to see patterns and understand connections that might not have been apparent to them before. By deconstructing the stories as narratives we could recognize personal growth over time, as well as story testing, decision testing, and sense-making. This beginning understanding of how narratives work for these "wounded storytellers" would have been difficult to come to via statistical analysis (Frank, 1995). Dissecting stories into small pieces (necessary for such quantitative interpretation) would hinder holistic integrity. The value of storytelling lies in its ability to integrate details into a whole. Understanding how that whole works in a person's life demands a broad look.

### Suggestions for Future Research

This study did not directly name the process of storytelling with the respondents. In future research, the topic of using stories could be approached more directly. Participants' personal reports of the usefulness of using stories could be solicited and probed. A drawback might be the transparency of storytelling, which could limit their ability to recognize its use and/or utility in their bereavement.

Another useful research strategy might be asking respondents to write about their bereavement or to deliberately tape-record stories from their bereavement experience. Research questions might include specific topics such as viewing the body, the funeral, incidents of supportive (nonsupportive) behavior from others, or cemetery experiences. They might also be in the form of writing prompts such as: the most difficult thing about my loss; effects of loss and how I'm managing them; or my current relationship with my deceased loved one. These methods might allow assessment of respondents' awareness of story rules and the elements they consider essential in telling a story.

Another approach might entail a second visit to the individuals involved in the current study. Besides providing an opportunity to compare and contrast the stories, such an approach could discuss the results of the current study and elicit personal reports from respondents that might verify or expand on the conclusions of this study.

This study has examined the use of storytelling by bereaved parents using the lens of Fisher's narrative paradigm. Further research might adopt another theoretical perspective, such as Schank and Abelson's (1977) plan–goal–theme–results–lesson chain with which to measure the use of narrative among respondents. Another study might also move from the context of bereavement to some other situation for looking at the use of narrative.

## CECILIA'S PERSONAL REFLECTIONS

Working with narrative data in this study provided a rich, deep look at the experiences of my respondents. However, a large amount of data could not easily be collapsed into convenient, manageable pieces. Sifting through the stories and looking for patterns was quite a task. I broke the data down by thinking about similarities between Fisher's work and the framework of other scholars regarding the nature and utility of storytelling. Finding the intersections between those ideas and then looking for evidence of their application in the stories of my respondents began to give me new ideas about the HOW of narrative's usefulness in processing grief. Doing the narrative analysis was almost like being a detective looking for clues, then building a new story out of the building blocks of theory and my respondents' stories.

The interviews were powerful and created an intimate space between myself and the respondents. I had a very strong feeling—and it was expressed or hinted at by several of the parents—that I would not have been granted the opportunity to interview had I not "earned" it by my own experience with the loss of a child, by my own grappling with the "octopus of grief."

Somewhere during the course of my research, I began to realize that a part of me wanted my thesis to say everything about grief that could be said, to allow me to so fully explore the subject that all of my questions about it would be answered. I wanted to do this as a final tribute to Teresa that would stand as a shining example of why she suffered—and why I suffered because of her suffering. I guess a part of me really believed that I would be finished with grief when I finished my research. Maybe that's why it took me so long to do it and why I tried so hard to make it my best effort. But, later, I also realized that those goals were futile. They were beyond the reach of this or any paper. My thesis is finished now. My diploma rests comfortably in my bookcase. And I still miss my little girl!—even 6 years later. There are still times my heart can't understand why she had to go. My eyes still well up with tears now and then (definitely not as often as they once did) and I long to hear others mention her name, saying that they miss her, too. My respondents' stories didn't "fix" my story any more than my listening to them "fixed" theirs. Our kids are all just as gone as ever!

I venture to say that my analysis might be a surprise to the parents whose stories I heard and examined. I am sure that they were largely unaware of doing any of the things I said that they did with their stories. Yet, I think, stories and poetry and plays—all narratives—have lives of their own. There is an intricacy to them that defies anyone to ever have the final word about what they contain. That's the special power of narrative—it connects to each hearer in its own way, interacting with that hearer's personality, perspectives, and specific stories to create ever new and living understandings of reality.

# 19

## Agency Through Narrative: Patients Managing Cancer Care in a Challenging Environment

∾

**Dan O'Hair**
**Denise Scannell**
**Sharlene Thompson**
*University of Oklahoma*

*I can't trust my body. It is no longer there for me. At this point, I may die this fall. I am sad about that. I am very aware of life's illusions—Joni Mitchell's song "Clouds"—everything seems in transition.*
—Female cancer patient, 56 years old

The newly diagnosed cancer patient faces an overwhelming and complex set of challenges as they navigate and negotiate the multiplex of caregiving processes. Upon receiving the news about their diagnosis, cancer patients often are devastated. The fear, dread, and terror that accompany the diagnostic message stem from multiple factors, especially those issues (a) situated in conceptions of self and (b) those perceived through social construction of reality. Traversing through multiple communication contexts involving self-identity, family members, providers, health care organizations, and environmental contingencies creates an overwhelming set of challenges for the cancer patient. The starts and stops along this journey may well determine the outcome of their cancer experience. This is not to say that this process determines the outcome of the chemotherapy treatment on the diseased cells, but rather it is to emphasize that it will determine how the cancer survivor fares after cancer. Some patients come through their cancer experience feeling empowered, strong and happy, whereas others feel disempowered, weak, and unhappy. Some cancer patients believe that cancer constitutes, in some way, a blessing, as they now truly appreciate life. What accounts for such discrepancies in the experience and outcomes of cancer? As contributions to this volume illustrate, a narrative perspective to understanding health care issues offers a powerful tool for both scholars and practitioners. This chapter emphasizes the need for patients to exercise agency through narrative in order to achieve a more successfully managed cancer care environment. Although narrative analysis in cancer-care is not a new phenomenon, neither is it a universal form of inquiry when investigating patient-care issues.

Three primary challenges facing cancer patients involve: (a) identity threats, (b) relating to close others, and (c) surviving, assimilating to, and managing a new and unfamiliar medical environment. While facing these challenges, patients simultaneously and continuously negotiate and renegotiate their self-identity, relationships with friends and family, their role in the medical environment (e.g. their patient role), and the patient–provider relationship. The manner in which patients face each of these challenges allows us to see the interface among patient, close others, and environment, as well as how patients make sense of and co-construct the cancer care process with players inherent to this environment. Our work seeks to explicate critical relationships among constituent parts of cancer care as a means for enhancing patient agency through narratives (ATN). We first examine narrative and the intersections with health communication. We then identify three challenges cancer patients face during their interaction with the health care delivery environment. It is during this discussion that patient narratives are employed to characterize the meaning patients give to their experiences.[1] In the following section, we turn the lens by which patients view narratives from one of description to one of agency, or how they can become choice-making communicators using narrative as a means of exerting voice and employing adaptation strategies for managing the cancer-care environment. In the final section, we offer some implications for research and practice for how narratives become a potential strategy in a patient's repertoire for negotiating and managing the cancer-care environment.

## NARRATIVE AND HEALTH COMMUNICATION

The phenomenon of narration is often explained as a human interaction, an activity, a genre, or simply a type of articulation that allows people to shift between the world of the unknown and the predictable (Bruner, 1990; Eggly 2002; Fisher, 1987; Mishler, 1984). Scholars from a broad spectrum of academic disciplines and social institutions use narrative data and structural methods of narrative analysis for understanding human expressions that go beyond objective evidence (Barthes, 1972; Bruner, 1990; Eggly, 2002; Ezzy, 1998; Fisher, 1987; Hunter, 1991; Labov, 1972; Langellier, 1989; Ricoeur, 1984b; Street, 2001). Although one may discover numerous interesting and compelling studies on narrative within scholarly inquiry, this chapter focuses on the study of narrative within the communication discipline and, in particular, in the context of cancer care.

Over the past 20 years, health-communication researchers has contributed to the understanding that patients should be active managers, interpreters, and creators of the meaning of their illness (J. K. Burgoon et al., 1987; Ellingson & Buzzanell, 1999; Thompson, 1990; Vanderford et al., 1997). A number of health research projects in recent years, however, have challenged this assumption by stressing that before implementing holistic methods it is necessary to understand the narrative practices that patients engage in before, during, and after the medical encounter (Eggly, 2002; Frank, 1995; Sharf & Vanderford, 2003). A patient's medical experience and discourse is fixed in the psychosocial context of the illness, which exceeds far beyond the realm of the medical environment (Engel, 1977; Goldberg, Haas, & Eaton, 1976; Houpt, Orleans, George, & Brodie, 1979; Spiro, 1996). In addition, it is not only the patient who is interpreting and negotiating meanings of their illnesses but also the people who interact with them everyday (Geist-Martin, Horsley, & Farrell, 2003; Goffman, 1963). Consequently, the inclusion of psychosocial factors positions patients as storytellers (Sharf & Vanderford, 2003). Accordingly, individuals use narration as a communicative means in order to become the active interpreter, organizer, and negotiator of the meaning of their illness. As a result, there has been a growing awareness of the value of narrative within the areas of health communication research and medicine (Eggly, 2002; Vanderford, Stein, Sheeler, & Skochelak, 2001).

A significant amount of health-communication research focuses on the socially constructed signs and symbols of narratives as linguistically articulated, restructured, and recorded in history (Berger & Luckman, 1996; Bochner, 1998; Bormann, 1985; Fisher, 1987; Mishler, 1984; Sharf & Vanderford, 2003). The social construction approach to health communication developed out of a need to counteract the biomedical model, which is criticized for identifying and treating the illness rather than acknowledging the patient as a whole person who exists beyond it (Frank, 1995; Sharf & Vanderford, 2003).

Nonetheless, the biomedical model, which is grounded in scientific reasoning, is the discourse needed to move the patient through the medical system and everyday life (i.e., diagnosis, treatment, insurance compensation, and time off from work, to name a few). In addition, the "patient role" within the biomedical model assumes an audience of medical professionals, such as physicians, nurses, lab technicians, and health care providers. Patients understand that medical professionals validate or judge the merits of their narration, so they often strive to be good storytellers for their audience (Fisher, 1987; Frank, 1995). Unfortunately, patients may respond to health-related questions according to how they perceive medical professionals would want them to answer (Robinson-Pant, 2001), inevitably leading them to enact their patient role in expected ways. As a result, many individuals continuously struggle against the linear structures of the biomedical narrative by seeking out spiritual, moral, and social elements that allow them to construct their own understanding about the personal and cultural significance of the illness, inevitably transcending science (Frank, 1995; Sharf & Vanderford, 2003).

This is not to say that all patients who seek to transcend science will achieve their goals. Certain factors, such as age, gender, income, and education can impede a patient's ability to achieve empowerment within the medical environment (Nussbaum, Ragan, & Whaley, 2003). Sharing stories with other patients and with family members, friends, co-workers, and acquaintances can provide individuals with a sense of empowerment. However, these narratives are not always harmonious with each other; conflict and tensions emerge between the interactional styles and values of the story. Indeed, narratives spring from a dialogue between multiple experiences embedded in the social context of the illness. Understanding emergent narratives becomes particularly important with cancer care where a host of providers and specialists participate. As a powerful mode of expression, these types of narratives allow individuals to transform their identity (Frank, 1995; McAdams, 1993; Sontag, 1977; Vanderford et al., 1997), assert control (Thompson, 2003), and gain a sense of community (Adelman & Frey, 1997).

## USING NARRATIVE TO EXPLAIN THE CHALLENGES FACING CANCER PATIENTS

This section addresses three primary challenges faced by cancer patients and the ways in which they negotiate and renegotiate these issues. Through cancer patient narratives, we explore how these challenges are understood.

### Identity Threats

Almost immediately, newly diagnosed cancer victims begin to question their self-concept (Colyer, 1996; Flannigan, 2000; Pedro, 2001), as the fear of the unknown (treatment, suffering, and death) instantly becomes a close companion in their lives. As cancer victims turn their thoughts outwardly, they confront the stigma associated with the disease (Colyer, 1996; Dakof & Taylor, 1990; Flannigan, 2000; Peters-Godman, 1982). Cancer patients face this stigma from both internal forces (their own perception that cancer is malevolent) as well as external cultural norms regarding the indignity of cancer (Pedro, 2001). As threats to self, ownership of stigma, and emotional distress intermingle, cancer patients may experience denial as a coping mechanism (Gattellari, Butow, Tattersall, Dunn, & MacLeod, 1999). Unfortunately, denial compromises communicative processes between the cancer patient and health care providers (Gattellari et al., 1999).

The initial difficulties already mentioned often produce a state of crisis or shock. Drawing upon scholarship from intercultural communication, this state of shock for cancer victims can be associated with the notion of cultural shock. *Culture shock* can be construed as the "anxiety that results from losing all of our familiar signs and symbols of social intercourse" (Oberg, 1960, p. 177) and as a loss of communication competence and distorted self-reflections based on interactions with others (Zaharna, 1989). This state of shock tends to move cancer victims from a state of low self-awareness to one of extreme self-awareness, similar to what occurs during culture shock (Adler, 1975; Villagran, Jones, & O'Hair, in press). This stage precipitates a great deal of cognitive and affective reflection that continues to reflexively agitate the affect system of a cancer patient creating occasions for, alterations of, and threats to the self-concept (Flannigan, 2000; O'Hair et al., 2003; Villagran et al., in press).

According to a number of scholars, the self is discovered in its own narrational acts, and self-identity is developed and maintained through narrative (Ezzy, 1998; Frank, 1995; Ricoeur, 1984b; Vanderford et al., 1997). Czarniawska-Joerges (1994) argued that identity construction becomes a "continuous process of narration where both the narrator and the audience formulate, edit, applaud, and refuse various elements of the ever-producing narrative" (p. 198). In addition, narrative construction occurs through a reflective process based on memory images of things that individuals have done in the past (Ezzy, 1998; Ricoeur, 1984b). Individuals constantly reconfigure the past and the future as part of an emergent present, and both the memories of the past and expectations of the future are symbolically organized and constructed to provide a congruent self-perception (Ezzy, 1998). Narrative identity reflects a person's life through a sequence of experiences, expectations, and memory categorized into a triad of past, present, and future. Because a narrative is an account of time, a listener can only witness movement through discourse. Movement, which semantically connects a sequence of events, illustrates temporal phrases that depict duration, frequency, and repetition. Consider these hypothetical examples, "My grandmother lived with diabetes for 30 years (duration) until she died"; or, "He went to the doctor three times (repetition) for the same symptoms"; and, "I felt a sharp pain in my chest every few hours (frequency)." Temporal phrases not only reveal a sequence of events within the medical narrative; they expose the enduring milestones of a person's life (Frank, 1995).

A patient's identity emerges and evolves out of many symbolic interactions between people, events, routines, expectations, imagination, and the discourse that shapes a person's story (Vanderford et al., 1997). For example, people seek out and use narratives like paths or illness maps that are consistent with their own expectations, values, and beliefs (Pentland, 1999; Sharf & Vanderford, 2003). Based on memory or stories of others' experiences, patients develop a general idea of what to expect when going to the doctor (O'Hair, Allman, & Moore, 1996). The typical office visit story line usually unfolds as "check in with a receptionist, sit down, wait, read magazines, get called in, enter room, undress, sit on table, talk to nurse, talk to doctor, get dressed, get medicine, make appointment, leave office" (O'Hair et al., 1996, p. 309). A health experience that violates the "normal" doctor–patient expectation changes the narrative. The patient will apply a new meaning or interpretation to an old story. A revised story will be told and retold. In order to tell the story in a socially acceptable way, the sick person must acquire a patient identity. However, Western society has stigmatized "being sick" and the patient role often is viewed as negative. Illness is perceived as an individualistic path that one must walk alone, taking full responsibly for his or her treatment. In some instances, such as HIV, society places blame on the victims of the disease (Sontag, 1977). Certain behavior traits also may be labeled as *disease prone*. For example, someone who is uptight, negative, and aggressive can be said to have a "cancer personality" (Fields, 1999). A successful doctor–patient relationship cannot be fully understood without exploring what the patient has to say about his or her own "health identity" (Frank, 1995).

Researchers often seek to understand how specific individuals use metaphor when talking or writing about their illness (Sontag, 1977). In arguing for the importance of metaphor in women's thinking about their experiences with cancer, Gibbs and Franks (2002) discovered multiple conceptual metaphors embodied in women's narratives, their understanding of their cancer, and their identity. The majority of metaphorical phrases concern the body, which is how patients often gauge normality. In the following narrative, a forty-nine year old female cancer patient expresses concern in her appearance. "I no longer feel beautiful. I had been morbidly obese for most of my adult life and then in 2000, I got a gastric bypass. I had lost down to my goal weight and felt beautiful. Now (after cancer), I feel skinny and ugly and bald and breastless and gray."

Medical narratives can function as indicators of how individuals define their illness and their identity, and ultimately the merging of the two. As demonstrated in a study conducted on pain and interpersonal relationships, Schlesinger (1996) reports:

> Sometimes I feel like, uh, my whole being, my whole identity is wrapped up in this pain.... I'm not Nan Fisch the computer programmer; I'm Nan the person with the problem with her hands ... I'm not Tom's wife; I'm that poor woman that's wearing those funny things on her arms ... sometimes I just feel like who I am is taking a back seat to this problem. (p. 253)

This excerpt reveals the inseparable nature of a patient's self-image and self-worth from illness and health.

Clearly, people assign meaning to illness in order to create and sustain personal identities. In addition, adapting to the patient role, depending on the severity of the illness, may evoke feelings of confusion and anxiety for all involved (Vanderford et al., 1997). Given such conflicts, how do individuals present their illnesses? Eventually, their feelings about illness slowly dominate their lives and their identities. The story, as a resource for empathy between the speaker and the audience, is inescapable. "How are you feeling?" works constantly to remind individuals of illness while simultaneously drawing attention to their difference, loss of control, and stigma of being sick (Geist-Martin et al., 2003; Goffman, 1963; Spiro, 1996). For example, Schlesinger (1996) writes, "Michelle expressed concern that she was 'sick and tired' of explaining herself: 'People don't understand. It's like a broken record ... I'd be so paranoid about someone calling me a hypochondriac' " (p. 251).

In this unique context, patients constantly renegotiate identities as evidenced by the narrative of a 53-year-old-female cancer patient who participated in our study.

> I was in severe pain and wanted to die and "get it over with" after being diagnosed. A friend came in and said "Don't die on me." Made me feel I was still of some use here. I started fighting. I "lost" myself and became severely depressed 3–4 months later. Then went through some therapy, became more open to positives/visits/etc. Scripture more comforting. Personal prayers from others comforting.

The cyclical nature of cancer care undoubtedly affects self-image (Granet, 2001). The threats posed by the disease, symptoms, and contraindications from treatment constitute substantial contributions to the identity-construction process. These threats provide an ever-present reminder that identity construction is a fluid and dynamic process. The following two statements from participants of this study demonstrate how they (re)negotiated their identities based on the threats posed. The first narrative demonstrates how this patient negotiated the complex process by focusing on what was left (the positive) after the cancer. The second narrative shows a possible difference in how males and females (re)negotiate their identity after it is threatened by cancer. The female patient allows the illness to have a positive meaning in order to create and sustain a self that is content, whereas the male patient allows the illness to be a crutch to lean on so that he no longer has to keep up a persona of invincibility.

> I recognized *every day* as a *gift* rather than an entitlement. I hope I'm a more loving person, a freer person. My senses are all heightened. My faith is stronger. My relationships are more meaningful. (Female cancer patient, 63 years old)

> Before I felt more invincible of course! I feel like I'm more patient with my children, and I am closer to God than I was. I do tend to think of myself as more sickly, which is very hard. (Male cancer patient, 43 years old)

No one expects to feel disconnected by his or her illness, a common experience with cancer (Frank, 1995). These feelings become burdensome, especially when the side effects of illness or medications, such as excessive weight loss or gain, hair loss, skin abrasions, continuously are providing evidence of falling behind. Being different is difficult, but the "undesired differentness from what we had anticipated" is even harder (Goffman, 1963, p. 73). Sontag (1977) explained that the body becomes an object from which the ill person feels disconnected. Even if the side effects are temporary, the impact from the disconnected feeling from one's body and identity can last longer than the actual illness. As a result, ill individuals acquire an identity that sets them apart from others. Such differences can lead to isolation, which may negatively affect the outcome of their treatment.

## Relating to Close Others

Patients have a tendency to incorporate various aspects or actors of their lives into stories because they perceive these features as closely related to their illness and their recovery (Ellingson & Buzzanell, 1999). Cancer patients we have worked with frequently discussed which family members or friends accompanied them to the doctor or assisted them with medication. The identities and relationships of the focal actors in the narrative can be friends, co-workers, family members, groups, organizations, to name a few (Pentland, 1999).

When a person deals with a health crisis (such as cancer), family support facilitates coping with stressors associated with the disease (Bauer, 2001). In many ways, family support can cushion the impact of the crisis. As one female patient explains, "My daughter is a great sounding board for my need to get back to a somewhat normal life." In our work with cancer patients, family members—spouses, parents, siblings, and children—often accompanied ill family members in the treatment room. In fact, the design of the cancer treatment room encouraged family members or friends to sit next to the individual while he or she received treatment. In addition, TVs, magazines, puzzles, and other types of media were available for the supporters who sat and waited for hours. Ellingson & Buzzanell (1999) claimed patients not only bring family members to gather information but also to help their physicians envision their lives. On many occasions, we observed family members talking with the nurses about treatment, medication, pain, diet, sleep, or other pertinent issues related to the patient's cancer care. Patients remain acutely aware of the disposition, comportment, and communication style of those close to them. Consider the narrative of an ovarian cancer patient from a study conducted by Ferrell, Smith, Ervin, Itano, and Melancon (2003), where she recounts how her husband shares her illness:

> I must give credit to my husband who without a doubt is the word's greatest "caregiver." So often they are the forgotten one. All concern is directed toward the patient. I heard my husband say "We were diagnosed with ovarian cancer last December." What a great expression of love and concern that was. (p. 658)

Caregivers, who use expressions like "We were diagnosed with cancer" instead of "My partner was diagnosed with cancer," show an incredible capacity to adapt their identity as well as their language in caring for their partner. Despite the difficulty of renegotiating close relationships after a cancer diagnosis, it can be done successfully. In large part, the extent of such renegotiation depends on how close others react to the cancer diagnosis (Kagawa-Singer & Wellisch, 2003; Langer, Abrams, & Syrjala, 2003).

It can be difficult to renegotiate relationships with close others even when they are not resistant to change. In spite of everything, when close others wish to be supportive, they may not know how. It then becomes the cancer patient's role to renegotiate this relationship. Furthermore, not all members can express support equally.

One female participant found her sisters to display more support than her husband:

> My husband has tried to be supportive, but he just doesn't have a clue about how to be supportive ... so I have to tell him. My sisters and friends have been supportive and allowed me to spew all my anxiety and pain, and I don't really know if I am doing well with this or not. (Female cancer patient, 53 years old)

Adapting to the patient role not only changes the health status for one's identity, but also for one's family and close friends (Vanderford et al., 1997). Any change can evoke feelings of confusion, impatience, timidity, anger, or denial (Vanderford et al., 1997). When an illness strikes, both patient and close others must simultaneously renegotiate previously established rules and norms of the relationship. One 48-year-old female participant stated, "My husband and son have been very supportive, but my daughter is very angry because I've been sick." Children of cancer victims experience a flux of emotion that can evoke overwhelming feelings of fear that a parent might "leave" them or anger because the parent–child role becomes reversed. In the narrative below, the cancer patient demonstrates that her renegotiation of the relationship with her husband forces her to manipulate her interactions with her doctor. In this narrative, the patient's metaphor reflects a weary warrior, battling not only the disease but also a resistant husband: "I first battle my husband who always goes into *denial* and does not hear the negatives. Then I have to get pointed with my doctor" (Female cancer patient, 56 years old).

The sick are frequently viewed as a burden by society because they cannot "keep up" with the rest of its members (Frank, 1995). Therefore, Goffman (1963) explained that individuals often try to pass as "being normal" in order not to humiliate themselves or others. Many patients construct identities that are multifaceted, and perhaps even recapitulated from identities of the past. Individuals may project the noncancerous self through narrative for various reasons, in particular appearing "normal" to audiences. By doing so, patients can use narratives about their noncancerous persona to reinforce in themselves an identity that cancer is only a part of who they are, not what they are. The following participant illustrates this when she discusses how she achieved a sense of normalcy:

> I lost some *friends* who could not deal with it, but the ones who supported me were great. I found that if I mixed in parts of my life that they were used to and not dwell on pancreatic cancer, they seemed more likely to want to talk. Like they used to. (Female cancer patient, 53 years old)

Regardless of whether they position themselves as either protagonist or antagonist in the person's life, significant others can weaken or strengthen patient compliance, health care decisions, treatment, and even recovery (Bauer, 2001; Pentland, 1999).

## Cancer-Care Environment

Anytime an environment metaphor is used to describe the context in which individuals interact, it necessitates an act of defining and operationalizing key elements that constitute such a phenomenon. We restrict our view of environment to three elements of cancer patients' experiences that we view as most salient for managing their care: provider communication, cancer-care delivery organizations (centers and hospitals), and the insurance industry.

We first address the most basic of patient issues—provider contact. Patients not only call on providers to help control (even conquer) cancer, but also to help manage symptoms. If pressed, they consider requests to address psychosocial concerns as well. In the following narrative, a 63-year-old female patient expressed aggravation with the manner in which her primary-care providers failed to meet her needs: "Most frustrating thing about my care? The busy schedule of the doctors—having to wait to talk to them. Having to talk to nurse's answering machines to get to the doctor or wait on a return call from the nurse, which usually comes when I'm gone."

Cancer patients also may object to the manner in which information is presented to them. In the following narrative, a 68-year-old male lung cancer patient complains about his oncologist:

> He spent more time talking about his other patients and how they were doing with this drug. When I asked him how long he thought I would last, he shrugged and said it would depend on my tolerance for the chemo. When my wife asked about side effects, he said it would be the normal type. Normal? What's normal about side effects? For the most part, he acted as if this was all a big secret that I didn't need to know about.

Our research, as well as that of others, reveals a general deficiency on the part of physicians in attending to patients' psychosocial, affective, and nonmedical needs (Gillotti, 2003; O'Hair, 1986; Thompson, 2000). Scholars conclude that although physicians have a great deal at stake in communicating with patients about their psychosocial concerns, physicians often fall short in meeting those needs. In the following narrative, one patient relates the frustration she experienced when her nonmedical needs went unmet by her providers:

I don't feel I have good communication with my doctors. I have had difficulty getting all the access I need because everyone is so busy with primary care of cancer needs. There is never time to talk about how I am
emotionally feeling or any of those issues. On a different note, none of my
doctors advised me of getting prostheses or breast reconstruction. I had
to ask for a prescription to look into a prosthesis, but I still have not received insurance approval. I have found a very lifelike prosthesis that is
made to match your skin color and shape—they do a plaster of paris
mold of your body to make it. None of my doctors knew about this; and
now I have to find out about this, too. I have been somewhat disappointed
in how little information is conveyed to me about any of the choices and
options I have in treatment before, during, or after my cancer treatment.
(Female cancer patient, 49 years old)

Although not commonplace, some cancer patients express their
suspicions and frustrations with physicians openly (O'Hair, Kreps, &
Sparks, in press; Robinson & Thorne, 1988). One patient who discovered potentially disreputable practices by an oncologist unnervingly
argued:

In my support group I learned something I suspected all along.
Oncologists will never give up. They will try everything and anything to
prolong your life even if that would deny you a peaceful ending with hospice care. It's personal with them that you don't die on them, even if it
means a dreadful existent for you. (Male cancer patient, 68 years old)

(Re)negotiating the medical system represents another challenge
facing cancer patients. For instance, the following narratives illustrate
how patients routinely experience frustrations related to insurance,
bureaucracy, and managed care. A 61-year-old female cancer patient
related the following narrative about the aggravation she experiences
with her health maintenance organization (HMO):

I fought tooth and nail to stay alive in spite of HMOs! I took matters into
my own hands and insisted upon referrals—some of my friends did the
same and were told to choose another primary! I would go to the media to
expose the lack of care if I had to—It just may come to that—the state I reside within is notoriously geriatric and the medical care is sloppy, hap-
hazard and as I expressed previously—I have a job to do—That is why I
am here after almost 5 years!!

Another 49-year-old female cancer patient recounts how she routinely
challenges her insurance company for coverage of benefits:

My insurance company has been awful. They routinely turn down any
bills, and then I have to appeal. For instance, the surgeon referred my bi-

opsy for analysis to a noninsurance group. Well, I had nothing to do with this; and yet, the company turned it down for payment. I had to call the company and then go through unbelievable bureaucratic paperwork about this ... and it's been ongoing since the start.

As mentioned earlier, cancer care involves a complex undertaking with numerous healthcare personnel, organizations, and "places." The breadth and depth of the cancer care system frequently appears unrelenting and uncompromising (Ledlow, O'Hair, & Moore, 2003). Patients often feel that they must face a bewildering and disorganized bureaucracy. A 54-year-old male patient shared, "Frustrations? One hand not knowing what the other hand is supposed to be doing. Having to wait so long when it comes to getting blood or platelets. Lack of concern that you're immune suppressed." Another 43-year-old patient suggests a strategy for the myriad of cancer services and obligations that many of his cancer cohorts would readily embrace: "I think they should all have a care coordinator to help them with all the information and questions and different doctors and providers they need to see."

Key components of the cancer care environment often do not act interdependently; rather, they work against one another, disillusioning and frustrating patients. Ultimately, these dynamics exert control over how patients experience cancer, chances of survival, and available treatment protocols. Medical narratives embody patient concerns, including relationships, power dynamics, diversions, resources, bureaucratic constraints, and decisionmaking (Vanderford et al., 1997). Patients who achieve agency through narrative likely navigate the complexities of this environment more smoothly.

## ACHIEVING AGENCY THROUGH NARRATIVE (ATN)

*Agency* provides choice for patients within the patient–health care contexts, empowering individuals to exert control over their health care. In previous work, we conceptualized the path to agency as one that occurs in phases beginning with the diagnosis of cancer (shock), moving to uncertainty, progressing to empowerment, and finally maturing to a level of agency (O'Hair et al., 2002; O'Hair et al., 2003). Although only a conceptual model, the introduction of narrative moves our goal of patient agency to a more realized, "practiced" level. We argue that patient agency can be achieved through two essential aspects of empowerment: Voice and adaptation.

### Voice

"One time I got three of my team to hold a conference call because I wrote a letter that there was no communication and I felt like I was in no man's land. The bad part was I would have liked to been included and wasn't" (Female cancer patient, 51 years old). Voice emerges as an especially salient issue in constructing a sense of agency. The medical narrative provides an outlet for the person's strength and voice within the story. For far too long, the biomedical model served as the primary testimony, or voice, by which individuals could compare their symptoms, suffering, challenges, and future expectations. Guttman (2003) referred to this social phenomenon as the medicalization of health care that increasingly becomes incorporated with medical definitions and control. Bakhtin (1981) explained that as human beings, we find meaning, identity, and freedom through a multilanguaged world. Just as we do not expect all people to wear the same shoe size, we cannot expect all people to place their individual health experiences into one mainstream story.

Within medical narratives, voices can be heard and vital information shared. As a natural source of therapeutic healing, narratives can provide people with a sense of control even when simple tasks, such as getting out of bed can be challenging or even impossible. In the following narrative, a 63-year-old female cancer patient engages voice through narratives as a means of achieving agency.

> Tell the doctor up front you *do not* want to hear predictions of your life expectancy and you *do* want to hear hopeful messages. If she cannot comply with this request, look for another doctor. Tell the doctor you want to be an informed patient, that you may not know the questions to ask, and that you want her to feed you lots of information. Ask what the office protocol is for getting questions answered by phone. Chat with the nurses. You may need them later. Express your feelings, fears, [and] concerns to a family member or friend. There's no virtue in being "brave." Say "I'm scared" if you are. Ask for help. Ask for prayer on your behalf.

Cancer patients often see themselves as marginalized and relegated to a standpoint of a "disease." The following narrative from a physician who participated in this study typifies this state of affairs. "Physicians are trained to be scientists. We rely on objective facts. We treat the disease, not the person. We expect the patients to help us treat the disease, but our role is in curing the disease. When that is achieved, the person obtains their goal as well."

Examining communication experiences of nondominant or marginalized groups provides opportunities to observe relationships among culture, power, and communication (Orbe, 1998). From this perspective, cancer patients may be understood as members of an underprivileged group (patients, cancer victims), unable to exert control or power in the medical care environment. However, by engaging in various communication strategies, ranging from aggressive to assertive to nonassertive approaches, disempowered cancer patients can challenge the dominant cancer delivery structure (Orbe, 1998). One 62-year-old female cancer patient offers poignant advice for other similarly affected patients:

> If you have questions—write them down so that you do not forget to ask about anything you are concerned about—Do not allow yourself to be treated as a second-class citizen by having your questions answered as though you may not understand—Insist upon laymen's terminology—Bring someone with you so the doctor will be sure to tell you the truth—Do not be satisfied with "You do not need a specialist"—Call your insurance companies and register a complaint—Remember, this is your body, your life, and we all have the right to proper treatment—And we all need a positive attitude.

Another patient recounted how she found her voice and challenged the dominant culture in order to receive better care: "Yes, I was raised to go to the doctor and do what he said to get better. I have learned it's okay to seek a second opinion, to feel good about your treatment by listening to your body, and to collect any information you can to help you make good decisions" (Female cancer patient, 51 years old).

### Adaptation

Kim (2001) positions *adaptation* as "the dynamic process by which individuals, upon relocating to a new, unfamiliar, or changed cultural environment, establish (or reestablish) and maintain relatively stable, reciprocal, and functional relationships with those environments" (p. 31). Given that patients have a stake in exerting influence over an unfamiliar (and sometimes unfriendly) cancer environment, processes of adaptation emerge as key factors in the agency process. One participant shared:

> I told myself after chemo began that I was not going to allow this to change me as a person. I lost hair, but I bought some wigs. I lost a lot of weight, but I had been overweight most of my life so that was a plus. I had been considering semiretirement for a few years and this was a reason to do so. (Female cancer patient, 63 years old)

One essential feature of adaptation theory involves the linear relationship of three concepts—*stress, adaptation,* and *growth.* For our purposes, this relationship can be reasoned in the following manner. As cancer patients grapple with multiple stressors that impinge upon their psyche from the cancer environment, they search for ways to adapt (communicatively, psychologically, emotionally, etc.) that lead to psychological and cross-cultural growth. Growth becomes a desirable outcome that empowers the patient. The following narrative reflects aspects of the adaptation process:

> I've learned the importance of asking the right questions and of partici-
> pating in my own care. I've learned to push for more information (They
> don't just volunteer it). It's important to me to see my doctors as just peo-
> ple and treat them that way. I try to laugh with them and give them hugs
> and praise. (Female cancer patient, 63 years old)

Another patient portrays the adaptation process when asked how she is different after cancer diagnosis:

> I see things differently now ... I see the beauty in things. I don't boil up in-
> side about things that really aggravate me (I let the steam out and then
> just move on). I wish I had learned to do that earlier. I routinely talk with
> God and have taught my children to talk with God. (Female cancer pa-
> tient, 49 years old)

## Agency Processes

Cancer patients often strive "for purposeful self-determination, at-tempting to make sense of, initiate, influence, and cope with events in line with personal values, goals, and expectations of the future in a con-text of cultural norms, traditions, and past experiences" (Fryer, 1998, p. 12). Agency opens the door of opportunity for choice within the pa-tient–health care context. As we argued in an earlier position:

> From our viewpoint then, agency might be described as a state of condi-
> tion where individuals become empowered to the extent that they under-
> stand the choices they want to make, advocate their own rights, take
> control of their own destiny, and demonstrate the competency necessary
> for acting in their own best interests. Agency is about having choice and
> the competencies to act on them. This definition does not limit the
> agent/patient from seeking help, support, or assistance. It does means
> that agent/patients know that those choices can be made and that they
> understand where such resources can be accessed. (O'Hair et al., 2003)

We understand that not all patients desire agency, and others may try and fail at such efforts of empowerment. Yet, it is our contention that for those so inclined, narrative represents an opportunity for real-izing agency. Our experiences with cancer patients, in fact, suggest that many have availed themselves of ATN. The following participant offers advice about dealing with the diagnosis of cancer and engaging the care environment in order to maximize the care process:

I suggest always getting a second opinion. Don't feel obligated to a doctor, if you are dissatisfied, get another. Talk with your insurance company—know the answer before you ask your doctor about tests, etc. (billing). Follow-up on everything!!! Keep your own records. Educate yourself to make good decisions. Take someone with you to appointments. Make a list of questions/concerns and communicate them to the doctor. Ask for a written plan of protocol, if possible, along with information on each chemo and other prescriptions. Join a support group and treat it as a doctor's appointment. Share concerns with the group—offer assistance to others if possible. Explore community resources if needed. Accept and appreciate offers of help from family and friends. Never hesitate to call the doctor's office with new symptoms or concerns. Let healthcare support people know if you want all info (statistics) or not—How much you want to know about disease, that is, "just what I need to know" or "everything." (Female cancer patient, 59 years old)

As patients come to understand the importance of narrative in recreating their identity, dealing with close others, and negotiating aspects of the cancer-care environment, they recognize opportunities for exerting agency into their lives. As their agency experiences grow, it is hoped and expected that they will learn the power of narrative as a means for taking an active role in their cancer care. Narratives not only become vehicles for agency, but a companion goal for cancer patients.

## IMPLICATIONS FOR THEORY AND PRACTICE

We conclude our analysis by articulating several implications for health communication scholars–practitioners. First, agency processes become more salient in light of the emerging state of health care delivery in this country. As managed care becomes commonplace, physicians who already demonstrate a tendency to limit their interaction with chronically or terminally ill patients (Addington & Wegescheide-Harris, 1995; Dunphy, 1976; Evans, 1971) may even have fewer incentives to act as advocates for their patients (Goldman, 1998; Walsh-Burke & Marcusen, 1999). Further, as the nursing shortage crisis continues to exacerbate an already overburdened delivery system (Morra, 2000), patients will have to turn to others as a means of support. Patients will recognize that ATN represents one of the few reliable strategies at their disposal for exerting control in their cancer care.

Second, for those health communication scholars who have suggested a groundswell of "patient empowerment," we have concerning news. The narratives from many of these patients confirm what we have feared for years—patients' timidity and eventual frustration in dealing with cancer-care delivery remains an unaddressed problem. Patient advocacy does not appear to be taking root at a level that many of us expected by now. The consumerism movement may have stalled in deference to an increasingly complex array of medical alternatives available to cancer patients and their providers. Increasing awareness of agency through narrative among principal actors (patients, families, providers) represents a critical next step in medical education and training, and health care-delivery.

Narrative also can become an especially important tool for patients with low literacy skills. Research indicates that people with language barriers or low literacy skills often lack the ability to read and comprehend prescription drugs, appointment slips, and other health-related materials, and misunderstand health information that is expressed through quantitative discourse (Bernhardt & Cameron, 2003). Because health literacy refers to patients' possessing the necessary skills to comprehend their medical condition, this condition can affect the decision-making process in two ways. First, people with low literacy skills may be more vulnerable to inaccurate health information, which can lead to irrational thoughts about their illness. Second, the shame and stigma that surrounds one's health literacy can prevent one from seeking out second opinions or alternative treatment. People with low health literacy may be more likely to respond to a doctor who encourages the co-construction of emergent health narratives.

Skelton & Hammond (1998) and Hunter (1991) contend that medical-school curriculum lends itself well to a narrative approach given the oral tradition of storytelling in medicine, and the ability of an individual story to act as the starting point for problem-based studies. Sharing medical knowledge through storytelling is evident in medical journals dating back to the late 1800s (Hunter, 1991). Eventually, the scientific interests of modern medicine reshaped the way doctors talked about their patients. The retelling or writing of the story became more objective, ultimately removing both the drama of the patient and the doctors' individual meanings (Skelton & Hammond, 1998). Nonetheless, the doctor narrative is still a powerful communicative technique that offers advice and teaches medical skills (Hunter, 1991). The medical narrative not only brings the patient to life, but also clarifies and contextualizes the doctor's experience (Borkan, Miller, & Reis, 1992). Communication research would benefit from understanding how providers' narratives function within the medical community in general and educational curriculums in particular.

Encouraging physicians to co-produce narratives with cancer patients involves much more than simply exchanging stories with patients. Eliciting patient narratives involves sensitivity toward and perceptual awareness of patients' needs. A strategy increasingly employed by cancer specialists involves *narrative emplotment* (Del Vecchio Good, Munakata, Kobayashi, Mattingly, & Good, 1994). Crossley (2003) described narrative emplotment as:

> encouraging the patient to focus on the immediate present and to place faith in the efficacy of specific treatments. However, it also explores how the attempt to live in the context of such a plot is fraught with anxiety for the patient, and how it co-exists with other largely "unspoken narratives" of uncertainty, fear and skepticism in relation to the power of medicine. (p. 439)

From this perspective, patients collaborate with providers in constructing narratives that chart a commitment for treatment options, optimistic thinking, and living in the moment. The latter of these can be especially important for purposes of avoiding obsessive thoughts about the future or potential endings of the narrative.

Physical, social, relational, and structural forces can enable and/or constrain patient agency. For example, an otherwise self-empowered patient may be constrained by a managed-care environment and/or by a domineering physician. The "wounded storyteller" (Frank, 1995) may be unable to exercise agency through narrative without support from other forces in the cancer-care environment. Wounded storytellers cannot exercise agency through narrative in isolation from other forces in the cancer-care environment. Further, already disempowered patients who receive a cancer diagnosis may have a harder time achieving agency. They simply may not possess the cognitive and emotional skills for exercising agency. Future analysis should examine the stories of patients who do not achieve agency by expanding the qualitative components used to measure or define agency. The integration and applicability of this analysis should not be limited to physician–patient interaction, but instead include the narrative considerations of the partial stories, the chaos stories (see Frank, 1995), and the stories that challenge our assumptions.

As a means of putting closure on our thoughts, we turn to a narrative that opens a book highlighting illness and communication by Richard Glass (2000), a prominent physician–researcher who joins with us in championing the cause of co-constructing the meaning of illness for patients. The Patient-Physician Covenant states that:

> Medicine is at its center, a moral enterprise grounded in a covenant of trust.... this moral enterprise surely includes the responsibility to communicate effectively with patients regarding explanations of the illness. I believe it also includes helping patients to struggle with the more difficult question of the meaning of illness for their life. (p. xiii)

Celebrating narrative processes in cancer care helps patients achieve agency, (re)define their identities, relate to close others, and manage the cancer-care environment.

## NOTES

1. Many of the narratives included in this chapter were produced by cancer patients in a study utilizing an open-ended survey conducted at multiple cancer-treatment centers in Oklahoma, California, and Tennessee. The study was approved by the Institutional Review Board at the University of Oklahoma. Patients were asked to respond to various demographic questions as well as questions pertaining to their experiences with the cancer-care environment. For example, patients responded to issues involving communication with providers, insurance carriers, and family members. Patients related stories about their coping strategies, interpersonal relationships, and thoughts on how cancer had affected their lives. Patients in Oklahoma were recruited from two cancer centers at a university-based hospital. The patients from Tennessee were recruited from two comprehensive cancer centers in the metropolitan area of Memphis. California patients were recruited through a cancer-advocacy network. When patients called in for information, counseling, or advice, they were invited to participate in our study. All questionnaires were completed anonymously and an informed-consent form was signed by all participants and then separated upon receipt by the principal investigator. Questionnaires were transcribed verbatim by a trained transcriptionist whereupon all questionnaires were destroyed. Data was identifiable only through code numbers and demographic information (e.g., "56-year-old-male").

# Afterword

# Continuing the Conversation: Reflections on Our Emergent Scholarly Narratives

ॐ

**Christina S. Beck**
**Lynn M. Harter**
*Ohio University*

**Phyllis M. Japp**
*University of Nebraska-Lincoln*

*On May 27, 1995, our life was, in an instant, inexplicably, unalterably changed ... We left an able-bodied existence full of privilege and ease and entered a life of disability, with all of its accompanying restrictions and challenges. We went from the "haves" to the "have nots." Or so we thought. What we had yet to discover were all the gifts that come out of sharing hardship, the hidden pleasures behind the pain, the simple joys revealed when the more obvious treats and diversions that life has to offer are taken away. Something miraculous and wonderful happened amidst terrible tragedy, and a whole new dimension of life began to emerge.*                                      —(Reeve, 1999, pp. 3–4)

As we crafted this book, we reflected on prior scholarly contributions to narrative as well as our own narrative co-constructions of health, wellness, sickness, and healing throughout our respective lives. Combined with our contributors, we pondered countless stories—stories of actual people who enact lives amid physical and emotional challenges; people who struggle with economic, political, relational, and societal constraints; people who try to live the best they can and to enrich the lives of their loved ones when possible; people like Christo-

433

pher Reeve's wife, Dana, who reframe overwhelming adversity into something positive and inspiring.

Through the editing process, we relived some of our own experiences, and we also savored the opportunity to learn from the narratives of others as we worked with our contributors, vicariously meeting their research co-participants as well. This book constitutes a collection of diverse voices, perspectives, and lived realities, and we believe that our chapter authors join us in making valuable theoretical and empirical contributions to the emergent scholarly narratives of narratives and health communication theory, research, and practice.

Notably, we do view our work as part of a continuing scholarly journey toward understanding the nature and implications of narrative, especially with regard to health communication scholarship—an ongoing, socially co-constructed story about this important line of inquiry. As we acknowledge in our introductory chapter, we interject our perspectives and analysis into a tradition of research that spans disciplines and decades. However, we hold that the chapters in this volume do more than echo those esteemed earlier authors. Instead, we strive to recast prior ways of discussing narrative (Babrow, Rawlins, & Kline, chap. 2, this volume; Harter, Japp, & Beck, chap. 1, this volume) and to highlight research that pushes the boundaries of narrative theorizing and empirical research.

Despite the scholarly value of this volume, we recognize that our book now becomes part of the trajectory of narrative research, hopefully, an integral part of the ongoing account of narrative scholarship. As such, we want to conclude by emphasizing four areas that we envision as ripe for future research—aspects of narrative work that we hint at in this volume but that warrant much deeper investigation and analysis in other subsequent projects.

## INTERSECTIONS BETWEEN CONCURRENT, CLASHING, COMPETING, CONTRADICTORY NARRATIVES

On May 19, 2004, the Associated Press published an article about mothers' childbirth rights. In one instance, staff members at a Wilkes-Barre, Pennsylvania hospital informed Amber Marlowe that she had to have a Cesarean section due to the size of her baby. Marlowe checked out of the hospital, and lawyers for the facility sued for guardianship of the unborn child. After she delivered the baby naturally at another hospital, Marlowe learned of the prior facility's legal action. She retorted, "They don't know me from anything, and they're making decisions about my body? It was terrifying" (Associated Press, May 19, 2004).

Amber Marlowe made a critical choice regarding her unborn child, confronting a challenging situation during a serious point in her pregnancy—a competing emergent narrative involving her life and the life of her child. The hospital treated Marlowe's choice about a vaginal birth (and the way in which she wanted to shape her child's entry into this world) as wrong, even irresponsible. Clearly, these two narrative constructions of the same health situation clashed, forcing one woman to leave a hospital and that hospital to seek legal assistance.

Although narrative researchers and health communication scholars acknowledge differing philosophical, social, cultural, economic, and spiritual orientations to lived realities, in general, and to wellness issues, in particular (see, e.g., Bosticco & Thompson, chap. 18, this volume), we need to do a better job of exploring the implications of contradictory narratives for health care participants. Gilda Radner powerfully articulated her struggle to sort through recommendations from diverse health care providers:

> On October 13, the acupuncturist stuck needles in my swollen stomach and gave me a special abdominal massage. Two days later, the holistic doctor suggested I have a colonic to clean out the bowel. I insisted that would be too weird for me. The next day, I saw my internist. He did blood work again—I was running a low-grade fever. He gave me a gamma globulin shot, which was working on some patients with this Epstein-Barr virus. He felt my stomach and told me I was literally "full of shit," and gave me a prescription for laxatives. He told me to come back in a week.
>
> Suddenly, I began to wonder how to please so many people. Do I take the magnesium citrate? What about the coffee enema? Do I do both? Do I do the abdominal massage or the colonic? Do I tell the doctors about each other? East meets West in Gilda's body: Western medicine down my throat, Eastern medicine up my butt. (Radner, 1989, p. 67)

Notably, this volume features empirical research that explores narratives shaped by philosophical, political, relational, and personal conflict (see, e.g., Buzzanell & Ellingson, chap. 13; Harter, Kirby, Edwards, & McClanahan, chap. 4; P. M. Japp & D. K. Japp, chap. 5; Sharf, chap. 15; Workman, chap. 6). However, we lack scholarly investigations into the dialogic co-constructions of these emergent narratives that would emerge from explorations of multiple perspectives of similar situations. The postmodern turn toward plurality of possibilities opens an ever-broadening range of alternatives (see related work by Gergen, 1991, 1994); however, sorting through options and reconciling incompatibilities can confuse health care seekers and frustrate health care providers and social support-system members, who may hold their own philosophical convictions about "right" or "wrong" choices.

Given that the previously mentioned Associated Press article did not share the hospital's "take" on the case, the legal, medical, moral, ethical, or economic positions that guided the hospital's reaction regarding Amber Marlowe remain a mystery to readers and likely to Marlowe. Yet, we propose that scholars should pursue those complexities that underscore conflicting narrative constructions as a means of fostering richer understandings of and contributions to discourses about health and wellness.

Particularly because narrative co-constructions contribute to our ways of knowing and being and enable us to sort through times of continuity as well as times of disruption (see Harter, Japp, & Beck, chap. 1, this volume), scholars could provide important insights (and perhaps, recommendations to health care participants) through rich analysis of complex competing narratives. Indeed, such conflicts can occur between (a) family members over the enactment of another family member's condition; (b) between co-workers who differ regarding the risk of contact with another co-worker with a certain illness, disability, or chronic condition; and (c) between members of a society who marginalize others due to illness or addiction. Without resolution or understanding, these clashing, concurrent narratives slash vast divides, perpetuating hurt and jeopardizing the potential for wellness and healing.

## UNSPOKEN UNDERCURRENTS

In chapter 7, Carabas and Harter explore "forbidden stories." Those narratives of oppression by Romanian citizens reflect the value of sharing narratives to commence healing and the societal barriers to such revelations. Although this case represents an extreme situation, Petronio (2002) observed that individuals may opt not to share important details about their lives due to potential stigma or relational consequences. Indeed, nearly 50 years ago, Goffman (1955, 1959) noted that people strive to protect and promote their social face, advancing aspects of themselves that fit with the preferred presentation of self.

Although these unspoken undercurrents stay beneath the surface during interactions, they remain critical dimensions of how participants respond to (and offer) recommendations, view choices, pursue information, and co-construct individual and relational identities. Yet, as narrative theorists and health communication scholars, we lack an adequate understanding of the implications of such private matters for health care interactions and for the emergent co-construction of health care narratives.

Miller, Geist-Martin, and Kristen Cannon Beatty (chap. 14, this volume) and Keeley and Kellas (chap. 17, this volume) note that narratives afford participants the creativity to actively shape their experiences. Yet, they also constrain the ways in which participants can legitimately express and enact their lived realities. Langellier and Peterson (2004) described the dominant political narrative of breast cancer as implicitly confining in terms of how women can legitimately explain their experiences. Building on Ehrenreich's (2001) critique, Langellier and Peterson (2004) explored the narrative of "Jane," a woman who overtly resists an emphasis on survivorship and cheerfulness, typical of breast cancer narratives. However, they argue:

> In performing a breast cancer story, a woman can function as an agent of mundane resistance. But because of the multileveled relations of power, resistance cannot be guaranteed by any particular text, even when it opposes the normative story; by any particular telling, even when it contributes to healing; by any particular hearing, even when it achieves personal and cultural witness to a life or death. Even had Jane chosen silence as a form of resistance to breast-cancer storytelling culture, that silence would resonate with ambiguities of embodiment and discourse. (p. 218)

As social actors in a particular location, social circle, and family at a given time, perhaps some thoughts or conditions may not be revealed without jeopardizing consistency with concurrent life narratives and identities as a certain type of person—a "good" patient, a "good" wife or child, a "survivor." The nature of the dominant societal narrative may preclude revelation of "inappropriate" perspectives or actions regarding disease or disability. For example, a recent Miss America (who happened to be deaf) confronted criticism for speaking instead of signing. Such pervasive discourse may also hinder disclosures regarding physical, emotional, or sexual abuse. Hunt (2000) revealed the story of Isabela, a woman who felt unable to refuse her husband's advances until she developed cervical cancer. She silently endured an abusive marital situation before her surgery for cancer afforded her a socially legitimate means of denying intercourse—pain. Hunt (2000) explained that "she has turned her suffering into a form of social empowerment ... She has thus managed to preserve her social identity as dutiful wife, while resisting the cultural mandated marital requirement for sexual submission" (p. 95).

Narratives implicitly get constrained by the choices that participants make, including the decision to omit details (e.g., smoking, drug, or alcohol practices) that may be critical to an effective diagnosis or treatment recommendation or details (such as knowledge of a sexually transmitted disease) that may endanger the wellness or life of a sexual partner. Withholding aspects of emergent narratives may also hinder healing (see Carabas & Harter, chap. 7, this volume) or effective treatment (see Beach & Mandelbaum, chap. 16, this volume).

Although difficult in design, narrative and health communication scholars should continue to pursue the implications of unspoken undercurrents for health care participants (including social support members and health care staff), especially with regard to mental, emotional, and spiritual health. Scholars have only recently explored issues such as stress in health care settings, mental health and wellness, and health and spirituality. For example, the recent special issue of *Health Communication* on religious faith, spirituality, and health communication highlights the salience of spirituality for health care participants (Parrott, 2004b). Yet, we continue to face a theoretical, empirical, and practical void in understanding and recommendations regarding these guarded, private matters, issues that may never come to the surface of interactions between health care providers and their patients or between family members.

Unspoken undercurrents and competing, clashing, and contradictory narratives raise, for us, questions about the politics of storytelling. Narratives often summon discourses of difference—in particular gender, race/ethnicity, sexuality, and class—and rely on these discursive affiliations to accomplish multiple forms of privilege and exclusion. Narrative constructions carry abstract, symbolic, structural, and normative force, cementing systems of "advantage and disadvantage, exploitation and coercion, action and emotion, meaning and identity" (Acker, 1990, p. 146). Narratives emerge embedded in systems of representation (see Singhal, Chitnis, & Sengupta, chap. 8, this volume), offering predictable yet elastic, clear yet contradictory subjectivities, relations among them, and attendant disciplinary practices (e.g., unspoken undercurrents and competing narratives).

As this volume concludes, we issue a call for further attention to narrative processes of ideological struggle and urge multiple, local ways of explaining dominance and representing resistance. For instance, how are societal and organizational narratives of gender invoked by individuals in particular situations, and how do these performances craft particular subjectivities, preserving and/or altering relations of domination? Gender, of course, exists as central to how we live our daily lives, but never works alone. Gender inevitably intersects with race, class, sexuality, organizational context, historical context, and so forth, influencing what stories are told, who tells the stories, and how audiences consume the stories. Narrative scholars ought to explore how competing, clashing, and concurrent narratives as well as unspoken undercurrents emerge as classed, gendered, and raced discourses and issues, and the subsequent material—psychological, and physiological outcomes.

## INTERSECTIONS OF NARRATIVE CO-CONSTRUCTIONS, PHYSIOLOGICAL EXPERIENCES, MATERIAL AND ENVIRONMENTAL CONDITIONS

As we reflected on Amber Marlowe's story, we wondered at her willingness to get up and leave a hospital while in labor. Sure, she was courageous to stick to her principles, but we also marvel at her physical ability to go somewhere else during labor. All too often, we fear, scholars focus on the beautiful construction of the narrative—the moving or inspiring story—without grappling with the physical realities of the participants' situations. Real people suffer through unimaginable difficulties—limitations in movement or awareness; nausea; decreased ability to see, hear, or breathe; loss of hair or other body parts; loss of control over bodily functions.

In her compelling study of a neonatal intensive-care unit, Renee Anspach tells the story of a premature infant who suffered a massive infection, seizures, internal bleeding, and decreased blood pressure. Doctors discussed the prognosis as well as possible courses of action, and they ultimately presented the understandably devastated parents with the news that their baby would likely die in spite of treatment. According to Anspach (1993), "Then, after several moments, she [the mother] asked, 'Is there nothing else you can do?' " (p. 95).

At such a point, the parents and doctors could opt to press on, to extend the health saga of this baby, its parents, and staff members. Each decision becomes consequential to how the drama will unfold as well as to the physical condition (and potential suffering) of the child. This case underscores the inherently physiological dimension of health narratives, even though our commitment to quest narratives (see Frank, 1995) could prompt us to gloss discomfort as we aspire to grander growth from medical situations.

In the passage at the beginning of this chapter, Dana Reeve (1999) wrote of the "whole new dimension of life" (p. 4) sparked by her husband's riding accident. Scholars note the preference for positives in breast cancer storytelling as opposed to complaints about the indignities of medical procedures and treatment protocols (see Couser, 1997; Ehrenreich, 2001; Langellier & Peterson, 2004). Yet, in aspiring for the "deeper meaning" of health setbacks, do we suppress voices that yearn to express frustration about pain or limitations? Do we construct a societal preference for muting attention to the countless challenges that accompany disease and disability?

Certainly, some of the chapters in this volume (such as Beck, chap. 3; P. M. Japp & D. K. Japp, chap. 5; Carabas & Harter, chap. 7; O'Hair, Scannell, & Thompson, chap. 19; Sharf, chap. 15; Sunwolf, Frey, &

Keranen, chap. 11) refer to physical struggles, as do other narrative scholars. Yet, as we considered this book, we believe that we could have pushed even harder to include the implications of physical challenges and constraints on narrative co-constructions. Further, we hold that future work would be well-served by featuring the implications of those challenges and constraints on caregivers and social support system members as well. How do people who suffer from such afflictions co-construct such experiences with loved ones in light of other relational realities?

Intersections between narrative co-constructions and physiological experiences also must be expanded to include environmental and material conditions. In 1994, Dana Cloud challenged communication scholars to recognize that symbols are not the only thing that matters. Of course, as chapters in this volume attest, discourses do matter—they have material effects and serve material interests in the world (see, e.g., Buzzanell & Ellingson, chap. 13, this volume). Moreover, narrative theory provides a repertoire of tools for understanding how political and economic power is mediated, reproduced, and resisted in texts under study. Yet, material practices of exploitation and oppression and environmental conditions also intertwine with (and take on meaning through) discursive formations that cannot be solely reduced to the socially constructed. Cloud (1994) poignantly argued:

> We ought not sacrifice the notions of practical truth, bodily reality, and material oppression to the tendency to render all of the experience discursive, as if no one went hungry or died in war. To say that hunger and war are rhetorical is to state the obvious; to suggest that rhetoric is all they are is to leave critique behind. (p. 159)

Communication scholars must come to terms with the material world. We agree with Cheney (2000) who argued that our discipline often engages in "symbol worship," occasionally to the point of denying that there are any other experiences. For example, employees develop illnesses because of exposure to chemicals in the workplace (see Gaither, 2004, for a discussion of a pending class-action lawsuit against IBM), toxic asbestos fibers (The Gazette, 2003), research animals and latex gloves (Farrar, 2004). Foregrounding intersections between the physiological, material, environmental, and symbolic would be a welcome development in narrative theorizing specifically and communication research more generally.

## EXPLORATIONS OF CHAOS STORIES

Amber Marlowe's story was easy to tell—it turned out well, and she is a proud mother for the seventh time. Her 11-pound, 9-ounce little girl looks quite healthy in the Associated Press photo ... How would the public 'retelling' of this narrative differ, though, if we altered the outcome—if the baby had died en route to another location?

Marlowe's narrative might have been worded more like that of another mother mentioned in the same article. In that case, a woman in Salt Lake City was charged with capital murder after she resisted a C-section. One of her twins died after she waited for 2 weeks before consenting to the procedure. (According to the Associated Press article, she subsequently bargained for a lesser offense, receiving probation as punishment.)

Consistent with a modernist, Western perspective of medicine, the hospital (and, eventually, the legal system) privileged and legitimized a singular "right" way to proceed. Although clear convictions about medical alternatives certainly reduce uncertainty (see Babrow, Kline, & Rawlins, chap. 2, this volume), stances that emphasize absolutism implicitly diminish the credibility of narratives that feature confusion about possibilities and frustration regarding medical failures.

"Jen," a beautiful, young, hairstylist with two small children, used to fix one of the co-editor's hair at a local styling salon. Over the course of a year, Jen spoke vaguely about a medical condition that annoyed her—never offering specific details about the nature of the condition, just casting it as an inconvenience, not life-threatening. Ultimately, Jen elected to pursue an optional surgery to correct her condition. She checked into a major regional hospital after interviewing physicians and selecting an expert who had completed the procedure on numerous other patients.

Unfortunately, the surgeon erred during the surgery, damaging her colon and bladder. That mistake propelled Jen on a new path—a journey of survival amid constant pain, recurrent infection, frequent trips to the emergency room, countless hospital stays, and additional medical procedures. She could not longer work, no more enjoy life in the ways that she had prior to the first surgery. Subsequent surgeries and treatments failed to heal Jen. Although she sued and obtained a sizable settlement, she suffered significantly, and sadly, she died in her early 30s within a few years of that original medical mistake, still searching in vain for a way to correct something that never should have occurred.

Borrowing Frank's (1995) terms, *chaos stories* receive far less attention than *restitution stories* by scholars. In the former, individuals (such as Jen) confront challenges without gaining positive resolution. Blurring the boundaries of public and private spheres, people now engage the media regarding personal matters, such as health. Yet, not all voices get heard; not everyone attains a response; not all cries for help get answered. Some launch like a "dud" firework that disappoints with a dull thud and a puff of smoke, only to disappear without consequence. No article ever appeared in the local newspaper about Jen, her struggle, her court case, or the medical mistake that devastated her life. Perhaps worse, near the end, health care workers began passing her around like a hot potato—dropping her in someone else's hands to avoid being held responsible for her current condition or even her death.

As scholars, we bring little focus to such stories, perhaps because they remain mere blips on our overall radar. Chapters in this book feature reflective and dedicated caregivers (Rawlins, chap. 9; Morgan-Witte, chap. 10), concerned medical educators (Ragan, Mindt, & Wittenberg, chap. 12), and committed family members (Bosticco & Thompson, chap. 18; Keeley & Kellas, chap. 17), not disgruntled or disenchanted health care providers or abusive parents or children. The Romanian narratives emerged after being published in a book (see Carabas & Harter, chap. 7); invisible diseases (or diseases that remain unclassified as such) lurk under the social surface until a famous person acknowledges the problem (see P. M. Japp & D. K. Japp, chap. 5). Would anyone know (or care) about Cathy Hainer's cancer if she wasn't Cathy Hainer, the *USA Today* reporter, especially because she failed to win her battle with this dread disease? (see Beck, chap. 3).

Notably, chaos stories hold the potential to enlighten us about the everyday challenges of actual people who face the physical, economic, social, and sometimes political ramifications of enacting health and wellness in contemporary society. We encourage future researchers to pursue such stories as a means of understanding narratives as partial and indeterminate, crafted by people who continue to struggle with a multiplicity of issues and who still lack the resolutions that they seek for their respective situations.

## SUMMARY

We believe that this book constitutes a compelling contribution to the literature on health communication and, in particular, health narratives. As this body of research continues to expand, we trust that the issues that have been detailed in this conclusion will be taken up by researchers and, ideally, shared with actual health care participants, people whose lives get crafted through the narratives that they co-construct with others.

In closing, we add one more expression of gratitude to the research co-participants who lent their voices to this work, and we thank the individuals who shared their stories with us in public and private settings, making them available as examples for this work. As we reflect on our journey, we remain quite aware of the trust that we hold with regard to those narratives. Ethically, we recognize the inherent risk in representing others' voices in our research endeavors, and we truly hope that we have presented them in ways in which others will be comfortable.

# Contributor Biographical Statements

࿓

**Austin S. Babrow** (PhD, University of Illinois) is a Professor in the Department of Communication at Purdue University. Author of many articles and chapters on health communication and communication theory and methods more generally, he is especially interested in the dynamic interrelationships among communication, beliefs, and values, an interest reflected in published works on the many meanings of uncertainty (with C. Kasch & L. Ford), the centrality of uncertainty and values to health communication (with M. Mattson), news constructions of the uncertainties of bio-terror (with M. Dutta-Bergman), coping with uncertainty in physical therapy (with D. Dinn), popular magazine constructions of breast cancer uncertainties (with E. Buenger), the "ideology of uncertainty reduction" in discourse on women's breast self-exams (with K. Kline), values and uncertainties in advance care planning (with S. Hines), social support and tensions between expectations and desires (with L. Ford and C. Stohl), and explaining illness (with S. Hines and C. Kasch).

**Wayne A. Beach** (PhD, University of Utah) is a Professor in the School of Communication at San Diego State University, Adjunct Professor in the Department of Surgery, and an Associate Member of the Rebecca and John Moores Cancer Center in the School of Medicine at the University of California, San Diego. His current research focuses on communication between cancer patients and oncologists, among family members talking through cancer diagnosis and treatment on the telephone, and a variety of interactional practices in ordinary conversations. Dr. Beach is currently working on two books: the first natural history of how family members work through cancer, and an edited volume focusing on routine problems that emerge as patients present and doctors respond to a wide range of health (biomedical and psychosocial) health issues. He has guest edited special issues focusing on "Lay Diagnosis" during medical interviews, the "Sequential Organization of Conversational Activities," and is author of *Conversations About Illness: Family Preoccupations With Bulimia* (1996, Mahwah, NJ: Lawrence Erlbaum Associates).

**Christina S. Beck** (PhD, University of Oklahoma) is an Associate Professor in the School of Communication Studies at Ohio University. The author of two award-winning books on health communication, Beck also co-edited a book on the Hill-Thomas hearings, and she has published numerous journal articles and invited book chapters. Her research interests span the areas of health communication and mass communication. Beck is currently the book review editor for *Journal of Health Communication: International Perspectives*, and she serves on the editorial boards of *Health Communication*, *Journal of Applied Communication Research*, and *Communication Studies*. She will begin her 3-year term as Editor of *Communication Yearbook* in 2005.

**Cecilia Bosticco** (MA, University of Dayton) is a mother and community volunteer who came to the study of communication at midlife. Her research interest in the role of communication in bereavement flows from her personal experience following the death of her youngest daughter while she was a Master's candidate. She has upcoming publications on bereavement issues in the journals *Omega* and *Journal of Family Communication*.

**Patrice M. Buzzanell** (PhD, Purdue University) is a Professor in the Department of Communication at Purdue University where she specializes in feminist organizational communication theorizing and gendered workplace practices, particularly those pertaining to careers. She has co-edited two books: *Rethinking Organizational and Managerial Communication from Feminist Perspectives* and *Gender in Applied Communication Contexts* and is working on a third, *Why Third Wave Feminisms? Shaping Contemporary Feminist Communication Theory*. She has published articles in journals including *Communication Monographs*, *Human Communication Research*, *Communication Theory*, and *Journal of Applied Communication Research*. She has edited *Management Communication Quarterly* and currently serves on 10 editorial boards.

**Kristen Cannon Beatty** (MA, San Diego State University) is a faculty member at the Art Institute of California-San Diego where she teaches

English composition, media literacy, and oral communication courses. Her research interests include health communication, intercultural communication, and community service-based learning.

**Teodora Carabas** (PhD, Ohio University) is a Visiting Assistant Professor at George Mason University. Her research interests focus on the rhetorical and political study of conflict as it emerges out of the interaction among various social groups or between citizens and the state. Her PhD dissertation investigated the enactment of citizenship and the formation of civil society in totalitarian contexts (with a focus on communist Eastern Europe). From January 2002 until August 2004 she also served as managing editor of *Explorations in Media Ecology*.

**Ketan Chitnis** (MA, University of Florida) is a doctoral candidate in the School of Telecommunications, Ohio University. Earlier he has worked in the field of advertising in India and as a communication consultant with UNICEF in Nepal. His research interest lies in Communication for Social Change. His previous research has been on male attitudes toward family planning in India. He is currently the team leader of Ohio University's online initiative on Communication and Development. Recently he has researched on Indian and American viewers' interpretation of health topics in the sitcom Friends. Presently he is pursuing his doctoral dissertation research on understanding participatory communicative practices used for organizing people for change in a health and development project in Jamkhed, India.

**Autumn Edwards** (MA, University of Kansas) is a doctoral candidate in the School of Communication Studies at Ohio University. Her research interests include interpersonal communication and communication theory as they relate to issues of community and social justice.

**Laura L. Ellingson** (PhD, University of South Florida) is an Assistant Professor in the Department of Communication at Santa Clara University. Her research interests include health care provider–patient communication, interdisciplinary communication, health care teamwork, and feminist theory and methodology. Her book, *Communicating in the Clinic: Negotiating Frontstage and Backstage Teamwork* (Hampton Press), mixes methods and genres to explore interdisciplinary healthcare teamwork through narrative ethnography, grounded theory, autoethnography, and feminist analysis. She also has published articles in *Health Communication, Journal of Aging Studies, Journal of Applied Communication Research, Women's Studies in Communication*, and *Communication Studies*. She has served as the Chair of the Ethnography Division of the National Communication Association. Currently, she is conducting an ethnography of team communication in a dialysis clinic.

**Arthur Frank** (PhD, Yale) is a Professor of Sociology at the University of Calgary, located in Alberta, Canada. He is the author of *At the Will of the Body* (1991), *The Wounded Storyteller: Body, illness, and ethics* (1995), and *The Renewal of Generosity: Illness, Medicine, and How To Live* (2004). He serves on the editorial boards of *Qualitative Health Research, Autobiography, Families, Systems & Health,* and *Body & Society,* and he is the book review editor of *Health*. His work attempts to link illness experience, narrative, bioethics, and social theory.

**Lawrence R. Frey** (PhD, University of Kansas) is a Professor and Associate Chair of the Department of Communication at The University of Colorado at Boulder. He teaches group communication, applied communication, and research methods courses, and his research focuses on how participation in collective communicative practices makes a difference in people's individual, relational, and collective life. He is the author/editor of 10 books, 3 special journal issues, and 55 book chapters and journal articles. He has received 10 distinguished scholarship awards, including the 2000 Gerald M. Phillips Award for Distinguished Applied Communication Scholarship from the National Communication Association (NCA); the 2003 and 2000 Ernest Bormann Research Award from NCA's Group Communication Division for the edited texts, *New Directions in Group Communication* and *The Handbook of Group Communication Theory and Research;* and the 1998 National Jesuit Book Award and 1988 Distinguished Book Award from NCA's Applied Communication Division for the coauthored text, *The Fragile Community: Living Together With AIDS*. He is a past president of the Central States Communication Association and a recipient of the Outstanding Young Teacher Award from that organization and the 2003 Master Teacher Award from the Communication and Instruction Interest Group of the Western States Communication Association.

**Patricia Geist Martin** (PhD, Purdue University) is a Professor in the School of Communication at San Diego State University where she teaches organizational communication, health communication, ethnographic research methods, and gender and organizational communication. Her research interests focus on negotiating identity, ideology, and control in organizations, particularly in health and illness. In 2003 her third book, *Communicating Health: Personal, cultural, and political complexities,* (co-authored with Eileen Berlin Ray and Barbara Sharf) was published by Wadsworth. Through stories this book captures the complexities of communicating in diverse health contexts ranging from provider–patient relationships to organizational health systems such as HMOs and media campaigns for preventative care. Her second book, co-edited with Linda A. M. Perry, is entitled *Courage of Conviction: Women's Words, Women's Wisdom*, published in 1997 by Mayfield. The volume presents the stories of women from all walks of life who, through courage and conviction, have broken silences and inspired others to speak, to listen, to be heard. Her first book, *Negotiating the Crisis: DRGs and the Transformation of Hospitals* (with Monica Hardesty) published in 1992 by Lawrence Erlbaum Associates examines communication among nurses, physicians, and hospital administrators as they negotiate a controversial change in hospital policy and structure. She has published over 50 articles and book chapters covering a wide range of topics including adaptation in a merging organization, decision making in medical groups, argument in teacher–administrator bargaining, empowerment for disabled persons, responding to sexual harassment, controversial television programming, social support strategies, and cross-cultural communication.

**Lynn M. Harter** (PhD, University of Nebraska) is an Assistant Professor in the School of Communication Studies at Ohio University. Her research and teaching interests focus on the discourses of health and healing and organizing processes, feminist and narrative theory and practice, communication and social justice. She has published numerous articles in outlets including *Management Communication Quarterly*, the *Journal of Applied Communication Research*, *Health Communication*, and *Qualitative Health Research*, and serves on multiple interdisciplinary and disciplinary editorial boards. She lives in Athens, Ohio, with husband Scott and daughter Emma Grace.

**Debra K. Japp** (PhD, University of Nebraska) is a Professor of Communication Studies at St. Cloud State University (Minnesota) and the Academic Affairs Coordinator for the Inter Faculty Organization, the faculty union for the Minnesota state universities. She teaches courses in persuasion and rhetorical criticism. Her research interests include media and popular culture, gender communication, and political communication.

**Phyllis M. Japp** (PhD, University of Nebraska) is an Associate Professor in the Department of Communication Studies at University of Nebraska-Lincoln where she teaches contemporary rhetorical theory and criticism, cultural studies, health communication, and communication ethics. She has authored a number of essays, most utilizing narrative theory and focusing on public and mediated discourses, especially those involving health, gender, ethics, or environmental issues. She is a co-editor of a recent book on environment and popular culture, is currently co-editing a book on communication ethics and popular culture, and has served on the editorial boards of a number of communication studies journals.

**Maureen Keeley** (PhD, University of Iowa) is an Associate Professor in the Department of Communication Studies at Texas State University-San Marcos. Her research focuses on the verbal and nonverbal communication that occurs within personal relationships in the midst of a health crisis. Most recently she is exploring the communication that occurs at the end-of-life from the survivors' perspectives. She has published a number of academic articles on this topic and is currently working on a popular press book titled: *Final Conversations: The Gifts We Are Left With.* She teaches in the areas of interpersonal/relational communication, nonverbal communication, gender communication, and family communication.

**Jody Koenig Kellas** (PhD, University of Washington) is an Assistant Professor in the Department of Communication Studies at the University of Nebraska-Lincoln. She specializes in relational communication, family communication, and narratives of personal relationships. Her research has explored the relationship between storytelling and individual adjustment, post-dissolutional communication, as well as attributions in marital relationships. She most recently has focused her research on the processes, identity negotiation, and relational qualities associated with joint storytelling in families.

**Lisa Keranen** (PhD, University of Pittsburgh) is an Assistant Professor in the Department of Communication at the University of Colorado at Boulder. She specializes in the rhetoric of medicine across interactional, institutional, and public contexts with emphases on end-of-life discourse, biomedical research controversies, and bioterrorism. Her primary publications appear in the *Journal of Medical Humanities* and the *Journal of Applied Communication Research.* She is currently working on a book that traces the construction of scientific character in a breast cancer research scandal.

**Erika L. Kirby** (PhD, University of Nebraska) is an Associate Professor in the Department of Communication Studies at Creighton University. Her teaching and research interests include organizational, applied and work-family communication and discourses as well as their intersections with gender and feminism. She has published articles in outlets such as the *Journal of Applied Communication Research,*

*Management Communication Quarterly* and *Communication Year-book*, and serves on the editorial boards of the *Journal of Applied Communication Research, Communication Studies and Communication Teacher.* She lives in Omaha, Nebraska with husband Bob and daughters Meredith and Samantha.

**Kimberly N. Kline** (PhD, University of Georgia) is an Assistant Professor in the Department of Speech Communication at Southern Illinois University in Carbondale. Her research focuses on the social construction of health, illness, and medicine, especially with regard to women's health issues. Her published studies have addressed topics such as the theoretical and methodological issues in the study of health and the mass media, the socially constructed understandings of illicit drug use during pregnancy and breast self-examination (BSE) including a focused study of "uncertainty reduction" and BSE (with Austin Babrow), and the use of textual analysis to evaluate the persuasive potential of breast cancer education materials (with Marifran Mattson). She is currently working on projects that use critical/interpretive methodologies to identify themes in television shows and feature films that reflect and constitute knowledge and ideologies related to health, illness, and medicine.

**Jenny Mandelbaum** (PhD, the University of Texas) is Associate Professor and Chair in the Department of Communication at Rutgers University. Her research examines the organization of everyday interaction, using video- and audio-tapes of naturally occurring conversations as a resource for describing, for instance, how we construct storytellings in conversation, and what we "do" through the stories we tell. Her published work focuses on various social interaction practices (particularly storytelling), and their implications for relationships and identity. She is co-editor of *Studies in Language and Social Interaction: In Honor of Robert Hopper,* (Lawrence Erlbaum Associates, 2003). She and her students are currently working on a large database of video-taped Thanksgiving, Easter, and Passover Dinners. She has received grant support for introducing web-based technologies to the University classroom, and serves regularly as a grant proposal reviewer for the National Cancer Institute. She serves on the Editorial Boards of *Communication Education* and *The Journal of Communication.*

**Andrea M. McClanahan** (PhD, Ohio University) is an Assistant Professor in the Department of Communication Studies at East Stroudsburg University of Pennsylvania. Her teaching and research areas include feminist rhetorical theory, critical/cultural studies, and alternative life choices of women.

**Magdalyn Z. Miller** (MA, San Diego State University) is currently an Instructor of English at the National University of Cajamarca in Cajamarca, Peru. Her research and teaching interests focus on interpersonal and intercultural communication and have led her to Peru where she is beginning a micro-enterprise small group gender project with the women of poverty in Northern Peru.

**Tiffany Mindt** (MA, University of Oklahoma) is currently a PhD student at the University of Oklahoma in the Department of Communication. She anticipates completing her PhD in 2006, under the direction of her chair, Dr. Sandy Ragan. Her areas of research include health communication, particularly those issues relevant to women's health.

**Jayne Morgan-Witte** (PhD, University of Nebraska) is an Associate Professor in the Department of Communication Studies at the University of Northern Iowa. Her teaching and research interests include emotion and workplace communication, particularly in health care contexts. She has published interpretive/critical studies in caregiver and manager emotionality, organizational identification, and metaphors of change in the workplace.

**Dan O'Hair** (PhD, University of Oklahoma) is a Professor in the Department of Communication at the University of Oklahoma. His teaching and research interests include organizational communication, health systems, and patient care communication processes. He has published more than 50 research articles and scholarly book chapters in communication, business management, and psychology journals and volumes, and has authored and edited 10 books in the areas of communication, business, and health. He is one of the founding directors of the Southwest Program for Pancreatic Cancer at the University of Oklahoma and was a co-chair of the Pancreatic Cancer Progress Group at the National Cancer Institute. He has served on the editorial boards of 18 research journals and is the immediate past editor of the *Journal of Applied Communication Research*, published by the National Communication Association.

**Sandra L. Ragan** (PhD, University of Texas) is a Professor in the Department of Communication at the University of Oklahoma. Her research in health communication began in the mid 1980's with an interest in women's health communication. This inquiry spawned a number of publications; perhaps more important, it helped launch the careers of two rising stars in the field—Athena duPre and Christina Beck (one of the co-editors of this volume). In the last several years, she has become interested in cancer and communication and is currently working on a book on palliative care.

**William K. Rawlins** (PhD, Temple University) is Stocker Professor in the School of Communication Studies at Ohio University. He teaches courses in interpersonal communication, dialogue and experience, interpretive and ethnographic inquiry, communication and narrative, Gregory Bateson and communication theory, and communication in friendships across the life course. He received the School of Liberal Arts Educational Excellence Award for 2002–2003 at Purdue University. His book, *Friendship Matters: Communication, Dialectics, and the Life Course*, was selected as an Outstanding Academic Book for 1993 by the editors of *Choice*, and received the Gerald R. Miller Book Award in 1994 from the Interpersonal and Small Group Interaction Division of NCA. In 2002 he received The Theory That Has Left a Legacy Award: "The Dialectical Perspective" from the Communication Theory Interest Group of the Central States Communication Association. He continues to study how communicating as friends serves the well-lived life for persons and societies.

**Denise Scannell** (MA, University of Oklahoma) is a PhD student in the Department of Communication at the University of Oklahoma who anticipates completing her degree in 2005. Her research in health communication focuses on narrative and identity. She currently has one book chapter on environmental communication published and two book chapters in press.

**Ami Sengupta** (MPS, Cornell University) is a doctoral student in the School of Communication Studies, Ohio University. Prior to joining Ohio University she has worked as a consultant for UNICEF Regional Office for South Asia and for the Nepal Country office. Her previous work has involved health communication campaigns and advocacy and research on violence against women and children. Her current research interests are non-Western feminist scholarship and role of communication in facilitating women's empowerment and health. Most recently her research is on how entertainment-education driven radio soap drama can spur changes in the performance of gender roles in Bihar, India.

**Barbara Sharf** (PhD, University of Minnesota) is a Professor and Director of Graduate Studies in the Department of Communication at Texas A & M. She is co-author of *Communicating Health: Personal, Cultural, and Political Complexities*, as well as *The Physician's Guide to Better Communication*. Her research has been published in *Health*

*Affairs, Health Communication, Journal of Health Communication, Communication Monographs, Literature & Medicine, Women & Health*, and elsewhere. She is an Associate Editor of *Health Communication* and consultant in qualitative research methodology and physician–patient communication to the EXCEED Program (Excellence Centers to Eliminate Ethnic/Racial Disparities) at Baylor College of Medicine Health Services Section and the Houston VA Center for Quality of Care and Utilization Studies.

**Arvind Singhal** (PhD, University of Southern California) is Professor and Presidential Research Scholar in the School of Communication Studies at Ohio University, where he teaches and conducts research in the areas of diffusion of innovations, mobilizing for change, design, and implementation of strategic communication campaigns, and the entertainment–education communication strategy. He is author of *Combating AIDS: Communication Strategies in Action* (2003, Sage Publications); *India's Communication Revolution: From Bullock Carts to Cyber Marts* (2001, Sage Publications); *Entertainment-Education: A Communication Strategy for Social Change* (1999, Lawrence Erlbaum Associates); and *India's Information Revolution* (1989, Sage Publications); and co-editor of *Entertainment-Education and Social Change: History, Research, and Practice* (2004, Lawrence Erlbaum Associates), and *The Children of Africa Confront AIDS: From Vulnerability to Possibility* (2003, Ohio University Press). His book, *Entertainment-Education: A Communication Strategy for Social Change*, received the National Communication Association's Applied Communication Division's Distinguished Book Award for 2000.

**Sunwolf** (PhD, University of California-Santa Barbara; J.D., University of Denver College of Law) is a former trial attorney and now an Associate Professor of Communication at Santa Clara University. Her research focuses on the effects of interpersonal storytelling, symbolic communication, and the social dynamics of inclusion/exclusion in childhood peer groups. A national storyteller, she teaches and publishes on multiple aspects of tale-telling (spirituality, ghostlore, multicultural tales, and healing). She serves on the editorial boards of the *Journal of Applied Communication Research, Communication Studies, Storytelling, Self, Society*, and *The Handbook of Applied Communication Research*. Taking both a symbolic and narrative perspective, her book, *Practical Jury Dynamics: From Individual Juror Reasoning to Group Decision Making* examines social and narrative sense-making by jurors, while *Gift-Giving Unwrapped: Strategies and Stresses While Giving or Receiving Gifts* describes the symbolic relational effects of giving less-than-perfect gifts.

**Sharlene Thompson** (MA, George Mason University) is a PhD student in the Department of Communication at the University of Oklahoma who anticipates completing her degree in 2005. Her interests include cancer communication, health campaigns, interpersonal health communication, and women's health issues. Her dissertation involves examining the communication of hope to terminally ill patients in initial bad news delivery interactions.

**Teresa L. Thompson** (PhD, Temple University) is Professor of Communication at the University of Dayton and editor of the journal *Health Communication*. She has published more than 50 journal articles and book chapters and has written or edited six books on various aspects of health communication. Her primary research interests focus on provider–patient interaction. She directed the Master's thesis on which the chapter included in this volume was based.

**Elaine M. Wittenberg-Lyles** (PhD, University of Oklahoma) is an Assistant Professor in the Department of Communication Studies at the University of Nevada, Las Vegas. Her research program entails a qualitative examination of the interpersonal processes occurring in the context of death and dying. This year she completed research on the role of hospice volunteers as well as examined the information sharing strategies of hospice case managers in IDT meetings. Overall, her research focuses on how communicative processes are affected by death and contact with dying persons. She currently has four articles and book chapters in press.

**Thomas A. Workman** (PhD, University of Nebraska) is the Assistant Director of Student Involvement for Information Strategies at the University of Nebraska-Lincoln. His duties include the strategic development and implementation of communication efforts surrounding student life issues, including social marketing and advocacy campaigns for NU Directions, a grant project funded by the Robert Wood Johnson Foundation to reduce high-risk drinking among UNL students. His research focuses on the investigation and critique of cultural texts surrounding collegiate alcohol use and the rhetoric of prevention. His work developing tools for college alcohol prevention has been utilized at institutions across the country. He is the author of several book chapters and journal articles on college alcohol prevention and communicating health messages to college students. He also serves as a Guest Lecturer in the Department of Communication Studies at the University of Nebraska-Lincoln and conducts workshops at a variety of conferences.

# References

*60 Minutes*. (2002, April 7). CBS Worldwide Inc.

Abma, T. A. (2001). Evaluating palliative care: Facilitating reflexive dialogues about an ambiguous concept. *Medicine, Health Care and Philosophy, 4*, 261–276.

Acker, J. (1990). Hierarchies, jobs, bodies: A theory of gendered organizations. *Gender & Society, 4*, 139–158.

Addington, T., & Wegescheide-Harris, J. (1995). Ethics and communication with the terminally ill. *Health Communication, 7*, 267–281.

Adelman, M. B., & Frey, L. R. (1997). *The fragile community: Living together with AIDS*. Mahwah, NJ: Lawrence Erlbaum Associates.

Adler, P. (1975). The transnational experience: An alternative view of culture shock. *Journal of Humanistic Psychology, 15*, 13–23.

Ahearn, L. M. (2001). Language and agency. *Annual Reviews in Anthropology, 30*, 109–137.

Ahlzen, R. (2002). The doctor and the literary text—potentials and pitfalls. *Medicine, Health Care, and Philosophy, 5*, 147–155.

Aiken, L. R. (2001). *Dying, death, and bereavement* (4th ed.). Mahwah, NJ: Lawrence Erlbaum Associates.

Albom, M. (2003). *The five people you meet in heaven*. New York: Hyperion Books.

Allison, J. M. (1994). Narrative and time: A phenomenological reconsideration. *Text and Performance Quarterly, 14*, 108–125.

Alvord, L. A., & Van Pelt, E. C. (1999). *The scalpel and the silver bear: The first Navajo woman surgeon combines western medicine and traditional healing*. New York: Bantam Books.

*Analele Sighet: Instaurarea comunismului—intre rezistenta si represiune. Comunicari prezentate la Simpozionul de la Sighetu Marmatiei (9–11 iunie 1995)*. [The Sighet files: The initial stages of communism—between resistance and repression. Testimonies presented at the Sighetu Marmatiei Convention, June 9–11, 1995]. Bucharest, Romania: Fundatia Academia Civica.

Andalao, P. (2003). Love, tears, betrayal ... and health messages. *Perspective in Health Magazine, 8*, 1–6.

Andersen, A. (1993a). Stories I tell my patients: Watering the roses when the house is on fire. *Eating Disorders, 1*, 79–82.

Andersen, A. (1993b). Stories I tell my patients: The Indian and the chessboard. *Eating Disorders, 1*, 167–169.

Anderson, C. (1998). "Forty acres of cotton waiting to be picked": Medical students, storytelling, and the rhetoric of healing. *Literature and Medicine, 17*, 280–297.

Anderson, J. A. (1996). *Communication theory: Epistemological foundations*. New York: Guilford.

Ang, I. (1996). *Living room wars: Rethinking media audiences for a postmodern world*. New York: Routledge.

Anspach, R. (1993). *Deciding who lives: Fateful choices in the intensive-care nursery*. Berkeley, CA: University of California Press.

Arendt, H. (1972). On violence. In H. Arendt (Ed.), *Crises of the republic* (pp. 103–198). San Diego, CA: Harcourt Brace Jovanovich. (Original work published 1969)

Arntson, P., & Droge, D. (1987). Social support in self-help groups: The role of communication in enabling perceptions of control. In T. Albrecht & M. Adelman (Eds.), *Communicating social support* (pp. 148–171). Newbury Park, CA: Sage.

Aronowitz, R. A. (1998). *Making sense of illness: Science, society, and disease*. Cambridge, England: Cambridge University Press.

Ashcraft, K. L. (1999). Managing maternity leave: A qualitative analysis of temporary executive succession. *Administrative Science Quarterly, 44*, 240–280.

Ashcraft, K. L., & Mumby, D. K. (2004). *Reworking gender: A feminist communicology of organization*. Thousand Oaks, CA: Sage.

Associated Press. (2004, May 19). Recent court cases revive debate about mothers' childbirth rights.

Associated Press. (2004, March 8). AMA ads warn of binge drinking. Retrieved March 8, 2004, from http://www.cnn.com/2004/EDUCATION/03/08/springbreak.ads.ap/index.html.

Atkinson, J. M., & Drew, P. (1979). *Order in court: The organization of verbal interaction in judicial settings*. London: Macmillan.

Atkinson, J. M., & Heritage, J. (Eds.). (1984). *Structures of social action*. Cambridge, England: Cambridge University Press.

Atkinson, P. (1995). *Medical talk and medical work*. London: Sage.

Atkinson, P. (1997). Narrative turn or blind alley? *Qualitative Health Research, 7*, 325–344.

Babrow, A. S. (1991). Tensions between health beliefs and desires: Implications for a health communication campaign to promote a smoking cessation program. *Health Communication, 3*, 93–112.

Babrow, A. S. (1992). Communication and problematic integration: Understanding diverging probability and value, ambiguity, ambivalence, and improbability. *Communication Theory, 2*, 95–130.

Babrow, A. S. (1993). The advent of multiple process theories of communication. *Journal of Communication, 43*, 110–118.

Babrow, A. S. (1995). Communication and problematic integration: Milan Kudera's 'Lost Letters' in the "Book of Laughter and Forgetting." *Communication Monographs, 62,* 283–300.

Babrow, A. S. (1998). Colloquy: Developing multiple-process theories of communication. *Human Communication Research, 25,* 152–155.

Babrow, A. S. (2001). Uncertainty, value, communication, and problematic integration. *Journal of Communication, 51,* 553–573.

Babrow, A. S. (in press). Problematic integration theory. In B. B. Whaley & W. Samter (Eds.), *Explaining communication: Contemporary theories and exemplars.* Mahwah, NJ: Lawrence Erlbaum Associates.

Babrow, A. S., & Dutta-Bergman, M. J. (2004). Constructing the uncertainties of bioterror: A case study of U.S. news reporting on the anthrax attack of Fall, 2001. In C. B. Grant (Ed.), *Rethinking communicative interaction: New interdisciplinary horizons* (pp. 295–315). Amsterdam: John Benjamins.

Babrow, A., Hines, S., & Kasch, C. (2000). Illness and uncertainty: Problematic integration and strategies for communicating about medical uncertainty and ambiguity. In B. B. Whaley (Ed.), *Explaining illness: Messages, strategies and contexts* (pp. 41–67). Mahwah, NJ: Lawrence Erlbaum Associates.

Babrow, A. S., Kasch, C. R., & Ford, L. A. (1998). The many meaning of 'uncertainty' in illness: Toward a systematic accounting. *Health Communication, 10,* 1–24.

Babrow, A., & Kline, K. N. (2000). From 'reducing' to 'coping with' uncertainty: Reconceptualizing the central challenge in breast self-exams. *Social Science & Medicine, 51,* 1805–1816.

Babrow, A., & Mattson, M. (2003). Theorizing about health communication. In T. Thompson (Ed.), *Handbook of health communication* (pp. 35–61). Mahwah, NJ: Lawrence Erlbaum Associates.

Baerger, D. R., & McAdams, D. P. (1999). Life story coherence and its relation to psychological well-being. *Narrative Inquiry, 9,* 69–96.

Bailyn, L. (1993). *Breaking the mold: Women, men, and time in the new corporate world.* New York: The Free Press.

Bakhtin, M. M. (1981). *The dialogic imagination: Four essays* (C. Emerson & M. Holquist, Trans.). Austin: University of Texas Press.

Bakhtin, M. M. (1984a). The hero, and the position of the author with regard to the hero, in Dostoevsky's art. In C. Emerson (Ed. & Trans.), *Problems of Dostoevsky's poetics* (pp. 47–77). Minneapolis: University of Minnesota Press.

Bakhtin, M. M. (1984b). *Speech genres and other late essays* (M. Holquist, Trans.). Austin: University of Texas Press.

Bakhtin, M. M. (1993). *Toward a philosophy of the act* (V. Liapunov, Trans.). Austin: University of Texas Press.

Balint, M. (1957). *The doctor, his patient, and the illness.* Madison, WI: International University Press, Inc.

Barbour, A. (1995). *Caring for patients: A critique of the medical model.* Stanford, CA: Stanford University Press.

Barker, J. R. (1999). *The discipline of teamwork: Participation and concertive control.* Thousand Oaks, CA: Sage.

Barker, K. (2002). Self-help literature and the making of an illness identity: The case of fibromyalgia syndrome (FMS). *Social Problems, 49,* 279–300.

Barnett, C. (2003). *Culture and democracy: Media, space, and representation.* Edinburgh, Scotland: Edinburgh University Press.

Barthes, R. (1972). *Mythologies* (A. Lavers, Trans.). New York: Hill & Wang. (Original work published 1957)

Basting, T. (1998). *The stages of age: Performing age in contemporary American culture.* Ann Arbor: University of Michigan Press.

Bateson, G. (1972). *Steps to an ecology of mind.* Chicago: University of Chicago Press.

Bauer, K. M. (2001). Networking, coping and communicating about a medical crisis: A phenomenonlogical inquiry of transplant recipient communication. *Health Communication, 13,* 141–161.

Bavelas, J., Coates, L., & Johnson, T. (2000). Listeners as co-narrators. *Journal of Personality and Social Psychology, 79,* 941–952.

Beach, W. A. (1993). Transitional regularities for 'casual' "Okay" usages. *Journal of Pragmatics, 19,* 325–352.

Beach, W. A. (1995). Preserving and constraining options: "Okays" and 'official' priorities in medical interviews. In G. H. Morris & R. Cheneil (Eds.), *The talk of the clinic: Explorations in the analysis of medical and therapeutic discourse* (pp. 259–289). Hillsdale, NJ: Lawrence Erlbaum Associates.

Beach, W. A. (1996). *Conversations about illness: Family preoccupations with bulimia.* Mahwah, NJ: Lawrence Erlbaum Associates.

Beach, W. A. (2000). Inviting collaborations in stories about a woman. *Language in Society, 29,* 379–407.

Beach, W. A. (Ed.). (2001). Introduction: Diagnosing 'lay diagnosis.' *Text, 21,* 13–18.

Beach, W. A. (2002). Between dad and son: Initiating, delivering, and assimilating bad cancer news. *Health Communication, 14,* 271–299.

Beach, W. A., & Dixson, C. (2001). Revealing moments: Formulating understandings of adverse experiences in a health appraisal interview. *Social Science & Medicine, 52,* 25–45.

Beach, W. A., Good, J. S., Pigeron, E., & Easter, D. W. (in press). Disclosing and responding to cancer "fears" during oncology interviews. *Social Science & Medicine.*

Beach, W. A., & LeBaron, C. (2002). Body disclosures: Attending to personal problems and reported sexual abuse during a medical encounter. *Journal of Communication, 52,* 617–639.

Beach, W. A., & Metzger, T. R. (1997). Claiming insufficient knowledge. *Human Communication Research, 23,* 562–588.

Beck, C. (2001). *Communicating for better health: A guide through the medical mazes.* Boston: Allyn & Bacon.

Beck, C. (1995). You make the call: The co-creation of media text through interaction in an interpretive community of "Giant" fans. *The Electronic Journal of Communication, 5*(1).

Beck, C. (with Ragan, S., & duPre, A.) (1997). *Partnership for health: Building relationships between women and health caregivers.* Mahwah, NJ: Lawrence Erlbaum Associates.

Beck, V. (2004). Working with daytime and prime-time television shows in the United States to promote health. In A. Singhal, M. Cody, E. M. Rogers, & M. Sabido (Eds.), *Entertainment-education and social change: History, research, and practice* (pp. 207–224). Mahwah, NJ: Lawrence Erlbaum Associates.

Becker, G. (1994). Metaphors in disrupted lives: Infertility and cultural constructions of continuity. *Medical Anthropological Quarterly, 8*, 383–410.

Becker, G., & Nachtigall, R. D. (1994). "Born to be a mother": The cultural construction of risk in infertility treatment in the U.S. *Social Science & Medicine, 39*, 507–518.

Beckman, H. B., & Frankel, R. M. (1984). The effect of doctor behavior on the collection of data. *Annals of Internal Medicine, 101*, 692–696.

Bell, S. (2000). Experiencing illness in/and narrative. In C. Bird, P. Conrad, & A. Fremont (Eds.), *Handbook of medical sociology* (5th ed., pp. 184–200). Upper Saddle River, NJ: Prentice Hall.

Bellah, R. N., Madsen, R., Sullivan, W. M., Swidler, A., & Tipton, S. M. (1985). *Habits of the heart: Individualism and commitment in American life.* Berkeley: University of California Press.

Bellet, P. S., & Maloney, M. J. (1991). The importance of empathy as an interviewing skill in medicine. *Journal of the American Medical Association, 266*, 1831–1832.

Berardo, D. H. (1988). Bereavement and mourning. In H. Wass, F. M. Berardo, & R. A. Neimeyer (Eds.), *Dying: Facing the facts* (pp. 279–300). New York: Hemisphere.

Berger, P., & Luckmann, T. (1966). *The social construction of reality: A treatise in the sociology of knowledge.* Garden City, NY: Doubleday.

Bergmann, J. R. (1992). Veiled morality: Notes on discretion in psychiatry interviews. In P. Drew & J. Heritage (Eds.), *Talk at work: Interaction in institutional settings* (pp. 137–162). Cambridge: Cambridge University Press.

Berne, K. H. (1992). *Running on empty.* Alameda, CA: Hunter House.

Bernhardt, J. M., & Cameron, K. A. (2003). Accessing, understanding and applying health communication messages: The challenge of health literacy. In T. L. Thompson, A. M. Dorsey, K. I. Miller, & R. Parrott (Eds.), *Handbook of health communication* (pp. 583–605). Mahwah, NJ: Lawrence Erlbaum Associates.

Bers, M. U., Gonzalez-Heydrich, J., Raches, D., & DeMaso, D. R. (2001). Zora: A pilot virtual community in the pediatric dialysis unit. In V. L. Patel, R. Rogers, & R. Haux (Eds.), *MEDINFO 2001: Proceedings of the 10th World Congress on Medical Informatics* (pp. 800–804). Washington, DC: IOA Press.

Best, J. (Ed.). (1995). *Images of issues: Typifying contemporary social problems*. New York: Aldine de Gruyter.

Billings, J., & Block, S. (1997). Palliative care in undergraduate medical education: Status report and future directions. *Journal of the American Medical Association, 278*, 733–738.

Biocca, F. A. (1988). Opposing conceptions of the audience: The active and passive hemispheres of mass communication theory. In J. Anderson (Ed.), *Communication yearbook 11* (pp. 51–80). Newbury Park, CA: Sage.

Blandiana, A. (1995). Un drum nu numai spre trecut, ci si spre viitor. [A path not only into the past but also into the future]. In *Analele Sighet: Instaurarea comunismului—intre rezistenta si represiune. Comunicari prezentate la Simpozionul de la Sighetu Marmatiei (9–11 iunie 1995)* (pp. 515–518). Bucharest, Romania: Fundatia Academia Civica.

Block, S. (2002). Medical education in end-of-life care: The status of reform. *Journal of Palliative Medicine, 5*, 243–248.

Blumer, H. (1969). *Symbolic interactionism: Perspective and method*. Englewood Cliffs, NJ: Prentice Hall.

Bochner, A. P. (1994). Perspectives on inquiry II: Theories and stories. In M. Knapp & G. R. Miller (Eds.), *Handbook of interpersonal communication* (2nd ed., pp. 21–41). Thousand Oaks, CA: Sage.

Bochner, A. P. (1998). Storied lives: Recovering the moral importance of social theory. In J. S. Trent (Ed.), *Communication: Views from the helm for the 21st century* (pp. 345–350). Boston: Allyn & Bacon.

Bochner, A. P. (2002). Perspectives on inquiry III: The moral of stories. In M. L. Knapp & J. A. Daly (Eds.), *Handbook of interpersonal communication* (3rd ed., pp. 73–101). Thousand Oaks, CA: Sage.

Bochner, A. P., & Ellis, C. (1995). Telling and living: Narrative co-construction and the practices of interpersonal relationships. In W. Leeds-Hurwitz (Ed.), *Social approaches to communication* (pp. 201–216). New York: Guilford Press.

Bochner, A. P., Ellis, C., & Tillman-Healy, L. M. (1997). Relationships as stories. In S. Duck (Ed.), *Handbook of personal relationships: Theory, research and interventions* (2nd ed., pp. 307–324). New York: John Wiley & Sons.

Boje, D. M. (1991). The storytelling organization: A study of story performance in an office-supply firm. *Administrative Science Quarterly, 36*, 106–126.

Boje, D. M. (2001). *Narrative methods for organizational and communication research*. Thousand Oaks, CA: Sage.

Book, P. L. (1996). How does the family narrative influence the individual's ability to communicate about death? *Omega, 33*, 323–341.

Borkan, J. M., Miller, W. L., & Reis, S. (1992). Medicine as story-telling. *Family Practice, 9*, 127–129.

Bormann, E. G. (1985). Symbolic convergence theory: A communication formulation. *Journal of Communication, 35*(6), 128–210.

Bormann, E. G. (1986). Symbolic convergence theory and communication in group decision-making. In R. Y. Hirokawa & M. S. Poole (Eds.), *Communication and group decision-making (pp. 219–236). Beverly Hills, CA: Sage.

Bosely, S. (2002, April 30). Women's fertility in decline by late 20s: Biological clock starts earlier, says scientists after surprise survey. *The Guardian* (London), p. 3.

Boyd, D. A. (1984). The Janus effect? Imported television entertainment programming in developing countries. *Critical Studies in Mass Communication, 1,* 379–391.

Brabant, S., Forsyth, C. J., & McFarlain, G. (1994). Defining the family after the death of a child. *Death Studies, 18,* 197–206.

Branch, W. T., & Malik, T. K. (1993). Using 'windows of opportunities' in brief interviews to understand patients' concerns. *Journal of the American Medical Association, 269,* 1667–1668.

Bridgman, T., & Barry, D. (2002). Regulation is evil: An application of narrative policy analysis to regulatory debate in New Zealand. *Policy Sciences, 35*(2), 141–162.

Bristow, T. (1997). Finding the healing story. *Storytelling Magazine, 9,* 18–20.

Britt, E. C. (2001). *Conceiving normalcy: Rhetoric, law, and the double binds of infertility.* Tuscaloosa: University of Alabama Press.

Brockelman, P. (1985). *Time and self: Phenomenological explorations.* New York: Crossroad Publishing.

Brockmeier, J., & Carbaugh, D. (2001). Introduction. In J. Brockmeier & D. Carbaugh (Eds.), *Narrative and identity: Studies in autobiography, self and culture* (pp. 1–22). Amsterdam: John Benjamins.

Brockmeier, J., & Harré, R. (1997). Narrative: Problems and promises of an alternative paradigm. *Research on Language and Social Interaction, 30,* 263–283.

Brody, H. (1980). The patient's role in clinical decision-making. *Annals of Internal Medicine, 93,* 718–722.

Brody, H. (1987). *Stories of sickness.* New Haven, CT: Yale University Press.

Brody, H. (1992). *The healer's power.* New Haven, CT: Yale University Press.

Brody, H. (2003). *Stories of sickness* (2nd ed.). New York: Oxford University Press.

Brown, M. H. (1985). That reminds me of a story: Speech action in organizational socialization. *Western Journal of Speech Communication, 49,* 27–42.

Brown, M. H. (1987). Sense making and narrative forms: Reality construction in organizations. In L. Thayer (Ed.), *Organizational communication: Emerging perspectives* (pp. 71–84). Norwood, NJ: Ablex.

Broyard, A. (1992). *Intoxicated by my illness and other writings on life and death.* New York: Fawcett Columbine.

Brummett, B. (1984). Burke's representative anecdote as a method in media criticism. *Critical Studies in Mass Communication, 1,* 161–176.

Bruner, J. (1986). *Actual minds, possible worlds.* Cambridge, MA: Harvard University Press.

Bruner, J. (1987). Life as narrative. *Social Research, 54,* 11–32.

Bruner, J. (1990). *Acts of meaning.* Cambridge, MA: Harvard University Press.

Bruner, J. (1991). The narrative construction of reality. *Critical Inquiry, 18,* 1–21.

Bruner, J. (1996). *The culture of education.* Cambridge, MA: Harvard University Press.

Bruner, J. (1997). A narrative model of self-construction. In J. G. Snodgrass & R. L. Thompson (Eds.), *The self across psychology: Self recognition, self-awareness, and self concept* (pp. 145–161). New York: New York Academy of Sciences.

Bruner, J. (2001). Self-making and world-making. In J. Brockmeier & D. Carbaugh (Eds.), *Narrative and identity: Studies in autobiography, self and culture* (pp. 25–38). Philadelphia: John Benjamins.

Bruner, J. (2002). *Making stories: Law, literature, life.* New York: Farrar, Straus, and Giroux.

Bruner, J., & Kalmar, D. A. (1998). Narrative and metanarrative in the construction of self. In M. Ferrari & R. J. Sternberg (Eds.), *Self-awareness: Its nature and development* (pp. 308–331). New York: Guilford Press.

Burgoon, J. K., Pfau, M., Parrott, R., Birk, T., Coker, R., & Burgoon, M. (1987). Relational communication, satisfaction, compliance-gaining strategies, and compliance in communication between physicians and patients. *Communication Monographs, 54,* 307–324.

Burke, K. (1950). *A rhetoric of motives.* Englewood Cliffs, NJ: Prentice-Hall.

Burke, K. (1957). *Philosophy of literary form: Studies in symbolic action* (3rd ed.). Berkeley: University of California Press.

Burke, K. (1965). *Permanence and change: An anatomy of purpose.* Indianapolis, IN: The Bobbs-Merrill Company.

Burke, K. (1966). *Language as symbolic action.* Berkeley: University of California Press.

Burke, K. (1969). *A grammar of motives.* Berkeley: University of California Press.

Burke, K. (1970). *The rhetoric of religion: Studies in logology.* Berkeley: University of California Press.

Burke, K. (1973). *The philosophy of literary form* (3rd ed.). Berkeley: University of California Press.

Burke, K. (1984). *Attitudes toward history.* Berkeley: University of California Press.

Burke, K. (1985). *Permanence and change* (3rd ed.). Berkeley: University of California Press.

Bury, M. (1982). Chronic illness as biographical disruption. *Sociology and Illness, 4,* 167–182.

Bury, M. (2000). On chronic illness and disability. In C. Bird, P. Conrad, & A. Fremont (Eds.), *Handbook of medical sociology* (5th ed., pp. 173–183). Upper Saddle River, NJ: Prentice Hall.

Butler, J. (1999). Bodies that matter. In J. Price & M. Shildrick (Eds.), *Feminist theory and the body: A reader* (pp. 235–245). New York: Routledge.

Buttny, R. (1993). *Social accountability in communication.* Newbury Park, CA: Sage.

Buzzanell, P. M. (1994). Gaining a voice: Feminist organizational communication theorizing. *Management Communication Quarterly, 7,* 339–383.

Buzzanell, P. M., Liu, M., Bowers, V. A., Remke, R., Meisenbach, R., & Conn, C. (2003, May). *Discourses of pink-collar maternity leaves: Standardization, strategic control, and disability.* Paper presented at the meeting of the International Communication Association, San Diego, CA.

Byrne, P. S., & Long, B. E. L. (1976). *Doctors talking to patients: A study of the verbal behaviors of doctors in the consultation.* London: Her Majesty's Stationery Office.

Calhoun, C. (Ed.). (1999). *Habermas and the public sphere.* Cambridge, MA: MIT Press.

Callanan, M., & Kelley, P. (1992). *Final gifts: Understanding the special awareness, needs, and communications of the dying.* New York: Bantam Books.

Callinicos, A. (1995). *Theories and narratives: Reflections on the philosophy of history.* Winston-Salem, NC: Duke University Press.

Capps, L., & Ochs, E. (1995). Out of place: Narrative insights into agoraphobia. *Discourse Processes, 19,* 407–439.

Carbaugh, D. (Ed.). (1990). *Cultural communication and intercultural contact.* Hillsdale, NJ: Lawrence Erlbaum Associates.

Carbaugh, D. (1996). *Situating selves: The communication of social identities in American scenes.* New York: State University of New York Press.

Carbaugh, D. (2001). 'The people will come to you': Blackfeet narratives as a resource for contemporary living. In J. Brockmeier & D. Carbaugh (Eds.), *Narrative and identity: Studies in autobiography, self and culture* (pp. 103–128). Amsterdam: John Benjamins.

Caresse, J., & Rhode, L. (1995). Western bioethics on a Navajo reservation: Benefit or harm? *Journal of the American Medical Association, 274,* 826–829.

Carr, D. (1986). *Time, narrative, and history.* Bloomington: Indiana University Press.

Carstairs, C. (1998). Innocent addicts, dope fiends and nefarious traffickers: Illegal drug use in 1920s English Canada. *Journal of Canadian Studies, 33*(3), 145–163.

Cashin, J. R., Presley, C. A., & Meilman, P. W. (1998). Alcohol use in the Greek system: Follow the leader? *Journal of Studies on Alcohol, 59,* 63–70.

Cassell, E. J. (1985). *Talking with patients: Volumes I & II.* Cambridge, MA: MIT Press.

Cassell, E. J. (1991). *The nature of suffering.* New York: Oxford University Press.

Centers for Disease Control and Prevention. (1997). *Fertility, family planning, and women's health: New data form the 1995 National Survey of Family Growth.* USA: U.S. Department of Health and Human Services.

Cesario, S. K. (2001). Care of the Native American woman: Strategies for practice, education, and research. *Journal of Obstetric, Gynecologic, and Neonatal Nursing, 30*, 13–19.

Chambers, T. (1999). *The fiction of bioethics: Cases as literary texts.* New York: Routledge.

Chambers, T., & Montgomery, K. (2002). Plot: Framing contingency and choice in bioethics. In R. Charon (Ed.), *Stories matter: The role of narrative in medical ethics* (pp. 77–84). New York: Routledge.

Chapman, R. (2003). Trying to think: A review of Henry Wechsler's 'Dying to Drink.' *The Report on Social Norms, 2,* 4.

Charmaz, K. (1991). *Good days, bad days: The self in chronic illness and time.* New Brunswick, NJ: Rutgers University Press.

Charmaz, K. (1995). The body, identity, and the self: Adapting to impairment. *Sociological Quarterly, 36,* 657–680.

Charon, R. (1993). Medical interpretation: Implications of literary theory of narrative for clinical work. *Journal of Narrative and Life History, 3,* 79–97.

Charon, R. (2001a). Narrative medicine: A model for empathy, reflection, profession, and trust. *The Journal of the American Medical Association, 286,* 1897–1902.

Charon, R. (2001b). Narrative medicine: Form, function, and ethics. *Annals of Internal Medicine, 134,* 83–87.

Charon, R., Greene, M. G., & Adelman, R. D. (1994). Multi-dimensional interaction analysis: A collaborative approach to the study of medical discourse. *Social Science & Medicine, 39,* 955–965.

Charon, R., Trautmann Banks, J., Connelly, J. E., Hunsaker Hawkins, A., Montgomery Hunter, K., Hudson Jones, A., Montellow, M., & Poierer, S. (1995). Literature and medicine: Contributions to clinical practice. *Annals of Internal Medicine, 122,* 599–606.

Cheney, G. (2000). Interpreting interpretive research: Toward perspectivalism without relativism. In S. R. Corman & M. S. Poole (Eds.), *Perspectives on organizational communication: Finding common ground* (pp. 17–45). New York: The Guilford Press.

Chitnis, K., Sengupta, A., & Singhal, A. (2004, May). *Tracking the global footprint of planet Hollywood: Narrative transparency, the sitcom Friends, and Indian viewers.* Paper presented at the meeting of the International Communication Association, New Orleans, LA.

Ciotti, J. R. (1998, March 13). Women are not alone in battle to fight breast cancer. [Letter to the editor]. *USA Today,* p. 14A.

Clair, R. P. (2001). Spirituality and aesthetics: Embracing narrative theory. In A. Rodriguez (Ed.), *Essays on communication and spirituality* (pp. 73–88). New York: University Press of America.

Clark, C. D. (1998). Childhood imagination in the face of chronic illness. In J. de Rivera & T. R. Sarbin (Eds.), *Believed-in imaginings: The narrative construction of reality* (pp. 87–100). Washington, DC: American Psychological Association.

Clark, W. (2000). *Activism in the public sphere: Exploring the discourse of political participation.* Aldershot, Burlington, VT: Ashgate.

Clayman, S., & Heritage, J. (2002). *The news interview.* Cambridge, England: Cambridge University Press.

Cleveland, A. (1999, December 9). Hainer's experience, journal brings gift of love. [Letter to the editor]. *USA Today*, p. 18A.

Cloud, D. (1994). The materiality of discourse as oxymoron: A challenge to critical rhetoric. *Western Journal of Communication, 58,* 141–163.

Cohen, A. (1997a, September 8). Battle of the binge. *Time, 150,* 54–57.

Cohen, A. (1997b, September 30). Death sparks campus-wide review of FSILGs, rush, and alcohol policies. *The (MIT) Tech* [Electronic Version]. Retrieved October 15, 2003, from http://www-tech.mit.edu.

Cohen, J. (1997). Dying patients need better doctoring. *Academic Medicine, 72,* 499–505.

Cohler, B. J. (1991). The life story and the study of resilience and response to adversity. *Journal of Narrative and Life History, 1,* 169–200.

Coles, R. (1989). *The call of stories: Teaching and the moral imagination.* Boston: Houghton Mifflin.

Colyer, H. (1996). Women's experience of living with cancer. *Journal of Advanced Nursing, 23,* 496–501.

Condit, C. M. (1994). Hegemony in a mass-mediated society: Concordance about reproductive technologies. *Critical Studies in Media Communication, 11,* 205–230.

Conquergood, D. (1986) "Is it real?": Watching television with Laotian refugees. *Directions, 2,* 1–5.

Conrad, C., & Millay, B. (2001). Confronting free market romanticism: Health care reform in the least likely place. *Journal of Applied Communication Research, 29,* 153–170.

Constantinescu, C., & Daescu, G. (1995). Deportarile din Mehedinti in Baragan. [The deportations from Mehedinti county to the Baragan fields]. In *Analele Sighet: Instaurarea comunismului—intre rezistenta si represiune. Comunicari prezentate la Simpozionul de la Sighetu Marmatiei (9–11 iunie 1995)* (pp. 442–448). Bucharest, Romania: Fundatia Academia Civica.

Coopman, S. J. (2003). Communicating disability: Metaphors of oppression, metaphors of empowerment. In P. J. Kalbfleisch (Ed.), *Communication Yearbook 27* (pp. 337–394). Mahwah, NJ: Lawrence Erlbaum Associates.

Corr, C. A. (1993). Coping with dying: Lessons that we should and should not learn from the work of Elisabeth Kubler-Ross. *Death Studies, 17,* 69–83.

Costin, A. (1995). O familie victima a represiunii comuniste. [A family that fell victim to communist repression]. In *Analele Sighet: Instaurarea comunismului—intre rezistenta si represiune. Comunicari prezentate la Simpozionul de la Sighetu Marmatiei (9–11 iunie 1995)* (pp. 90–94). Bucharest, Romania: Fundatia Academia Civica.

Cotter, M. (1998). Can stories heal? *Storytelling World, 14,* 4.

Cottle, M. (2002, April 28). Dads are parents, too. *Pittsburgh Post-Gazette*, p. E-1e.

Coulehan, J. (1995). Tenderness and steadiness: Emotions in medical practice. *Literature and Medicine, 14,* 222–236.

Couto, R. A. (1993). Narrative, free space, and political leadership in social movements. *The Journal of Politics, 55*, 57–79.

Creswell, J. W. (1998). *Qualitative inquiry and research design: Choosing among five traditions*. Thousand Oaks, CA: Sage.

Cronon, W. (1992). A place for stories: Nature, history, and narrative. *The Journal of American History, 78*, 1347–1376.

Crossley, M. (2003). 'Let me explain': Narrative emplotment and one patient's experience of oral cancer. *Social Science & Medicine, 56*, 439–448.

Currie, G., & Brown, A. D. (2003). A narratological approach to understanding processes of organizing in a UK hospital. *Human Relations, 56*, 563–586.

Curtis, J., Wenrich, M., Carline, J., Shannon, S., Ambrozy, D., & Ramsey, P. (2001). Understanding physicians' skills at providing end-of-life care: Perspectives of patients, families, and health care workers. *Journal of General Internal Medicine, 16*, 41–49.

Czarniawska, B. (1998). *A narrative approach to organization studies*. Thousand Oaks, CA: Sage.

Czarniawska, B., & Gagliardi, P. (Eds.). (2003). *Narratives we organize by*. Amsterdam: John Benjamins.

Czarniawska-Joerges, B. (1994). Narratives of individual and organizational identities. In S. Deetz (Ed.), *Communication Yearbook 17* (pp. 193–221). Beverly Hills, CA: Sage.

Dakof, G., & Taylor, S. (1990). Victim's perception of social support: What is helpful and from whom? *Journal of Personality and Social Psychology, 58*, 80–89.

Daly, J. (1989). Innocent murmurs: Echocardiography and the diagnosis of cardiac normality. *Sociology of Health and Illness, 11*, 99–116.

Danis, M., Federman, D., Fins, J., Fox, E., Kastenbaum, B., Lanken, P., Long, K., Lowenstein, E., Lynn, J., Rouse, F., & Tulsky, J. (1999). Incorporating palliative care into critical care education: Principles, challenges, and opportunities. *Critical Care Medicine, 27*, 2005–2013.

Davis, K. (1997). Embodying theory: Beyond modernist and postmodernist readings of the body. In K. Davis (Ed.), *Embodied practices: Feminist perspectives on the body* (pp. 1–26). London: Sage.

Deem, M. (2002). Stranger sociability, public hope, and the limits of political transformation. *Quarterly Journal of Speech, 88*, 444–454.

Deetz, S. A. (1995). *Transforming communication, transforming business: Building responsive and responsible workplaces*. Cresskill, NJ: Hampton.

Degner, L., & Gow, C. (1988). Evaluations of death education in nursing: A critical review. *Cancer Nursing, 11*(3), 151–159.

Del Vecchio Good, M., Munakata, T., Kobayashi, Y., Mattingly, C., & Good, B. (1994). Oncology and narrative time. *Social Science & Medicine, 38*, 855–862.

Delaney, B. (1998, November 23). Alcohol still top health risk to college students. *CNN News*.

DeLuca, K., & Peeples, J. (2002). From public sphere to public screen: Democracy, activism, and the 'violence' of Seattle. *Critical Studies in Media Communication, 19*, 125–151.

Demers, D. (1999). *Global media: Menace or Messiah.* Cresskill, NJ: Hampton Press.

Dennis, M. R. (2001). *Effects of judgmental orientation on use of qualitative and quantitative information for health-related inference.* Unpublished doctoral dissertation, Purdue University, West Lafayette, IN.

deTocqueville, A. (1956). Democracy in America (R. D. Heffner, Ed.). New York: New American Library. (Original work published 1835)

Dewey, J. (1922). *Human nature and culture.* New York: Hart, Holt, & Co.

DiClemente, R. J., Hansen, W. B., & Ponton, L. E. (1996). Adolescents at risk: A generation in jeopardy. In R. J. DiClemente, W. B. Hansen, & L. E. Ponton (Eds.), *Handbook of adolescent health risk behavior* (pp. 1–4). New York: Plenum Press.

Donnelly, W. (1988). Righting the medical record: Transforming chronicle into story. *Journal of the American Medical Association, 260*, 823–825.

Doorenbos, A., Briller, S., & Chapleski, E. (2003). Weaving cultural context into an interdisciplinary end-of-life-curriculum. *Educational Gerontology, 29*, 405–416.

Dougherty, K. (2003, October 30). Asbestos alarm sounded: Linked to cancer. Fatal lung disease more prevalent here. *The Gazette (Montreal, Quebec)*, p. A1.

Dozier, D. (2003, June). *Impact evaluation of the Tariq Khamisa Foundation's PeaceWorks Program at Kroc Middle School.* Unpublished report, San Diego, CA.

Drew, P. (1978). Accusations: The use of religious geography in describing events. *Sociology, 12*, 1–22.

Drew, P. (1984). Speakers' reportings in invitation sequences. In J. M. Atkinson & J. Heritage (Eds.), *Structures of social action: Studies in conversation analysis* (pp. 129–151). Cambridge, England: Cambridge University Press.

Drew, P. (1985). Analyzing the use of language in courtroom interaction. In T. van Dijk (Ed.), *Handbook of discourse analysis* (pp. 133–147). London: Academic Press.

Drew, P. (1992). Contested evidence in courtroom cross-examination: The case of a trial for rape. In P. Drew & J. Heritage (Eds.), *Talk at work: Interaction in institutional settings* (pp. 470–52). Cambridge: Cambridge University Press.

Drew, P., & Heritage, J. (Eds.). (1992). *Talk at work: Interaction in institutional settings.* Cambridge, England: Cambridge University Press.

Duck, S. W. (1994). *Meaningful relationships: Talking, sense, and relating.* Thousand Oaks, CA: Sage Publications.

Duck, S., Rutt, D. J., Hurst, M. H., & Strejc, H. (1991). Some evident truths about conversations in everyday relationships: All communications are not created equal. *Human Communication Research, 18*, 228–267.

Duff, K. (2001, November). The stigma of CFS. *Townsend Letter for Doctors and Patients*, pp. 100–104.

Dunphy, J. E. (1976). Annual discourse: On caring for the patient with cancer. *New England Journal of Medicine, 295,* 313–319.

Dunson, D. B., Colombo, B., & Baird, D. D. (2002). Changes with age in the level and duration of fertility in the menstrual cycle. *Human Reproduction, 17,* 1399–1403.

Durand, M. F. (2000, September 18). A major turning point: MIT case causes repercussions throughout nation. *ABC News.*

Durgahee, T. (1997). Reflective practice: Nursing ethics through story telling. *Nursing Ethics, 4,* 135–146.

Eadie, W. F. (1990). Hearing what we ought to hear. *Journal of the International Listening Association, 4,* 1–4.

Eastland, L. S. (1993). The dialectical nature of ethnography: Liminality, reflexivity, and understanding. In S. L. Herndon & G. L. Kreps (Eds.), *Qualitative research: Applications in organizational communication* (pp. 121–138). Cresskill, NJ: Hampton Press.

Eco, U. (1994). *Six walks in a fictional woods.* Cambridge, MA: Harvard University Press.

Eggly, S. (2002). Physician-patient co-construction of illness narratives in the medical interview. *Health Communication, 14,* 330–360.

Ehrenfeld, T. (2002, March 25). Infertility: A guy thing. *Newsweek, 60.*

Ehrenreich, B. (2001, November). Welcome to cancerland: A mammogram leads to a cult of pink kitsch. *Harper's Magazine,* pp. 43–53.

Eisenberg, E., & Goodall, H. L. (2004). *Organizational communication* (4th ed.). Boston: Bedford/St. Martin's.

Ellingson, L. L. (2003). Interdisciplinary health care teamwork in the clinic backstage. *Journal of Applied Communication Research, 31,* 93–117.

Ellingson, L. L., & Buzzanell, P. M. (1999). Listening to women's narratives of breast cancer treatment: A feminist approach to patient satisfaction with physician-patient communication. *Health Communication, 11,* 153–185.

Elliott, C. (2003). *Better than well: American medicine meets the American dream.* New York: Norton.

Ellis, C. (1995). *Final negotiations: A story of love, loss, and chronic illness.* Philadelphia: Temple University Press.

Ellis, C. (1997). Evocative autoethnography: Writing emotionally about our lives. In W. G. Tierney & Y. S. Lincoln (Eds.), *Representation and the text: Re-framing the narrative voice* (pp. 115–139). Albany: State University of New York Press.

Ellis, C., & Bochner, A. (2000). Autoethnography, personal narrative, reflexivity. In N. K. Denzin & Y. S. Lincoln (Eds.), *Handbook of qualitative research* (2nd ed., pp. 733–768). Thousand Oaks, CA: Sage.

Ellis, C., & Bochner, A. (2001). Writing from the periphery. In S. Cole (Ed.), *What's wrong with sociology?* (pp. 341–372). Princeton, NJ: Transactions Press.

Elwyn, G., & Gwyn, R. (1999). Stories we hear and stories we tell: Analyzing talk in clinical practice. *British Medical Journal, 318,* 323–325.

Engel, G. L. (1977). The need for a new medical model: A challenge for biomedicine. *Science, 196,* 129–136.

Equal Employment Opportunity Commission. (2000). *The Family and Medical Leave Act, the Americans with Disabilities Act, and Title VII of the Civil Rights Act of 1964*. Retrieved February 25, 2003, from http://www.eeoc.gov/docs/fmlaada.html.

Equal Employment Opportunity Commission. (2003). *The Pregnancy Discrimination Act of 1978*. Retrieved July 3, 2003, from http://www.eeoc.gov/35th/thelaw/pregnancy_discrimination-1978.html.

Erlandson, D. A., Harris, E. L., Skipper, B. L., & Allen, S. D. (1993). *Doing naturalistic inquiry: A guide to methods*. Newbury Park, CA: Sage.

Evans, J. (1971). *Living with a man who is dying: A personal memoir*. New York: Taplinger.

Ezzy, D. (1998). Theorizing narrative identity: Symbolic interactionism and hermeneutics. *The Sociological Quarterly, 39,* 239–253.

Fackelmann, K. (2003, August 4). "Seabiscuit" author puts a face on chronic fatigue syndrome. *USA Today,* p. D8.

Fadiman, A. (1998). *The spirit catches you and you fall down*. New York: Farrar, Straus and Giroux.

Fairhurst, G., & Putnam, L. (2004). Organizations as discursive constructions. *Communication Theory, 14,* 5–26.

Faludi, S. (1991). *Backlash: The undeclared war against American women*. New York: Anchor Books.

Farrar, S. (2004, May 28). Staff at risk in hazardous labs. *The Times Higher Education Supplement,* p. 11.

Felitti, V. J., Anda, R. F., Nordenberg, D., Williamson, D. F., Spitz, A. M., Edwards, V., Koss, M. P., & Marks, J. S. (1998). Relationship of childhood abuse and household dysfunction to many of the leading causes of death in adults: The adverse childhood experiences (ACE) study. *American Journal of Preventive Medicine, 14,* 245–255.

Fergus, M. A. (2002, June 30). In the struggle to balance career and motherhood, many women are left wondering if they waited too long; Is time running out? *The Houston Chronicle.* p. L–1.

Ferraro, G. (2001, June 21). Blood cancers. *Testimony before the Subcommittee on Labor, Health and Human Services, Education, and Related Agencies*. Washington, DC: U.S. Government Printing Office.

Ferrell, B., Smith, S., Ervin, K., Itano, J., & Melancon, C. (2003). A qualitative analysis of social concerns of women with ovarian cancer. *Psychooncology, 12,* 647–663.

Fields, R. (1999, Fall). Cancer as metaphor [Review of the book *Illness as metaphor*]. *Whole Earth,* p. 19.

Fine, G. A. (1988). Letting off steam? Redefining a restaurant's work environment. In M. D. Moore & R. C. Snyder (Eds.), *Inside organizations: Understanding the human dimension* (pp. 119–127). Newbury Park, CA: Sage.

Fineman, S. (1996). Emotion and organizing. In S. Clegg, C. Hardy, & W. Nord (Eds.), *Handbook of organization studies* (pp. 543–564). London: Sage.

Fink, L. O. (1970). History and fiction as modes of comprehension. *New Literary History, 1,* 551–558.

Fins, J., & Nilson, E. (2000). An approach to educating residents about palliative care and clinical ethics. *Academic Medicine, 75*, 662–665.

Fisher, S. (1991). A discourse of the social: Medical talk/power talk/oppositional talk? *Discourse and Society, 2,* 157–182.

Fisher, W. R. (1984). Narration as a human communication paradigm: The case of public moral argument. *Communication Monographs, 51*, 1–22.

Fisher, W. R. (1985a). The narrative paradigm: An elaboration. *Communication Monographs, 52*, 347–367.

Fisher, W. R. (1985b). The narrative paradigm: In the beginning. *Journal of Communication, 35*(4), 74–89.

Fisher, W. R. (1987). *Human communication as narration: Toward a philosophy of reason, value, and action.* Columbia: University of South Carolina Press.

Fisher, W. R. (1989). Clarifying the narrative paradigm. *Communication Monographs, 56*, 55–58.

Fiske, J. (1986). Television: Polysemy and popularity. *Critical Studies in Mass Communication, 3,* 391–409.

Flannigan, J. (2000). Social perceptions of cancer and their impacts: Implications for nursing practice arising from the literature. *Journal of Advanced Nursing, 32*, 740–749.

Fletcher, P. N. (2002). Experiences in family bereavement. *Family Community Health, 25*, 57–70.

Forester, J. (1980). Listening: The social policy of everyday life. *Social Praxis, 7,* 219–232.

Foucault, M. (1975). *The birth of the clinic: An archeology of medical perception.* New York: Vintage.

Foucault, M. (1995). *Discipline and punish: The birth of the prison* (A. Sheridan, Trans.). New York: Vintage Books. (Original work published 1975)

Frank, A. W. (1991). *At the will of the body: Reflections on illness.* Boston: Houghton Mifflin Co.

Frank, A. W. (1993). The rhetoric of self-change: Illness experience as narrative. *The Sociological Quarterly, 34,* 39–52.

Frank, A. W. (1995). *The wounded storyteller: Body, illness, and ethics.* Chicago: University of Chicago.

Frank, A. W. (1997). Enacting illness stories: When, what, and why. In H. L. Nelson (Ed.), *Stories and their limit: Narrative approaches to bioethics* (pp. 31–49). New York: Routledge.

Frank, A. W. (2000a). Illness and the interactionist vocation. *Symbolic Interaction, 23,* 321–333.

Frank, A. W. (2000b). The standpoint of storyteller. *Qualitative Health Research, 10,* 354–365.

Frank, A. W. (2002a). *At the will of the body: Reflections on illness* [With a new Afterword]. Boston: Houghton Mifflin.

Frank, A. W. (2002b). The extrospection of suffering: Strategies of first-person illness narratives. In W. Patterson (Ed.), *Strategic narrative: New perspectives on the power of personal and cultural stories* (pp. 165–178). New York: Lexington.

Frank, A. W. (2002c). What's wrong with medical consumerism? In S. Henderson & A. Petersen (Eds.), *Consuming health: The commodification of health care* (pp. 13–30). London: Routledge.

Frank, A. W. (2004). *The renewal of generosity: Illness, medicine, and how to live.* Chicago: University of Chicago Press.

Frankel, R. M., & Beckman, H. B. (1988). The pause that refreshes. *Hospital Practice, 71,* 62–67.

Frankenberg, R. (1993). *White women, race matters: The social construction of whiteness.* Minneapolis: University of Minnesota Press.

Freedman, L. (2001, December 13). For Peterson competing is the easy part. *Knight Ridder/Tribune News Service.*

Freeman, M. (1991). Therapeutic use of storytelling for older children who are critically ill. *Children's Health Care, 20,* 208–215.

Freeman, M. (1997). Why narrative? Hermeneutics, historical understanding, and the significance of stories. *Journal of Narrative and Life History, 7,* 169–176.

Freeman, M. (1998). Mythical time, historical time, and the narrative fabric of the self. *Narrative Inquiry, 8,* 27–50.

Freeman, M., & Brockmeier, J. (2001). Narrative integrity: Autobiographical identity and the meaning of the "good life." In J. Brockmeier & D. Carbaugh (Eds.), *Narrative and identity: Studies in autobiography, self and culture* (pp. 75–99). Amsterdam: John Benjamins.

Friend, R. (1993). Drinking practices and expectancies in undergraduate males as a function of ethnicity and fraternity membership. *Dissertation Abstracts International, 54*(2), 1095B.

Fryer, D. (1998). Agency restriction. In N. Nicholson (Ed.), *The Blackwell encyclopedic dictionary of organizational behavior* (p. 12). Malden, MA: Blackwell Business.

Gadamer, H. G. (1975). *Truth and method.* New York: Crossroad.

Gadamer, H. G. (1991). *Truth and method* (2nd ed.). New York: Continuum.

Gaither, C. (2004, June 10). Ex-IBM workers' case sent to jury. *Los Angeles Times,* 3C.

Garfinkel, H. (1967). *Studies in ethnomethodology.* Englewood Cliffs, NJ: Prentice-Hall.

Garro, L. C. (1992). Chronic illness and the construction of narratives. In M. J. Good, P. Brodwin, B. Good, & A. Kleinman (Eds.), *Pain as human experience* (pp. 100–137). Berkeley: University of California Press.

Garro, L. C. (1994). Narrative representations of chronic illness experience: Cultural models of illness, mind and body in stories concerning the temporomandibular joint (TMJ). *Social Science & Medicine, 38,* 775–788.

Garro, L. C., & Mattingly, C. (2000). Narrative as construct and construction. In C. Mattingly & L. C. Garro (Eds.), *Narrative and the cultural construction of illness and healing* (pp. 1–49). Berkeley: University of California Press.

Gatrad, A., Brown, E., Notta, H., & Sheikh, A. (2003). Palliative care needs of minorities. *British Medical Journal, 327,* 176–178.

Gattellari, M., Butow, P. N., Tattersall, M. H., Dunn, S. M., & MacLeod, C. A. (1999). Misunderstanding in cancer patients: Why shoot the messenger? *Annals of Oncology, 10*, 39–46.

Geertz, C. (1973). *Interpretation of cultures*. New York: Basic Books.

Geertz, C. (1988). *Works and lives: The anthropologist as author*. Stanford, CA: Stanford University Press.

Geist, P., & Dreyer, J. (1993). The demise of dialogue: A critique of medical encounter ideology. *Western Journal of Communication, 57*, 233–246.

Geist, P., & Gates, L. (1996). The poetics and politics of re-covering identities in health communication. *Communication Studies, 47*, 218–228.

Geist-Martin, P., Cannon, K., Ngampornchai, A., Zimmerman, A., Goehring, C., & Olejnik, L. (2003, June). *Touchstones and lessons: Assessing PeaceWorks' community of learners*. Unpublished report, San Diego, CA.

Geist-Martin, P., & Dreyer, J. (2001). Accounting for care: Different versions of different stories in the health care context. In S. L. Herndon & G. L. Kreps (Eds.), *Qualitative research: Applications in organizational life* (2nd ed., pp. 121–149). Cresskill, NJ: Hampton Press.

Geist-Martin, P., Horsley, K., & Farrell, A. (2003). Working-well: Communicating individual and collective wellness initiatives. In T. L. Thompson, A. M, Dorsey, K. I. Miller, & R. Parrott (Eds.), *Handbook of health communication* (pp. 423–448). Mahwah, NJ: Lawrence Erlbaum Associates.

Geist-Martin, P., Ray, E. B., & Sharf, B. F. (2003). *Communicating health: Personal, cultural, and political complexities*. Belmont, CA: Wadsworth.

Gergen, K. J. (1991). *The saturated self: Dilemmas of identity in contemporary life*. New York: Basic Books.

Gergen, K. J. (1994). *Realities and relationships: Soundings in social construction*. Cambridge, MA: Harvard University Press.

Gergen, K. J. (1999). *An invitation to social construction*. London: Sage.

Gerstel, N., & McGonagle, K. (1999). Job leaves and the limits of the Family and Medical Leave Act: The effects of gender, race, and family. *Work & Occupations, 26*, 510–534.

Gibbs, R. W., & Franks, H. (2002). Embodied metaphor in women's narratives about their experiences with cancer. *Health Communication, 14*, 139–166.

Giddens, A. (1979). *Central problems in social theory*. Berkeley: University of California Press.

Giddens, A. (1984). *Modernity and self-identity: Self and society in the late modern age*. Stanford, CA: Stanford University Press.

Gill, V. T. (1998). Doing attributions in medical interaction: Patients' explanations for illness and doctors' responses. *Social Psychology Quarterly, 61*, 342–360.

Gill, V. T., Halkowski, T., & Roberts, F. (2001). Accomplishing a request without making one: A single case analysis of a primary care visit. *Text, 21*, 55–82.

Gillotti, C. (2003). Medical disclosure and decision-making: Excavating the complexities of physician-patient information exchange. In T. L.

Thompson, A. M, Dorsey, K. I. Miller, & R. Parrott (Eds.), *Handbook of health communication* (pp. 163–181). Mahwah, NJ: Lawrence Erlbaum Associates.

Glass, R. (2000). Foreword. In B. Whaley (Ed.), *Explaining illness* (pp. xi–xiii). Mahwah, NJ: Lawrence Erlbaum Associates.

Goffman, E. (1955). On face-work. *Psychiatry, 18,* 213–231.

Goffman, E. (1959). *The presentation of self in everyday life.* New York: Doubleday.

Goffman, E. (1961). *Asylums.* Garden City, NY: Doubleday.

Goffman, E. (1963). *Stigma: Notes on the management of spoiled identity.* Englewood, NJ: Prentice-Hall.

Goffman, E. (1967). *Interaction ritual: Essays on face-to-face behavior.* New York: Pantheon Books.

Goffman, E. (1974). *Frame analysis: An essay on the organization of experience.* New York: Harper and Row.

Goldberg, R. L., Haas, M. R., & Eaton, J. S. (1976). Psychiatry and the primary care physician. *Journal of the American Medical Association, 236,* 994–995.

Goldman, E. (1998). Protecting patient welfare in managed care: Six safeguards. *Journal of Health Politics, Policy & Law, 23,* 635–659.

Goldstein, M. S. (1999). The origins of the health movement. In K. Charmaz & D. A. Paterniti (Eds.), *Health, illness, and healing: Society, social context, and self* (pp. 31–41). Los Angeles: Roxbury Publishing.

Good, B. J. (1994). *Medicine, rationality, and experience.* Cambridge, England: University of Cambridge Press.

Goodwin, C. (2003). Embedded context. *Research on Language and Social Interaction, 36,* 323–350.

Goodwin, L. (1989). Explaining alcohol consumption and related experiences among fraternity and sorority members. *Journal of College Student Development, 30,* 448–458.

Goodwin, M. H. (1990). *He said she said: Talk as social organization among black children.* Bloomington: Indiana University Press.

Goranson, N. (1996). *Silent trespass: Learning to live with chronic fatigue syndrome.* Retrieved February 1, 2004, from www.wwcoco.com/cfids/nadine/tresp.html.

Gough, M. L. (1999). Remembrance photographs: Caregiver's gift for families of infants who die. In S. L. Bertman (Ed.), *Grief and the healing arts: Creativity as therapy* (pp. 205–216). Amityville, NY: Baywood.

Granet, R. (2001). *Surviving cancer emotionally.* New York: John Wiley & Sons.

Greenhalgh, T. (1998). Narrative based medicine in an evidence based world. In T. Greenhalgh & B. Hurwitz (Eds.), *Narrative based medicine: Dialogue and discourse in clinical practice* (pp. 247–265). London: British Medical Journal Publishers.

Greenhalgh, T. (1999). Narrative based medicine in an evidence based world. *British Medical Journal, 318,* 323–325.

Greenhalgh, T., & Hurwitz, B. (Eds.). (1998). *Narrative based medicine: Dialogue and discourse in clinical practice.* London: BMJ Publishers.

Greenhalgh, T., & Hurwitz, B. (1999). Narrative based medicine: Why study narrative? *British Medical Journal, 318,* 48–50.

Grosz, E. (1999). Psychoanalysis and the body. In J. Price & M. Shildrick (Eds.), *Feminist theory and the body: A reader* (pp. 267–271). New York: Routledge.

Gugelberger, G. M. (Ed.). (1996). *The real thing: Testimonial discourse and Latin America.* Durham, NC: Duke University Press.

Gullette, M. M. (1997). *Declining to decline: Cultural combat and the politics of midlife.* Charlottesville: University Press of Virginia.

Gunter, B. (1988). Finding the limits of audience activity. In J. Anderson (Ed.), *Communication Yearbook 11* (pp. 108–126). Newbury Park, CA: Sage.

Gusdorf, G. (1980). Conditions and limits of autobiography. In J. Olney (Ed.), *Autobiography: Essays theoretical and critical* (pp. 28–48). Princeton, NJ: Princeton University Press.

Gusfield, J. R. (1996). *Contested meanings: The construction of alcohol problems.* Madison: The University of Wisconsin Press.

Guttman, N. (2003). Ethics in health communication interventions. In T. L. Thompson, A. M. Dorsey, K. I. Miller, & R. Parrott (Eds.), *Handbook of health communication* (pp. 651–680). Mahwah, NJ: Lawrence Erlbaum Associates.

Gwyn, R. (2002a). *Communicating health and illness.* Thousand Oaks, CA: Sage.

Gwyn, R. (2002b). Narrating and the voicing of illness. In *Communicating health and illness* (pp. 139–165). Thousand Oaks, CA: Sage.

Haakana, M. (2001). Laughter as a patient's resource: Dealing with delicate aspects of medical interaction. *Text, 21,* 187–219.

Haas, J., & Shaffir, W. (1982). Taking on the role of doctor: A dramaturgical analysis of professionalization. *Symbolic Interaction, 5,* 187–203.

Habermas, J. (1987). *The theory of communicative action* (Vol. 2). Boston, MA: Beacon Press.

Hafferty, F. W. (1988). Cadaver stories and the emotional socialization of medical students. *Journal of Health and Social Behavior, 29,* 344–356.

Hager, J. (1995). Deportarea svabilor satmareni in U.R.S.S. [The deportation of German ethnics from the North of Romania to the Soviet Union]. In *Analele Sighet: Instaurarea comunismului—intre rezistenta si represiune. Comunicari prezentate la Simpozionul de la Sighetu Marmatiei (9–11 iunie 1995)* (pp. 426–428). Bucharest, Romania: Fundatia Academia Civica.

Hahn, M. L. (1998, March 13). Women are not alone in battle to fight breast cancer. [Letter to the editor]. *USA Today,* p. 14A.

Hahn, P. (1996). *Changing my act.* Retrieved February 1, 2004, from http://www.wwcoco.com/cfids/pamh.html.

Hainer, C. (1998, March 10). My battle against cancer. *USA Today,* p. 1A.

Hainer, C. (1998, March 26). 'Mind makes the magic' against cancer. *USA Today,* p. 6D.

Hainer, C. (1998, April 15). Praying for deliverance amid plagues of chemo. *USA Today,* p. 9D.

Hainer, C. (1999, April 20). Learning to live after cancer comes back. *USA Today*, p. 1D.

Hainer, C. (1998, May 13). Where to go after chemo. *USA Today*, p. 1D.

Hainer, C. (1998, June 22). Another battle won, but war's still on, for cancer survivor. *USA Today*, p. 1D.

Hainer, C. (1999, July 19). A lesson learned outside the lab: To keep living. *USA Today*, p. 7D.

Hainer, C. (1999, September 27). A new attack at summer's end. *USA Today*, p. 7D.

Hainer, C. (1998, October 1). At nine months, a reprieve from illness. *USA Today*, p. 1D.

Hainer, C. (1999, November 4). Painfully aware of life, death. *USA Today*, p. 6D.

Hainer, C. (1999, December 6). 'In effect, I am a virtual prisoner in my body.' *USA Today*, p. 9D.

Hales, D. (2003, October 12). When the body attacks itself. *Parade Magazine*, pp. 4–6.

Halkowski, T. (2000). *Patients' alcohol counts and accounts*. Unpublished manuscript.

Hall, S. (1980). *Culture, media, language: Working papers in cultural studies*. London: University of Birmingham.

Halpern, J. (2001). *From detached concern to empathy: Humanizing medical practice*. New York: Oxford University Press.

Hanh, T. N. (1988). *The heart of understanding: Commentaries on the Prajnaparamita Heart sutra*. Berkeley, CA: Parallax Press.

Hanh, T. N. (1998). *Interbeing: Fourteen guidelines for engaged Buddhism* (3rd ed.). Berkeley, CA: Parallex Press.

Hanne, M. (1994). *The power of the story: Fiction and political change*. Providence, RI: Berghahn Books.

Hansen, C. D., & Kahnweiler, W. M. (1993). Storytelling: An instrument for understanding the dynamics of corporate relationships. *Human Relations, 46*, 1391–1410.

Hansen, D. J. (1995). *Preventing alcohol abuse: Alcohol, culture and control*. Westport, CT: Praeger.

Haraway, D. (1988). Situated knowledges: The science question in feminism and the privilege of partial perspective. *Feminist Studies, 14*, 575–599.

Hardwig, J. (1997). Autobiography, biography, and narrative ethics. In H. Nelson (Ed.), *Stories and their limits: Narrative approaches to bioethics*. (pp. 50–64). New York and London: Routledge.

Hart, B. (2003, March 23). Some single women are convinced of their 'right' to have a child. *The Athens Messenger*, p. A8.

Hart, J. (1992). Cracking the code: Narrative and political mobilization in the Greek Resistance. *Social Science History, 16*, 631–668.

Harter, L. M. (2004). Masculinity, the agrarian frontier myth, and cooperative forms of organizing: Contradictions and tensions in the experience and enactment of democracy. *Journal of Applied Communication Research, 34*, 89–118.

Harter, L. M., & Japp, P. M. (2001). Technology as representative anecdote in popular discourses of health and medicine. *Health Communication, 13*, 409–425.

Harter, L. M., Stephens, R. J., & Japp, P. M. (2000). President Clinton's apology for the Tuskegee syphilis experiment: A narrative of remembrance, redefinition, and reconciliation. *The Howard Journal of Communication, 11*, 19–34.

Harvey, J. H. (2000). *Give sorrow words: Perspectives on loss and trauma.* Philadelphia: Brunner/Mazel.

Harvey, J. H., Orbuch, T. L., Weber, A. L., Merbach, N., & Alt, R. (1992). House of pain and hope: Accounts of loss. *Death Studies, 16*, 99–124.

Hassard, J. (1996). Images of time in work and organization. In S. R. Clegg, C. Hardy, & W. R. Nord (Eds.), *Handbook of organization studies* (pp. 581–598). Thousand Oaks, CA: Sage.

Hawkins, A. H. (1993). *Reconstructing illness: Studies in pathography.* West Lafayette, IN: Purdue University Press.

Hawkins, A. H. (1999). Pathography: Patient narratives of illness. *Western Journal of Medicine, 171*, 127–134.

Hayes, K. (1997, October 19). Bridgewater State College weighs alcohol restrictions. *Boston Globe*, p. 1.

Heath, C. (1986). *Body movement and speech in medical interaction.* Cambridge, England: Cambridge University Press.

Heath, C. (1988). Embarrassment and interactional organization. In P. Drew & T. Wootton (Eds.), *Erving Goffman: Exploring the interaction order* (pp. 136–160). Boston: Northeastern University Press.

Heath, C. (2002). Demonstrable suffering: The gestural (re)embodiment of symptoms. *Journal of Communication, 52*, 597–616.

Hedtke, L. (2002). Reconstructing the language of death and grief. *Illness, Crisis & Loss, 10*, 285–293.

Heidegger, M. (1972). *On time and being* (J. Stambaugh, Trans.). New York: Harper & Row.

Heinz, B., & Lee, R. (1998). Getting down to the meat: The symbolic construction of meat consumption. *Communication Studies, 49*, 86–100.

Heinz, D. (1999). *The last passage.* New York: Oxford University Press.

Helmer, J. (1993). Storytelling in the creation and maintenance of organizational tension and stratification. *Southern Communication Journal, 59*, 34–44.

Heritage, J. (1983). Accounts in action. In G. N. Gilbert & P. Abell (Eds.), *Accounts and action* (pp. 117–131). Aldershot, England: Gower.

Heritage, J. (1984). A change-of-state token and aspects of its sequential placement. In J. M. Atkinson & J. Heritage (Eds.), *Structures of social action: Studies in conversational analysis* (pp. 299–345). Cambridge, England: Cambridge University Press.

Heritage, J. (1998). Oh-prefaced responses to inquiry. *Language in Society, 27*, 291–334.

Heritage, J., & Maynard, D. W. (Eds.). (in press). *Practicing medicine: Structure and process in primary care consultations*. Cambridge, England: Cambridge University Press.

Herper, M. J. (1999). Binge and purge. *Reason*. Retrieved October 5, 2000, from reason.com/9911/fe.mh. binge.html

Herzlich, C., & Pierret, J. (1987). *Illness and self in society*. Baltimore: Johns Hopkins University Press.

Hill, L. (1992). Fairy tales: Visions for problem resolution in eating disorders. *Journal of Counseling and Development, 70*, 584–587.

Hillenbrand, L. (2003, July 7). A sudden illness: How my life changed. *The New Yorker*, pp. 56–65.

Hinchman, L. P., & Hinchman, S. K. (1997). *Memory, identity, community: The idea of narrative in the human sciences*. Albany, NY: State University of New York Press.

Hochschild, A. R. (1983). *The managed heart*. Berkeley: University of California Press.

Hochschild, A. R. (1997). *The time bind: When work becomes home and home becomes work*. New York: Metropolitan Books.

Holcomb, L., Neimeyer, R., & Moore, M. (1993). Personal meanings of death: A content analysis of free response narratives. *Death Studies, 17*, 299–318.

Holleman, W. L. (1991). Death education in American medical schools: Tolstoy's challenge to Kubler-Ross. *The Journal of Medical Humanities, 12*, 11–18.

Holquist, M. (2002). *Dialogism: Bakhtin and his world* (2nd ed.). London: Routledge.

Holstein, J. A., & Gubrium, J. F. (2000). *The self we live by: Narrative identity in a postmodern world*. New York: Oxford University Press.

Holstein, J. A., & Miller, G. (1993). *Constructionist controversies: Issues in social problems theory*. New York: Aldine de Gruyter.

Home Alone in Europe. (1997, March 22). *The Economist, 342*(8009), 74.

hooks, b. (2000). *Feminist theory: From margin to center*. Cambridge, MA: South End Press Classics. (Original work published 1984)

Houpt, J. L., Orleans, C. S., George, L. K., & Brodie, H. K. (1979). *The importance of mental health services to general health care*. Cambridge, MA: Ballinger.

Hunt, L. (2000). Strategic suffering: Illness narratives as social empowerment among Mexican cancer patients. In C. Mattingly & L. Garro (Eds.), *Narrative and the cultural construction of illness and healing* (pp. 88–107). Berkeley, CA: University of California Press.

Hunter, K. M. (1991). *Doctors' stories: The narrative structure of medical knowledge*. Princeton, NJ: Princeton University Press.

Hunter, K. M., Charon, R., & Coulehan, J. (1995). The study of literature in medical education. *Academic Medicine, 70*, 787–793.

Hyde, J. S., Essex, M. J., Clark, R., Klein, M. H., & Byrd, J. E. (1996). Parental leave: Policy and research. *Journal of Social Issues, 52*, 91–109.

Hyde, M. (2004). The ontological workings of dialogue and acknowledgment. In R. A. Anderson, L. A. Baxter, & K. N. Cissna (Eds.), *Dialogue: Theorizing difference in communication studies* (pp. 57–74). Thousand Oaks, CA: Sage.

Ibarra, P. R., & Kitsuse, J. I. (1993). Vernacular constituents of moral discourse: An interactionist proposal for the study of social problems. In G. Miller & J. A. Holstein (Eds.), *Constructivist controversies: Issues in social problems theory* (pp. 131–152). New York: Walter De Gruyter.

Imber-Black, E. (1991). Rituals and the healing process. In F. Walsh & M. McGoldrick (Eds.), *Living beyond loss* (pp. 164–175). New York: Norton.

Irwin, H. (1991). Depiction of loss: Uses of clients' drawings in bereavement counseling. *Death Studies, 15,* 481–497.

Jacobs, R. N. (2002). The narrative integration of personal and collective identity in social movements. In M. C. Green, J. S. Strange, & T. C. Brock (Eds.), *Narrative impact: Social and cognitive functions* (pp. 205–229). Mahwah, NJ: Lawrence Erlbaum Associates.

Jefferson, G. (1978). Sequential aspects of storytelling in conversation. In J. Schenkein (Ed.), *Studies in the organization of conversational interaction* (pp. 219–247). New York: Academic Press.

Jefferson, G. (1988). On the sequential organization of troubles talk in ordinary conversation. *Social Problems, 35,* 418–441.

Jefferson, G. (1990). List construction as a task and resource. In G. Psathas (Ed.), *Interaction competence* (pp. 63–92). Lanham, MD: University Press of America.

Johnstone, B. (2000). The individual voice in language. *Annual Reviews in Anthropology, 29,* 405–424.

Jones, A. H. (1999). Narrative based medicine: Narrative in medical ethics. *British Medical Journal, 318,* 253–256.

Jones, C. M., & Beach, W. A. (in press). "I just wanna know why": Patient's attempts and doctors' responses to premature solicitation of diagnostic information. In M. Maxwell (Ed.), *Diagnosis as a cultural practice.* New York: Mouton de Gruyter.

Jones, J. H. (1993). *Bad blood: The Tuskegee syphilis experiment.* New York: Free Press.

Joseph, A. E., & Kearns, R. A. (1999). Unhealthy acts: Interpreting narratives of community mental health care in Waikato, New Zealand. *Health and Social Care in the Community, 7,* 1–8.

Jurgensen, K. (1999). The Cathy Hainer journals: A story of courage. *USA Today.*

Kagawa-Singer, M., & Wellisch, D. K. (2003). Breast cancer patients' perceptions of their husbands' support in a cross-cultural context. *Psycho-Oncology, 12,* 24–37.

Kalb, C., Springen, K., Scelfo, J., & Pierce, E. (2001, August 13). Should you have your baby now? *Newsweek, 40.*

Karasik, M. (1998). *Why CFIDS advocacy?* Retrieved February 1, 2004, from http://www.wwcoco.com/ cfids/melwhy.html.

Katz, I. (1981). *Stigma: A social psychological analysis*. Hillsdale, NJ: Lawrence Erlbaum Associates.

Kellog, K. (1999). *Binge drinking on college campuses*. Washington, DC: Clearinghouse on Higher Education. (ERIC Document Reproduction Service, No. ED436110).

Khamisa, A. (2002). *Azim's bardo: A father's journey from murder to forgiveness*. La Jolla, CA: ANK Publishing.

Kim, Y. Y. (2001). *Becoming intercultural. An integrative theory of communication and cross-cultural adaptation*. Thousand Oaks, CA: Sage.

Kirkwood, W. G. (1992). Narrative and the rhetoric of possibility. *Communication Monographs, 59*, 30–47.

Kitzinger, C. (2000). Doing feminist conversation analysis. *Feminism & Psychology, 10*, 163–193.

Kleinman, A. (1988). *The illness narratives: Suffering, healing, and the human condition*. New York: Basic Books.

Kleinman, A. (1992). Pain and resistance: The de-ligitimation and re-ligitimation of local worlds. In M. J. Good, P. Brodwin, B. Good, & A. Kleinman (Eds.), *Pain as human experience* (pp. 169–197). Berkeley: University of California Press.

Kleinman, A. (1995). *Writing at the margin: Discourse between anthropology and medicine*. Berkeley: University of California Press.

Kleinman, A. F., Eisenberg, L., & Good, B. (1978). Culture, illness, and care: Clinical lessons from anthropologic and cross-cultural research. *Annals of Internal Medicine, 88*, 251–258.

Klingler, A. (1997). The storyteller in healthcare settings. *Storytelling Magazine, 9*, 21–23.

Koenig Kellas, J. (2003, November). *Family ties: Communicating identity through jointly told family stories*. Paper presented at the meeting of the National Communication Association, Miami, FL.

Kreps, G. L. (1990). Stories as repositories of organizational intelligence: Implications for organizational development. *Communication yearbook, 13*, 191–202.

Krylova, A. (2001). "Healers of wounded souls": The crisis of private life in Soviet literature, 1944–1946. *The Journal of Modern History, 73*, 307–331.

Kubler-Ross, E. (1969). *On death and dying*. New York: Macmillan.

Kubler-Ross, E. (1997). *Living with death and dying*. New York: Simon & Schuster.

Kvale, S. (1996). *InterViews: An introduction to qualitative research interviewing*. Thousand Oaks, CA: Sage.

La Pastina, A. C., Patel, D. S., & Schiavo, M. (2004). Social merchandizing in Brazilian telenovelas. In A. Singhal, M. Cody, E. M. Rogers, & M. Sabido (Eds.), *Entertainment education and social change: History, research, and practice* (pp. 261–280). Mahwah, NJ: Lawrence Erlbaum Associates.

Labov, W. (1972). *Language and the inner city*. Philadelphia: University of Pennsylvania.

Lancaster, T., Hart, R., & Gardner, S. (2002). Literature and medicine: Evaluating a special study module using the nominal group technique. *Medical Education, 36,* 1071–1076.

Lang, F., Floyd, M. R., & Beline, K. L. (2000). Clues to patients' explanations and concerns about their illnesses: A call for active listening. *Journal of the American Medical Association, 9,* 222–227.

Langellier, K. M. (1989). Personal narratives: Perspectives on theory and research. *Text and Performance Quarterly, 9,* 243–276.

Langellier, K. M. (2001). 'You're marked': Breast cancer, tattoo, and the narrative performance of identity. In J. Brockmeier & D. Carbaugh (Eds.), *Narrative and identity: Studies in autobiography, self and culture* (pp. 145–184). Amsterdam: John Benjamins.

Langellier, K. M., & Peterson, E. E. (2004). *Storytelling in daily life: Performing narrative.* Philadelphia: Temple University Press.

Langer, S. (1942). *Philosophy in a new key: A study in the symbolism of reason, rite and art.* Cambridge, MA: Harvard University Press.

Langer, S., Abrams, J., & Syrjala, K. (2003). Caregiver and patient marital satisfaction and affect following hematopoietic stem cell transplantation: A prospective, longitudinal investigation. *Psycho-Oncology, 12,* 239–253.

Larson, D. G. (1993). *The helper's journey: Working with people facing grief, loss, and life-threatening illness.* Champaign, IL: Research Press.

Lazarus, R. S. (1991). *Emotion and adaptation.* New York: Oxford University Press.

Ledlow, G., O'Hair, D., & Moore, S. (in press). Environmental influences on cancer care and communication. In D. O'Hair, G. Kreps, & L. Sparks (Eds.), *Cancer care and communication.* Cresskill, NJ: Hampton Press.

Lee, R. E., & Dwyer, T. (1995). Co-constructed narratives around being "sick": A minimalist model. *Contemporary Family Therapy, 17,* 65–83.

Leondar, B. (1977). Hatching plots: Genesis of storymaking. In D. Perkins & B. Leondar (Eds.), *The arts and cognition* (pp. 172–191). Baltimore: Johns Hopkins University Press.

Levi-Strauss, C. (1966). *The savage mind.* Chicago: University of Chicago Press.

Levinson, W., Gorawara-Baht, R., & Lamb, J. (2000). A study of patient cues and physician responses in primary care and surgical settings. *Journal of the American Medical Association, 284,* 1021–1027.

Levy-Warren, M. H. (1996). *The adolescent journey: Development, identity formation, and psychotherapy.* Northvale, NJ: Jason Aronson.

Lief, H. I., & Fox, R. C. (1963). Training for "detached concern" in medical students. In H. I. Lief, V. F. Lief, & N. R. Lief (Eds.), *The psychological bases of medical practice* (pp. 12–35). New York: Harper & Row.

Linde, C. (1993). *Life stories: The creation of coherence.* New York: Oxford University Press.

Lindemann-Nelson, H. (1996). Sophie doesn't. *Hypatia, 11,* 91–104.

Lindemann-Nelson, H. (1997). How to do things with stories. In H. Lindemann-Nelson (Ed.), *Stories and their limits. Narratvie approaches to bioethics* (pp. vvii–xx). New York: Routledge.

Lindemann-Nelson, H. (2001). *Damaged identities, narrative repair.* Ithaca, NY: Cornell University Press.

Lindlof, T. R. (1988). Media audiences as interpretive communities. In J. Anderson (Ed.), *Communication Yearbook 11* (pp. 81–107). Newbury Park, CA: Sage.

Lindlof, T. R. (1995). *Qualitative communication research methods.* Thousand Oaks, CA: Sage.

Lindlof, T. R., & Meyer, T. P. (1987). Mediated communication as ways of seeing, acting, and constructing culture: The tools and foundations of qualitative research. In T. R. Lindlof (Ed.), *Natural audiences: Qualitative research of media effects* (pp. 1–32). Norwood, NJ: Ablex Publishing Company.

Locke, J. (1975). An essay concerning human understanding (P. H. Nidditch, Ed.), Oxford: Clarendon Press. (Original work published 1690)

Loftus, L. (1998). Student nurses' lived experience of the sudden death of their patients. *Journal of Advanced Nursing, 27,* 641–649.

Lorber, J. (1994). *The paradoxes of gender.* New Haven, CT: Yale University Press.

Lorde, A. (1980). *The cancer journals.* Argyle, NY: Spinsters Ink.

Loseke, D. R. (1999). *Thinking about social problems: An introduction to constructionist perspectives.* New York: Walter de Gruyter, Inc.

Loya, O. (1997). Special audiences. *Storytelling World, 12,* 10.

Lucaites, J. L., & Condit, C. M. (1985). Re-constructing narrative theory: A functional perspective. *Journal of Communication, 35,* 90–108.

Lupton, D. (1994). *Medicine as culture: Illness, disease and the body in Western societies.* London: Sage.

Lyotard, J. F. (1984). *The postmodern condition: A report on knowledge.* Minneapolis: University of Minnesota Press.

MacIntyre, A. (1981). *After virtue: A study in moral theory* (2nd ed.). Notre Dame, IN: University of Notre Dame Press.

Mahan, C. K., & Calica, J. (1997). Perinatal loss: Considerations in social work practice. *Social Work in Health Care, 24,* 141–152.

Mail call. (2001, September 3). *Newsweek, 14.*

Maher, L. (2002, July). More than memory: The ancient art of storytelling can liberate the voices and imaginations of those with Alzheimer's disease. *Contemporary Long Term Care, 25*(7), 16–18.

Mahoney, D. B. (2001). A normative construction of Gulf War syndrome. *Perspectives in Biology and Medicine, 44,* 575–584.

Maines, D. R. (2001). *The faultline of consciousness: A view of interactionism in sociology.* Hawthorne, NY: Aldine de Gruyter.

Malhotra, S., & Rogers, E. M. (2000). Satellite television networks and the new Indian women. *Gazette, 62,* 407–429.

Man being robbed of mind. (2004, May 23). *Omaha World Herald,* p. 9A.

Mandelbaum, J. (1989). Interpersonal activities in conversational storytelling. *Western Journal of Speech Communication, 53,* 114–126.

Mandelbaum, J. (1996). Constructing social identity in the workplace: Interaction in bibliographic database searches. In H. B. Mokros (Ed.), Information and behavior, Vol. 6: Interaction and identity (pp. 145–169), New Brunswick, NJ: Transaction Press.

Mangan, K. (2000, February 13). Behind every symptom, a story. *The Chronicle of Higher Education,* p. A48.

Martin, E. (2001). *The woman in the body: A cultural analysis of reproduction.* Boston: Beacon.

Martin, J. (1990). Deconstructing organizational taboos: The suppression of gender conflict in organizations. *Organization Science, 1,* 339–357.

Martin, K. A. (1996). *Puberty, sexuality, and the self: Boys and girls at adolescence.* New York: Routledge.

Martin, S. (1993). Altered states. *Storytelling Magazine, 5,* 20–23.

Marvel, M. K., Epstein, R. M., Flowers, K., & Beckman, H. B. (1999). Soliciting the patient's agenda: Have we improved? *Journal of the American Medical Association, 281,* 283–287.

Mattingly, C. (1991). The narrative nature of clinical reasoning. *The American Journal of Occupational Therapy, 45,* 998–1005.

Mattingly, C. (1994). The concept of therapeutic 'emplotment.' *Social Science & Medicine, 38,* 811–822.

Mattingly, C. (1998). *Healing dramas and clinical plots: The narrative structure of experience.* Cambridge, England: Cambridge University Press.

Mattingly, C. (2000). Emergent narratives. In C. Mattingly & L. Garro (Eds.), *Narrative and the cultural construction of illness and healing* (pp. 181–211). Berkeley: University of California Press.

Mattingly, C. (2001). *Healing dramas and clinical plots: The narrative structure of experience.* Cambridge, England: Cambridge University Press.

May, E. T. (1995). *Barren in the promised land.* Cambridge, MA: Harvard University Press.

Maynard, D. W. (1991). Interaction and asymmetry in clinical discourse. *American Journal of Sociology, 97,* 448–495.

Maynard, D. W. (1997). The news delivery sequence: Bad news and good news in conversational interaction. *Research on Language and Social Interaction, 30,* 93–130.

Maynard, D. W. (2003). *Bad news, good news, and the structure of everyday life.* Cambridge: Cambridge University Press.

McAdams, D. P. (1990). Unity and purpose in human lives: The emergence of identity as a life story. In A. I. Rabin, R. A. Zucker, R. E. Emmons, & S. Frank (Eds.), *Studying persons and lives* (pp. 148–200). New York: Springer.

McAdams, D. P. (1993). *The stories we live by: Personal myths and the making of the self.* New York: Morrow.

McAdams, D. P., & Bowman, P. (2001). Narrating life's turning points: Redemption and contamination. In D. P. McAdams, R. Josselson, & A. Lieblich (Eds.), *Turns in the road: Narrative studies of lives in transition* (pp. 3–34). Washington, DC: American Psychological Association.

McCafferty, D. (2004, May 28–30). You can't let the disease paralyze you. *USA Weekend,* pp. 14–15.

McChesney, R. W. (1997). *The global media giants: The nine firms that dominate the world.* Retrieved January 7, 2001, from http://www.fair.org/extra/9711/gmg.html.

McCormick, J., & Kalb, C. (1998, June 15). Dying for a drink. *Newsweek,* 30–35.

McCracken, G. (1988). *The long interview.* Newbury Park, CA: Sage.

McFadden, C. (1999, August 1). Why did Scott die? Binge drinking—a life and dream cut short. *ABC News 20/20.*

McGee, M. C. (1975). In search of "the people": A rhetorical alternative. *Quarterly Journal of Speech, 61,* 235–249.

McGee, M. C., & Nelson, J. S. (1985). Narrative reason in public argument. *Journal of Communication, 35,* 139–155.

McGinn, D. (2000, November 27). Scouting a dry campus. *Newsweek.*

McGuire, W. J. (1960). A syllogistic analysis of cognitive relationships. In C. I. Hovland & M. J. Rosenberg (Eds.), *Attitude organization and change* (pp. 65–111). New Haven, CT: Yale University Press.

McMillin, D. C. (2002). Choosing commercial television's identities in India: A reception analysis. *Journal of Media and Cultural Studies, 16,* 123–136.

McQuail, D. (1997). *Audience analysis.* Thousand Oaks, CA: Sage.

McQuellon, R. P., & Cowan, M. A. (2000). Turning toward death together: Conversation in mortal time. *American Journal of Hospice and Palliative Care, 17,* 312–318.

Mead, G. (1934). *Mind, self, and society.* Chicago: University of Chicago Press.

Meade, E. M. (1995). *Tell it by heart: Women and the healing power of a story.* Chicago: Open Court.

Metzger, T. R., & Beach, W. A. (1996). Preserving alternative versions: Interactional techniques for organizing courtroom cross-examination. *Communication Research, 23,* 749–765.

Meyrowitz, J. (1985). *No sense of place: The impact of electronic media on social behavior.* New York: Oxford University Press.

Miller, V. D., Jablin, F. M., Casey, M. K., Lamphear-Van Horn, M., & Ethington, C. (1996). The maternity leave as a role negotiation process. *Journal of Managerial Issues, 8,* 286–309.

Minow, M. (1990). *Making all the difference: Inclusion, exclusion and the American law.* Ithaca, NY: Cornell University Press.

Mishara, A. L. (1995). Narrative and psychotherapy: The phenomenology of healing. *American Journal of Psychotherapy, 49,* 180–195.

Mishler, E. G. (1984). *The discourse of medicine: Dialectics of medical interviews*. Norwood, NJ: Ablex.

Mishler, E. G. (in press). Narrative and identity: The double arrow of time. In A. D. Fina, D. Schiffrin, & M. Bamberg (Eds.), *The discursive construction of identities*. Cambridge, England: Cambridge University Press.

Mitchell, J. (1999, September 30). *USA Today* reporter's brave struggle against cancer. *USA Today*, p. 18A.

Mock, C., & Bruno, A. (1994). The expectant executive and the endangered promotion. *Harvard Business Review, 72*, 16–25.

Mohanty, C. T. (2003). *Feminism without borders: Decolonizing theory, practicing solidarity*. Durham, NC: Duke University Press.

Moller, D. W. (1996). *Confronting death: Values, institutions, and human morality*. New York: Oxford University Press.

Monk, G., Winslade, J., Crocket, K., & Epston, D. (1997). *Narrative therapy in practice: The archaeology of hope*. San Francisco: Jossey-Bass/ Pfeiffer.

Montello, M. (1997). Narrative competence. In H. L. Nelson (Ed.), *Stories and their limits: Narrative approaches to bioethics* (pp. 185–197). New York: Routledge.

Moonsage. (1998). *Supermom has a tear in her cape*. Retrieved February 1, 2004, from http://www.wwcoco.com/cfids/moonsage-supermom.html.

Morgan, J. M. (2002, November). *Walking the wire of detached concern: Emotional involvement and distance in the ER*. Paper presented at the meeting of the National Communication Association, New Orleans, LA.

Morgan, J. M., & Krone, K. J. (2001). Bending the rules of "professional" display: Emotional improvisation in caregiver performances. *Journal of Applied Communication Research, 29*, 317–340.

Morgan, J. M., Reynolds, C. M., Nelson, T. J., Johanningmeier, A. R., Griffin, M., & Andrade, P. (2004). Tales from the fields: Sources of employee identification in agribusiness. *Management Communication Quarterly, 17*, 360–395.

Morra, M. E. (2000). New opportunities for nurses as patient advocates. *Seminars in Oncology Nursing, 16*, 57–64.

Morris, D. B. (1998). *Illness and culture in the postmodern age*. Berkeley: University of California Press.

Moyers, J. D., & O'Neill, J. D. (Producers), & Mannes, E. (Director). (2000). *On our own terms: Moyes on dying*. [Documentary]. (Available from Films of the Humanities. Princeton, NJ 08543)

Mumby, D. K. (1987). The political function of narrative in organizations. *Communication Monographs, 54*, 113–127.

Mumby, D. K. (1988). *Communication and power in organizations: Discourse, ideology, and domination*. Norwood, NJ: Ablex.

Mumby, D. K. (Ed.). (1993). *Narrative and social control: Critical perspectives*. Newbury Park, CA: Sage.

Mumby, D. K. (2000). Power and politics. In F. M. Jablin & L. L. Putnam (Eds.), *The new handbook of organizational communication* (pp. 585–623). Thousand Oaks, CA: Sage.

Mumby, D. K. (2004). Discourse, power, and ideology: Unpacking the critical approach. In D. Grant, C. Hardy, C. Oswick, N. Phillips, & L. Putnam (Eds.), *The handbook of organizational discourse* (pp. 237–258). Thousand Oaks, CA: Sage.

Mumby, D. K., & Stohl, C. (1996). Disciplining organizational communication studies. *Management Communication Quarterly, 10*, 50–72.

Murphy, M. (1999, April 30). Reporter battling breast cancer an inspiration. [Letter to the editor]. *USA Today,* P. 12A.

Nadeau, J. W. (1998). *Families making sense of death.* Thousand Oaks, CA: Sage.

Nadesan, M. H., & Trethewey, A. (2000). Performing the enterprising subject: Gendered strategies for success. *Text & Performance Quarterly, 20*, 223–250.

Narayan, U. (1997). *Dislocating cultures: Identities, traditions, and third-world feminism.* New York: Routledge.

National Cancer Institute. (1993). *Native American monograph 1: Documentation of the cancer research needs of American Indians and Alaska Natives* (National Institute of Health No. 94–3603). Bethesda, MD: U.S. Government Printing Office.

National Center for Juvenile Justice. (1999). *Juvenile offenders and victims: 1999 national report.* Retrieved March 23, 2002, from http://www.ncjrs.org/html/ojjdp/nationalreport99/toc.html.

National Institute of Alcohol Abuse and Alcoholism Task Force on College Drinking. (2002, April). *A call to action: Changing the culture of drinking at U.S. colleges.* NIH Publication Number: 02-5010

Nelson, H. L. (1996). Sophie doesn't. *Hypatia, 11*, 91–104.

Nelson, H. L. (1997). How to do things with stories. In H. Lindemann-Nelson (Ed.), *Stories and their limits: Narrative approaches to bioethics* (pp. vvii–xx). New York: Routledge.

Nelson, H. L. (2001). *Damaged identities, narrative repair.* Ithaca, NY: Cornell University Press.

Newcomb, H. M. (1984). On the dialogic aspects of mass communication. *Critical Studies in Mass Communication, 1*, 34–50.

Norris, M. (2002a, April 10). Deadly drinking. *ABC World News Tonight.*

Norris, M. (2002b, March 21). Out of control? Medical experts worry spring break ads promote binge drinking. *ABC World News Tonight.*

Nussbuam, J. F., Ragan, S., & Whaley, B. (2003). Children, older adults, and women: Impact on provider–patient interaction. In T. Thompson, A. M. Dorsey, K. I. Miller, & R. Parrot (Eds.), *Handbook of health communication* (pp. 183–204). Mahwah, NJ: Lawrence Erlbaum Associates.

Oberg, K. (1960). Cultural shock: Adjustment to new cultural environments. *Practical Anthropology, 7*, 170–179.

Oceanna. (1998). The healing power of story listening. *Storytelling World, 14*, 20.

Ochs, E. (1997). Narrative. In T. van Dijk (Ed.), *Discourse as structure and process* (pp. 185–207). Thousand Oaks, CA: Sage.

Ochs, E., & Capps, L. (1996). Narrating the self. *Annual Reviews in Anthropology, 25*, 19–43.

O'Hair, D. (1986). Patient preferences for physician persuasion strategies. *Theoretical Medicine, 7*, 147–164.

O'Hair, D., Allman, J., & Moore, S. D. (1996). A cognitive-affective model of relational expectations in the provider–patient context. *Journal of Health Psychology, 1*, 307–322.

O'Hair, D., Kreps, G., & Sparks, L. (in press). Conceptual issues in cancer care and communication. In D. O'Hair, G. Kreps, & L. Sparks (Eds.), *Cancer care and communication.* Cresskill, NJ: Hampton Press.

O'Hair, D., Villagran, M., Wittenberg, E., Brown, K., Hall, T., & Doty, T. (2002). *Cancer advocacy and liaison model (C.A.L.M.): Implications for patient decision making.* Paper presented at the meeting of the National Communication Association, New Orleans, LA.

O'Hair, D., Villagran, M., Wittenberg, E., Brown, K., Hall, T., Doty, T., & Ferguson, M. (2003). Cancer survivorship and agency model (CSAM): Implications for patient decision making. *Health Communication, 15*, 193–202.

Olson, S. R. (1999). *Hollywood planet: Global media and the competitive advantage of narrative transparency.* Mahwah, NJ: Lawrence Erlbaum Associates.

Oprah. (2002, May 1). Harpo Productions Inc.

Orbe, M. (1998). From the standpoint(s) of traditionally muted groups: Explicating a co-cultural communication theoretical model. *Communication Theory, 8*, 1–26.

Parens, E. (Ed.). (1998). *Enhancing human traits: Ethical and social implications.* Washington, DC: Georgetown University Press.

Park-Fuller, L. (1995). Narration and narratization of a cancer story: Composing and performing a clean breast of it. *Text and Performance Quarterly, 15*, 60–67.

Parrott, R. L. (2004a). "Collective amnesia": The absence of religious faith and spirituality in health communications research and practice. *Health Communication, 16*, 1–5.

Parrott, R. L. (Ed.). (2004b). Special issue: Religious faith, spirituality, and health communication. *Health Communication, 17*.

Pedro, L. W. (2001). Quality of life for long-term survivors or cancer: Influencing variables. *Cancer Nursing, 24*, 1–11.

Pennebaker, J. W. (2000). Telling stories: The health benefits of narrative. *Literature and Medicine, 19*, 3–18.

Pennebaker, J. W., & Beall, S. K. (1986). Confronting a traumatic event: Toward an understanding of inhibition and disease. *Journal of Abnormal Psychology, 95*, 274–281.

Pennebaker, J. W., & O'Heeron, R. C. (1984). Confiding in others and illness rate among spouses of suicide and accidental-death victims. *Journal of Abnormal Psychology, 93*, 473–476.

Pentland, B. T. (1999). Building process theory with narrative: From description to explanation. *Academy of Management Review, 24*, 711.

Peräkylä, A. (2002). Agency and authority: Extended responses to diagnostic statements in primary care encounters. *Research on Language and Social Interaction, 35,* 219–247.

Perkins, H. W. (Ed.). (2003). *The social norms approach to preventing school and college age substance abuse: A handbook for educators, counselors, and clinicians.* San Francisco: Jossey-Bass.

Perlman, S. E. (1997, December 1). Searching for solutions. *New York Newsday,* p. A23.

Perlow, L. A. (1998). Boundary control: The social ordering of work and family time in a high-tech corporation. *Administrative Science Quarterly, 43,* 328–357.

Peseschkian, N. (2000). *Positive psychotherapy: Theory and practice of a new method.* New Delhi, India: Sterling Publishers.

Peters-Godman, H. (1982). Breast cancer: Varied perceptions of social support in the illness experience. *Social Science & Medicine, 16,* 483–491.

Peterson, K. (1999), December 16). Thank you, Cathy, for all you taught us. USA Today, p. 9D.

Petrie, K. (1995). Disclosure of trauma and immune response to hepatitis B vaccination program. *Journal of Consulting and Clinical Psychology, 63,* 787–792.

Petronio, S. (2002). *Boundaries of privacy: Dialectics of disclosure.* Albany: State University of New York Press.

Phelan, S. (2001). *Sexual strangers: Gays, lesbians, and dilemmas of citizenship.* Philadelphia: Temple University Press.

Polkinghorne, D. E. (1988). *Narrative knowing and the human sciences.* Albany: State University of New York.

Pollman, L. (1997). *A letter to friends in medical school.* Retrieved February 1, 2004, from http://www.wwcoco.com/cfids/robynletter.html

Pollock, D. (1999). *Telling bodies, performing birth: Everyday narratives of childbirth.* New York: Columbia University Press.

Pomerantz, A. (1984a). Pursuing a response. In J. F. Atkinson & J. Heritage (Eds.), *Structures of social action: Studies in conversation analysis* (pp. 152–163). Cambridge, England: Cambridge University Press.

Pomerantz, A. (1986). Extreme case formulations: A way of legitimizing claims. *Human Studies, 9,* 219–229.

Pomerantz, A., & Fehr, B. J. (1997). Conversation analysis: An approach to the study of social action as sense making practices. In T. A. van Dijk (Ed.), *Discourse: A multidisciplinary introduction* (pp. 64–92). Thousand Oaks, CA: Sage.

Pop, V., & Nicoara, A. (1995). Tragedia unei familii, victima a deportarii si domiciliului obligatoriu. [The tragedy of a family who was victim of deportation and forced residence]. In *Analele Sighet: Instaurarea comunismului—intre rezistenta si represiune. Comunicari prezentate la Simpozionul de la Sighetu Marmatiei (9–11 iunie 1995)* (pp. 411–415). Bucharest, Romania: Fundatia Academia Civica.

Putnam, L. L., Phillips, N., & Chapman, P. (1996). Metaphors of communication and organization. In S. R. Clegg, C. Hardy, & W. Nord (Eds.), *Handbook of organization studies* (pp. 375–408). London: Sage.

Query, J. L., Kreps, G. L., Arneson, P. A., & Caso, N. S. (2001). Towards helping organizations manage interaction: The theoretical and pragmatic merits of the critical incident technique. In S. L. Herndon & G. L. Kreps (Eds.), *Qualitative research: Applications in organizational life* (2nd ed., pp. 91–119). Cresskill, NJ: Hampton Press.

Rabinow, P., & Sullivan, W. M. (Eds.). (1987). *Interpretive social science: A second look*. Berkeley: University of California Press.

Radford, S. (2003, February). The challenge of myalgic encephalomyelitis. *Student British Medical Journal, 3–6*.

Radner, G. (1989). *It's always something*. New York: Simon & Schuster.

Ragan, S. L., Wittenberg, E., & Hall, H. T. (2003). The communication of palliative care for the elderly cancer patient. *Health Communication, 15*, 219–226.

Râpeanu, M. (1995). Deportari si confiscari in baza decretului 83/1949. [Deportatations and property confiscations in basis of Decree 83/1949]. In *Analele Sighet: Instaurarea comunismului—intre rezistenta si represiune. Comunicari prezentate la Simpozionul de la Sighetu Marmatiei (9–11 iunie 1995)* (pp. 406–410). Bucharest, Romania: Fundatia Academia Civica.

Ratiu, V. (1995). Revolta de la Ocnita (Bistrita Nasaud), 1961. Marturie de Aurel Catineanu. [The Ocnita (Bistrita Nasaud) rebellion, 1961. A testimony given by Aurel Catineanu]. In *Analele Sighet: Instaurarea comunismului—intre rezistenta si represiune. Comunicari prezentate la Simpozionul de la Sighetu Marmatiei (9–11 iunie 1995)* (pp. 142–149). Bucharest, Romania: Fundatia Academia Civica.

Rawlins, W. K. (2003). Hearing voices/learning questions. In R. P. Clair (Ed.), *Expressions of ethnography: Novel approaches to qualitative methods* (pp. 119–125). Albany: State University of New York Press.

Reeve, D. (1999). *Care packages: Letters to Christopher Reeve from strangers and other friends*. New York: Random House.

Reifler, D. (1996). "I actually don't mind the bone saw": Narratives of gross anatomy. *Literature and Medicine, 15*, 183–199.

Remen, R. N. (1996). *Kitchen table wisdom: Stories that heal*. New York: Riverhead Books.

Reynolds, T. A. (2003). Editor's note: Once upon a time. *Medical Student Journal of the American Medical Association, 289*, 612.

Richman, J., & Jason, L. (2001). Gender biases underlying the social construction of illness states: The case of chronic fatigue syndrome. *Current Sociology, 49*(3), 15–29.

Richman, J., Jason, L., Taylor, R., & Jahn, S. (2000). Feminist perspectives on the social construction of chronic fatigue syndrome. *Health Care for Women International, 21*(3), 173–186.

Ricoeur, P. (1981a). The narrative function (J. B. Thompson, Trans.). In J. B. Thompson (Ed.), *Hermeneutics and the human sciences* (pp. 274–305). Cambridge, England: Cambridge University Press.

Ricoeur, P. (1981b). Narrative time. In W. J. T. Mitchell (Ed.), *On narrative* (pp. 165–186). Chicago: University of Chicago Press.

Ricoeur, P. (1984a). Narrative time. *Critical Inquiry, 7,* 169–190.

Ricoeur, P. (1984b). *Time and narrative* (K. McLaughlin & D. Pellaver, Trans.). Chicago: University of Chicago Press.

Ricoeur, P. (1988). *Time and narrative* (Vol. 3). Chicago: University of Chicago Press.

Riessman, C. (2000). 'Even if we don't have children [we] can live': Stigma and infertility in South India. In C. Mattingly & L. Garro (Eds.), *Narrative and the cultural construction of illness and healing* (pp. 128–152). Berkeley: University of California Press.

Rifkin, J. (1995). *The end of work: The decline of the global labor force and the dawn of the post-market era.* New York: Jeremy P. Tarcher/Putnam.

Rislove, A. (1998, March 30). Sharing anti-cancer battle. [Letter to the editor]. *USA Today,* p. 14A.

Robbins, P. R. (1998). *Adolescent suicide.* Jefferson, NC: McFarland & Company.

Robinson, C., & Thorne, S. (1988). Health care relationships: The chronic illness perspective. *Research in Nursing & Health, 11,* 293–300.

Robinson, J. A., & Hawpe, L. (1986). Narrative thinking as a heuristic process. In T. R. Sarbin (Ed.), *Narrative psychology* (pp. 111–125). New York: Praeger.

Robinson, J. D. (2001). Asymmetry in action: Sequential resources in the negotiation of a prescription request. *Text, 21,* 19–54.

Robinson-Pant, A. (2001). Women's literacy and health: Can an ethnographic researcher find the links? In B. Street (Ed.), *Literacy and development: Ethnographic perspectives* (pp. 152–171). New York: Routledge.

Rogers, E. M., Singhal, A., Vasanti, P. N., Thombre, A., Chitnis, K., Sengupta, A., Kumar, S., & Chatterjee, A. (2003). *Audience interpretations of health-related content in two American television programs broadcast in India.* Report presented to the Centers for Disease Control and Prevention, Atlanta, GA.

Rogers, L. (2002). Both sides of the stethoscope where science meets life. *Humanities, 23,* 32–35.

Rosen, M. (2003, May). Living with pain: She visited top docs and quacks, took drugs, and tried surgery. One woman's quest for a cure. *Good Housekeeping,* 100–102.

Roter, D. L., & Hall, J. A. (1992). *Doctors talking with patients/Patients talking with doctors.* Westport, CT: Auburn House.

Rothman, B. K. (1991). *In labor: Women and power in the birthplace.* New York: Norton.

Rothman, E. L. (1999). *White coat: Becoming a doctor at Harvard Medical School.* New York: William Morrow & Company.

Rothman, S. M., & Rothman, D. (2004). *The pursuit of perfection: The promise and perils of medical enhancement.* New York: Pantheon Books.

Rueveni, U. (1995). Stories and metaphors as interventions with headache sufferers. *Contemporary Family Therapy, 17,* 39–46.

Russo, K. (1998, September 17). MIT fraternity indicted. Associated Press. Retrieved January 10, 2001, from http://www.ABCNEWS.com.

Sacks, H. (1992). *Lectures on conversation.* Oxford: Blackwell.

Sage, A. (2004, May 25). Woman lives without part of skull due to insurance snag. *Lincoln Journal Star,* p. 2D.

Sarbin, T. R. (1986). *Narrative psychology: The storied nature of human conduct.* New York: Praeger.

Sarbin, T. R. (1998). Believed-in imaginings: A narrative approach. In J. de Rivera & T. R. Sarbin (Eds.), *Believed-in imaginings: The narrative construction of reality* (pp. 15–30). Washington, DC: American Psychological Association.

Schafhütl, J. (1995). Krasnodon—Lagarul 1210. [Krasnodon—Concentration Camp 1210]. In *Analele Sighet: Instaurarea comunismului— intre rezistenta si represiune. Comunicari prezentate la Simpozionul de la Sighetu Marmatiei (9–11 iunie 1995)* (pp. 421–425). Bucharest, Romania: Fundatia Academia Civica.

Schank, R. C. (1990). *Tell me a story: A new look at real and artificial memory.* New York: Scribner.

Schank, R. C., & Abelson, R. P. (1997). *Scripts, plans, goals, and understanding: Inquiry into human knowledge structures.* Hillsdale, NJ: Lawrence Erlbaum Associates.

Schegloff, E. A. (1980). Preliminaries to preliminaries: "Can I ask you a question?" *Sociological Inquiry, 50,* 104–152.

Schlesinger, L. (1996). Chronic pain, intimacy, and sexuality: a qualitative study of women who live with pain. *The Journal of Sex Research, 33,* 249–256.

Schon, D. A. (1979). Generative metaphor: A perspective on problem-setting in social policy. In A. Ortony (Ed.), *Metaphor and thought* (pp. 284–324). Cambridge, England: Cambridge University Press.

Schutz, A. (1962). *Collected papers I: The problem of social reality.* The Hague, Netherlands: Martinus Nijhoff.

Schwartz, F. N. (1989). Management women and the new facts of life. *Harvard Business Review, 67*(1), 65–76.

Schwartz, F. N. (1992). Women as a business imperative. *Harvard Business Review, 70*(2), 105–113.

Schwartzman, H. B. (1993). *Ethnography in organizations.* Newbury Park, CA: Sage.

Schwartzman, R. (2001). Recovering the lost canon: Public memory and the Holocaust. *Rhetoric and Public Affairs, 4,* 543–558.

Schwartzstein, R. M. (1998, June 29). A preventable tragedy: Alcohol and the death of Scott Krueger. *The Wellesley Townsman.* Retrieved November 18, 2003, from http://phoenix.edc.org/hec/thisweek/tw980629.html

Scott, M., & Lyman, S. (1968). Accounts. *American Sociolgocial Review, 33,* 46–62.

Scott, W. G., & Hart, D. K. (1989). *Organizational values in America.* New Brunswick, NJ: Transaction.

Searle, J. R. (1995). *The construction of social reality*. New York: Free Press.

Sedney, M., Baker, J. E., & Gross, E. (1994). "The story" of a death: Therapeutic considerations with bereaved families. *Journal of Marital and Family Therapy, 20*, 287–296.

Shaderowfsky, E. (1996). *My doctor*. Retrieved February 1, 2004, from http://www.wwcoco.com/cfids/esdoctor.html.

Shapiro, C. H. (1993). *When part of the self is lost: Helping clients heal after sexual and reproductive losses*. San Francisco: Jossey-Bass.

Sharf, B. F. (1990). Physician–patient communication as interpersonal rhetoric: A narrative approach. *Health Communication, 2*, 217–231.

Sharf, B. F. (1997). Communicating breast cancer on-line: Support and empowerment on the Internet. *Women and Health, 26*, 63–82.

Sharf, B. F. (2001). Out of the closet and into the legislature: The impact of communicating breast cancer narratives on health policy. *Health Affairs, 20*, 213–218.

Sharf, B. F., & Freimuth, V. S. (1993). The construction of illness on entertainment television: Coping with cancer on *thirtysomething*. *Health Communication, 5*, 141–160.

Sharf, B. F., Freimuth, V. S., Greenspon, P., & Plotnick, C. (1996). Confronting cancer on *thirtysomething*: Audience response to health content on entertainment television. *Journal of Health Communication: International Perspectives, 1*, 157–172.

Sharf, B. F., Haidet, P., & Kroll, T. L. (2005). "I want you to put me in the grave with all my limbs": The meaning of active health participation. In E. B. Ray (Ed.), *Health communication in practice* (2nd ed., pp. 39–51). Mahwah, NJ: Lawrence Erlbaum Associates.

Sharf, B. F., & Vanderford, M. L. (2003). Illness narratives and the social construction of health. In T. L. Thompson, A. M. Dorsey, K. I. Miller, & R. Parrott (Eds.), *Handbook of health communication* (pp. 9–34). Mahwah, NJ: Lawrence Erlbaum Associates.

Sharlet, R. (1983). Varieties of dissent and regularities of repression in the European communist states: An overview. In J. L. Curry (Ed.), *Dissent in Eastern Europe* (pp. 1–19). New York: Praeger.

Shave, L. (2003, February). Former nursing student Laura Shave has ME: She shares her views. *Student British Medical Journal, 4*.

Shaw, G. D. (2000). Planning and communicating using stories. In M. J. Hatch, M. H. Larsen, & M. Schultz (Eds.), *The expressive organization: Linking identity, reputation, and the corporate brand* (pp. 182–196). Oxford, England: Oxford University Press.

Shaw, R. (1999, December 17). Farewell, Cathy Hainer. [Letter to the editor]. *USA Today*, p. 30A.

Shellenbarger, S. (2003, January 23). A downside of taking family leave; getting fired while you're gone. *Wall Street Journal*, p. D1.

Sheppard, D. L. (1989). Organizations, power and sexuality: The image and self-image of women managers. In J. Hearn, D. L. Sheppard, P. Tancred-Sheriff, & G. Burrell (Eds.), *The sexuality of organization* (pp. 139–157). London: Sage.

Shorter, E. (1992). *From paralysis to fatigue: A history of psychosomatic illness in the modern era.* New York: Free Press.

Shorts, B. (1999, April 23). Brave reporter, battler. [Letter to the editor]. *USA Today,* p. 14A.

Showalter, E. (1997). *Hystories: Hysterical epidemics and the modern media.* New York: Columbia University Press.

Sicher, E. (2001). The future of the past: Countermemory and postmemory in contemporary American post-Holocaust narratives. *History and Memory, 12,* 56–91.

Silko, L. (1977). *Ceremony.* New York: Viking Press.

Silverman, P. R. (1988). In search of new selves: Accommodating to widowhood. In L. A. Bond & B. M. Wagner (Eds.), *Families in transition: Primary prevention programs that work* (pp. 200–220). Newbury Park, CA: Sage.

Singhal, A., & Rogers, E. M. (1999). *Entertainment-education: A communication strategy for social change.* Mahwah, NJ: Lawrence Erlbaum Associates.

Singhal, A., & Rogers, E. M. (2001). *India's communication revolution: From bullock carts to cyber marts.* Thousand Oaks, CA: Sage.

Singhal, A., & Rogers, E. M. (2002). A theoretical agenda for entertainment education. *Communication Theory, 14,* 117–135.

Singhal, A., Cody, M., Rogers, E. M., & Sabido, M. (Eds.). (2004). *Entertainment-education and social change: History, research, and practice.* Mahwah, NJ: Lawrence Erlbaum Associates.

Sitton, J. (2003). *Habermas and contemporary society.* New York: Palgrave Macmillan.

Skelton, J., & Hammond, P. (1998). Medical narratives and the teaching of communication in context. *Medical Teacher, 20,* 548–551.

Skelton, J., Macleod, J., & Thomas, C. (2000). Teaching literature and medicine to medical students, part II: Why literature and medicine. *The Lancet, 356,* 2001–2003.

Slater, M. D. (2002). Entertainment education and the persuasive impact of narratives. In M. C. Green, J. J. Strange, & T. C. Brock (Eds.), *Narrative impact: Social and cognitive foundations* (pp. 157–182). Mahwah, NJ: Lawrence Erlbaum Associates.

Smith, A. C., & Kleinman, S. (1989). Managing emotions in medical school: Students' contacts with the living and the dead. *Social Psychology Quarterly, 52,* 56–69.

Smith, D. (2003, October 11). Diagnosis goes low tech. *The New York Times,* p. 9B1.

Smith, R. (2002, April 13). In search of 'non-disease.' *British Medical Journal, 324,* 834.

Smith, S. (1994). Identity's body. In K. Ashley, L. Gilmore, & G. Peters (Eds.), *Autobiography & postmodernism* (pp. 266–292). Amherst: The University of Massachusetts Press.

Snyder, K. (Director). (2001). *I remember me* [Documentary film]. United States: Zeitgeist Video.

Solomon, M. (1985). The rhetoric of dehumanization: An analysis of medical reports of the Tuskegee syphilis project. *Western Journal of Speech Communication, 49*, 233–247.

Somers, M. R. (1994). The narrative constitution of identity: A relational and network approach. *Theory and Society, 23*, 605–649.

Sontag, S. (1977). *Illness as metaphor.* New York: Vintage.

Sontag, S. (1988). *AIDS and its metaphors.* New York: Farrar Straus Giroux.

Spiegel, J. (1999). Healing words: Emotional expression and disease outcome. *Journal of the American Medical Association, 277*, 1328–1329.

Spiro, H. (1996). The wounded storyteller: Body, illness, and ethics [Review of the book *The wounded storyteller: Body, illness, and ethics*]. *The Journal of the American Medical Association, 275*, 1933–1935.

Star Wars. (1997, March 22). *The Economist, 342*(8009), 15–16.

Sterk, H. M. (1996). Contemporary birthing practices: Technology over humanity? In R. L. Parrott & C. M. Condit (Eds.), *Evaluating women's health messages: A resource book* (pp. 124–134). Thousand Oaks, CA: Sage.

Sterk, H. M., Hay, C. H., Kehoe, A. B., Ratcliffe, K., & VandeVusse, L. G. (2002). *Who's having this baby? Perspectives on birthing.* Lansing: Michigan State University Press.

Stewart, C. J., & Cash, W. B. (2000). *Interviewing: Principles and practices* (9th ed.). Boston: McGraw Hill.

Stewart, J. (1991). A postmodern look at traditional communication postulates. *Western Journal of Speech Communication, 55*, 354–379.

Stivers, T. (2002). "Symptoms only" versus "candidate diagnosis": Presenting the problem in pediatric encounters. *Health Communication, 14*, 299–339.

Stivers, T., & Heritage, J. (2001). Breaking the sequential mould: Answering "more than the question" during comprehensive history taking. *Text, 21*, 151–186.

Stolting, J. (1998, August). Reaching her goal. *The Exceptional Parent, 28*(8), 69–71.

Stone, R. (1996). *The healing art of storytelling: A sacred journey of personal discovery.* New York: Hyperion.

Stotland, E., Mathews, K. E., Sherman, S. E., Hansson, R. O., & Richardson, B. Z. (1978). *Empathy, fantasy, and helping.* Beverly Hills, CA: Sage.

Straus, R., & Bacon, S. D. (1953). *Drinking in college.* New Haven: Yale University Press.

Strauss, A., & Corbin, J. (1990). *Basics of qualitative research: Grounded theory procedures and techniques.* Newbury Park, CA: Sage.

Street, B. (Ed.). (2001). *Literacy and development: Ethnographic perspectives.* New York: Routledge.

Strickland, C. J., Chrisman, N. J., Yallup, M., Powell, K., & Squeoch, M. D. (1996). Walking the journey of womanhood: Yakama Indian women and papanicolaou (pap) test screening. *Public Health Nursing, 13*, 141–150.

Struck, J. J. (2000, September). True grit. *Today's Christian Woman*, *22*(5), 36–46.

Sturgeon, M. (1999, December 17). Farewell, Cathy Hianer. [Letter to the editor]. *USA Today*, p. 30A.

Suchman, A., Markakis, K., Beckman, H. B., & Frankel, R. (1997). A model of empathic communication in the medical interview. *Journal of the American Medical Association*, *277*, 678–682.

Sullivan, A., Lakoma, M., & Block, S. (2003). The status of medical education in the end-of-life care. *Journal of General Internal Medicine*, *18*, 685–696.

Sunwolf. (1999). The pedagogical and persuasive effects of Native American lesson stories, African dilemma tales, and Sufi wisdom tales. *Howard Journal of Communications*, *10*, 47–71.

Sunwolf. (2003). Grief tales: The therapeutic power of folktales to heal bereavement and loss. *Diving in the Moon: Honoring Story, Facilitating Healing*, *4*, 36–42.

Sunwolf. (in press). Empathic attunement facilitation: Stimulating immediate task engagement in zero-history training groups of helping professionals. In L. R. Frey (Ed.), *Innovations in group facilitation: Applications in natural settings* (2nd ed.). Cresskill, NJ: Hampton Press.

Sunwolf, & Frey, L. R. (2001). Storytelling: The power of narrative communication and interpretation. In W. P. Robinson & H. Giles (Eds.), *The new handbook of language and social psychology* (pp. 119–135). London: Wiley.

Tangherlini, T. R. (2000). Heroes and lies: Storytelling tactics among paramedics. *Folklore*, *111*, 43–66.

Taniguchi, H. (1999). The timing of childbearing and women's wages. *Journal of Marriage and the Family*, *61*, 1008–1019.

Tannen, D. (1988). Hearing voices in conversation, fiction, and mixed genres. In D. Tannen (Ed.), *Linguistics in context: Connecting observation and understanding* (pp. 89–113). Norwood, NJ: Ablex.

Tariq Khamisa Foundation. [On-line]. Available at: http://www.tkf.org

Tavris, C. (1992). *The mismeasure of woman: Why women are not the better sex, the inferior sex, or the opposite sex*. New York: Simon & Schuster.

Taylor, C. (1991). *The ethics of authenticity*. Cambridge, MA: Harvard University Press.

Taylor, E. J. (1997). The story behind the story: The use of storytelling in spiritual caregiving. *Seminars in Oncology Nursing*, *13*, 252–254.

Taylor, S. E., Aspinwall, L. G., Giuliano, T. A., Dakof, G. A., & Reardon, K. K. (1993). Storytelling and coping with stressful events. *Journal of Applied Social Psychology*, *23*, 703–733.

Terasaki, A. K. (1976). Pre-announcement sequences in conversation. *Social Science Working Paper*, No. 99. School of Social Science, University of California, Irvine.

Tester, K. (1994). *Media, culture, and morality*. New York and London: Routledge.

Thomas, A. G. (1997). *The women we become: Myths, folktales, and stories about growing older*. Rocklin, CA: Prima Publishing.

Thompson, T. L. (1990). Patient health care: Issues in interpersonal communication. In E. B. Ray & L. Donohew (Eds.), *Communication and health: Systems and applications* (pp. 27–50). Hillsdale, NJ: Lawrence Erlbaum Associates.

Thompson, T. L. (2000). The nature and language of illness explanations. In B. Whaley (Ed.), *Explaining illness: Research, theory, and strategies* (pp. 3–40). Mahwah, NJ: Lawrence Erlbaum Associates.

Thompson, T. L. (2003). Introduction. In T. Thompson, A. M. Dorsey, K. I. Miller, & R. Parrot (Eds.), *Handbook of health communication* (pp. 1–5). Mahwah, NJ: Lawrence Erlbaum Associates.

Thomson, R. G. (1997). *Extraordinary bodies: Figuring physical disability in American culture and literature.* New York: Columbia University Press.

Tiggemann, M., & Pennington, B. (1990). The development of gender differences in body-size dissatisfaction. *Australian Psychologist, 25,* 306–313.

Totka, J. P. (1996). Exploring the boundaries of pediatric practice: Nurse stories related to relationships. *Pediatric Nursing, 22,* 191–197.

Trautman, J. (1982). The wonders of literature in medical education. *Mobius, 2,* 23–31.

Trethewey, A. (2000). Revisioning control: A feminist critique of disciplined bodies. In P. M. Buzzanell (Ed.), *Rethinking organizational and managerial communication from feminist perspectives* (pp. 107–127). Thousand Oaks, CA: Sage.

Trethewey, A. (2001). Reproducing and resisting the master narrative of decline: Midlife professional women's experiences of aging. *Management Communication Quarterly, 15,* 183–226.

Treweek, G. L. (1996). Emotion work, order, and emotional power in care assistant work. In V. James & J. Gabe (Eds.), *Health and the sociology of emotions* (pp. 114–132). Oxford, England: Blackwell.

Turner, V. (1980). Social dramas and stories about them. *Critical Inquiry, 7,* 141–168.

TV Globo. (2003). *The Camilla effect.* San Paola, Brazil: TV Globo.

U.S. Department of Labor. (2003). *Compliance assistance—Family and Medical Leave Act* (FMLA). Retrieved July 3, 2003, from http://www.dol.gov/esa/whd/fmla/.

Usdin, S., Singhal, A., Shongwe, T., Goldstein, S., & Shabalala, A. (2004). No short cuts in entertainment education. Designing Soul City step-by-step. In A. Singhal, M. Cody, E. M. Rogers, & M. Sabido (Eds.), *Entertainment education and social change: History, research, and practice* (pp. 153–176). Mahwah, NJ: Lawrence Erlbaum Associates.

Vanderford, M. L., Jenks, E. B., & Sharf, B. F. (1997). Exploring patients' experiences as a primary source of meaning. *Health Communication, 9,* 13–26.

Vanderford, M. L., & Smith, D. H. (1996). *The silicone breast implant story: Communication and uncertainty.* Mahwah, NJ: Lawrence Erlbaum Associates.

Van Maanen, J. (1992). Drinking our troubles away: Managing conflict in a British police agency. In D. M. Kolb & J. M. Bartunek (Eds.), *Hidden conflict in organizations* (pp. 32–62). Newbury Park, CA: Sage.

Van Slant, P. (2002, April 17). Spring break exposed. *CBS News 48 Hours.*

Vest, C. M. (1997). Statement on death of MIT student Scott Krueger. Retrieved December 10, 2003, from http://web.mit.edu/newsoffice/nr/1997/krueger930.html.

Villagran, M., Jones, L., & O'Hair, D. (in press). Agency-identity theory in cancer care. In D. O'Hair, G. Kreps, & L. Sparks (Eds.), *Cancer care and communication.* Cresskill, NJ: Hampton Press.

Von Gunten, C. F., Ferris, F. D., & Emanuel, L. L. (2000). Ensuring competency in end-of-life care: Communication and relational skills. *Journal of the American Medical Association, 284,* 3051–3057.

Waitzkin, H. (1991). *The politics of medical encounters.* New Haven, CT: Yale University Press.

Walsh-Burke, K., & Marcusen, C. (1999). Self-advocacy training for cancer survivors: The cancer survival toolbox. *Cancer Practice, 7,* 297–301.

Walton, D. (2003, August 6). Hagel visits with cancer patients. *Lincoln Journal Star,* 1B, 3B.

Ware, N. C. (1992). Suffering and the social construction of illness: The delegitimation of illness experience in chronic fatigue syndrome. *Medical Anthropology Quarterly, 6,* 347–361.

Ware, N. C., & Kleinman, A. (1992). Culture and somatic experience: The social course of illness in neurasthenia and chronic fatigue syndrome. *Psychosomatic Medicine, 54,* 546–560.

Warner, M. (2002). Publics and counterpublics [Abbreviated version]. *Quarterly Journal of Speech, 88,* 413–425.

Watt, R. (Producer), & Schuermann, P. (Writer, Director). (2002). *Tell me something I don't know* [Motion picture and facilitator guide]. Available from the International Fraternity of Phi Gamma Delta, P.O. Box 4599, Lexington, KY 49544–4599. Produced by Watt Imagination Video Production.

Wear, D., & Nixon, L. L. (2002). Literary inquiry and profession development in medicine against abstractions. *Perspectives in Biology and Medicine, 45,* 104–124.

Weber, A. L., Harvey, J. H., & Stanley, M. A. (1989). The nature and motivations of accounts for failed relationships. In R. Burnett, P. McGhee, & D. D. Clarke (Eds.), *Accounting for relationships: Explanation, representation, and knowledge* (pp. 114–133). London: Methuen.

Weber, M. (1996). What is a state? In B. E. Brown & R. C. Macridis (Eds.), *Comparative politics: Notes and readings* (8th ed., pp. 43–46). Belmont, CA: Wadsworth Publishing Company.

Wechsler, H., Dowdall, G. W., Davenport, A., & DeJong, W. (1993). *Binge drinking on campus: Results of a national study.* Bulletin produced by the Higher Education Center for Alcohol and Other Drug Prevention, U.S. Department of Education, Washington, DC.

Wechsler, H., Dowdall, G. W., Davenport, A., & DeJong, W. (1994). Health and behavioral consequences of binge drinking in college. *Journal of the American Medical Association, 272*(21), 1672–1677.

Wechsler, H., Dowdall, G. W., Maener, G., Gledhill-Hoyt, J., & Lee, H. (1998). Changes in binge drinking and related problems among American college students between 1993 and 1997: Results of the Harvard School of Public Health College Alcohol Study. *Journal of American College Health, 47*, 57–69.

Wechsler, H., Isaac, N., Grodstein, F., & Sellers, D. E. (1994). Continuation and initiation of alcohol use from the first to the second year of college. *Journal of Studies on Alcohol, 55*, 41–46.

Wechsler, H., Kuh, G., & Davenport, A. (1996). Fraternities, sororities and binge drinking: Results from a national study of American Colleges. *NASPA Journal, 33*(4), 260–279.

Wechsler, H., Lee, J. E., Kuo, M., Seibring, M., Nelson, T. F., & Lee, H. (2002). Trends in college binge drinking during a period of increased prevention efforts: Findings from 4 Harvard School of Public Health college alcohol surveys. *Journal of American College Health, 50*(5), 203–217.

Wechsler, H., Molnar, B. E., Davenport, A. E., & Baer, J. S. (1999). College alcohol use: A full or empty glass? *Journal of American College Health, 47*, 247–252.

Wechsler, H., & Wuetrich, B. (2002). *Dying to drink: Confronting binge drinking on college campuses.* New York: Rodale, Inc.

Weick, K. E. (1995). *Sensemaking in organizations.* Thousand Oaks, CA: Sage.

Weinstein, N. D. (1987). Unrealistic optimism about susceptibility to health problems: Conclusions from a community-wide sample. *Journal of Behavioral Medicine, 10*, 481–500.

Welch, K. (2000). Interdisciplinary communication in a literature and medicine course: Personalizing the discourse of medicine. *Technical Communication Quarterly, 9*, 311–329.

Werner, A., & Malterud, K. (2003). It is hard work being a credible patient: Encounters between women with chronic pain and their doctors. *Social Science & Medicine, 57*, 1409–1419.

White, H. (1980). The value of narrativity in the representation of reality. *Critical Inquiry, 5–28.*

White, H. (1981). On the value of narrativity in the representation of reality. In W. J. T. Mitchell (Ed.), *On narrative* (pp. 1–23). Chicago: University of Chicago Press.

White, H. (1987). *The content of the form: Narrative discourse and historical representation.* Baltimore: Johns Hopkins University Press.

White, M., & Epston, D. (1990). *Narrative means to therapeutic ends.* New York: W. W. Norton.

Wieder, D. L., & Pratt, S. (1990). On being a recognizable Indian among Indians. In D. Cargaugh (Ed.), *Cultural communication and intercultural contact.* Hillsdale, NJ: Lawrence Erlbaum Associates.

Wigren, J. (1994). Narrative completion in the treatment of trauma. *Psychotherapy, 31*, 415–423.

Williams, G. (1997). The genesis of chronic illness: Narrative reconstruction. In L. P. Hinchman & S. K. Hinchman (Eds.), *Memory, identity, community: The idea of narrative in the human sciences* (pp. 185–212). Albany: State University of New York Press.

Williams, J. (2000). *Unbending gender: Why work and family conflict and what to do about it.* New York: Oxford University Press.

Williams-Brown, S., Baldwin, D. M., & Bakos, A. (2002). Storytelling as a method to teach African American women breast health information. *Journal of Cancer Education, 17,* 227–230.

Wilson, C. (1999, December 16). A final farewell, but forever a friend. *USA Today,* p. 1D.

Wilson, M. (1999, November 8). Hainer battle offers life, death insight. [Letter to the editor]. *USA Today,* p. 26A.

Wittenberg, D. (2002). Going out in public: Visibility and anonymity in Michael Warner's 'Publics and Counterpublics.' *Quarterly Journal of Speech, 88,* 426–444.

Wittenberg, E., & Ragan, S. L. (in press). Narrative research in palliative care: Exploring the benefits. In G. Kreps & H. D. O'Hair (Eds.), *Cancer care and communication.* Cresskill, NJ: Hampton Press.

Wittgenstein, L. (1953). *Philosophical investigations.* New York: McMillan.

Wolf, M. J. (1999). *The entertainment economy.* New York: Times Books.

Wood, J. T. (2003). *Gendered lives: Communication, gender, and culture* (5th ed.). Belmont, CA: Wadsworth.

Woolf, V. (2002). *On being ill.* Ashfield, MA: Paris Press.

Worden, J. W. (2002). *Grief counseling and grief therapy: A handbook for the mental health practitioner* (3rd ed.). New York: Springer.

Workman, T. A. (2001a). Finding the meanings of college drinking: An analysis of fraternity drinking stories. *Health Communication, 13,* 427–447.

Workman, T. A. (2001b). *An intertextual analysis of the collegiate drinking culture.* Unpublished doctoral dissertation, University of Nebraska–Lincoln.

Yam, B., Rossiter, J., & Cheung, K. (2001). Caring for dying infants: Experiences of neonatal intensive care nurses in Hong Kong. *Journal of Clinical Nursing, 10,* 651–659.

Yoo, D. (1996). Captivating memories: Museology, concentration camps, and Japanese American history. *American Quarterly, 48,* 680–699.

Young, K. (1987). *Taleworlds and storyrealms: The phenomenology of narrative.* Dordrecht, Netherlands: Martinus Nijhoff Publishers.

Zaharna, R. (1989). Self-shock: The double-binding challenge of identity. *International Journal of Intercultural Relations, 13,* 501–525.

Zavestoski, S., Brown, P., McCormick, S., Mayer, B., D'Ottavi, M., & Lucove, J. (2004). Patient activism and the struggle for diagnosis: Gulf War illnesses and other medically unexplained physical symptoms in the U.S. *Social Science & Medicine, 58,* 161–175.

Zook, E. (1994). Embodied health and constitutive communication: Toward an authentic conceptualization of health communication. In S. A. Deetz (Ed.), *Communication Yearbook 17* (pp. 344–377). Thousand Oaks, CA: Sage.

Zukier, H. (1986). The paradigmatic and narrative modes in goal-guided inference. In R. M. Sorrentino & E. T. Higgins (Eds.), *Handbook of motivation and cognition: Foundations of social behavior* (pp. 456–502). New York: Guilford Press.

# Author Index

**503**

# Subject Index